Differential Diagnosis in Computed Tomography

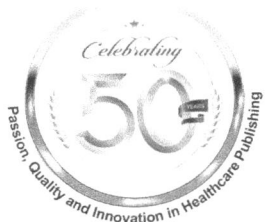

Differential Diagnosis in Computed Tomography

Third Edition

Sumeet Bhargava MBBS DNB (Radiodiagnosis)
FCGP FICRI FIAMS MNAMS FCCP FIMSA
Associate Professor
Department of Radiology and Imaging
MS Medical College
Hapur, Uttar Pradesh, India

Satish K Bhargava MBBS MD (Radiodiagnosis)
MD (Radiotherapy) DMRD FICRI FIAMS FCCP FUSI FIMSA FAMS
Former Professor and Head
Department of Radiology and Imaging
School of Medical Sciences and Research, Sharda Hospital
Sharda University, Greater Noida, Uttar Pradesh
Former Professor and Head
Department of Radiology and Imaging
University College of Medical
Sciences (University of Delhi) and
Guru Teg Bahadur Hospital, New Delhi
Former Head, Department of Radiology
JN Medical College, Aligarh Muslim University
Aligarh, Uttar Pradesh, India

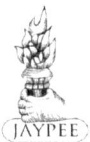

JAYPEE BROTHERS MEDICAL PUBLISHERS
The Health Sciences Publisher
New Delhi | London

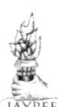 **Jaypee Brothers Medical Publishers (P) Ltd**

Headquarters

Jaypee Brothers Medical Publishers (P) Ltd
4838/24, Ansari Road, Daryaganj
New Delhi 110 002, India
Phone: +91-11-43574357
Fax: +91-11-43574314
E-mail: jaypee@jaypeebrothers.com

Overseas Office

JP Medical Ltd
83 Victoria Street, London
SW1H 0HW (UK)
Phone: +44 20 3170 8910
Fax: +44 (0)20 3008 6180
E-mail: info@jpmedpub.com

Website: www.jaypeebrothers.com
Website: www.jaypeedigital.com

© 2021, Jaypee Brothers Medical Publishers

The views and opinions expressed in this book are solely those of the original contributor(s)/author(s) and do not necessarily represent those of editor(s) of the book.

All rights reserved. No part of this publication may be reproduced, stored or transmitted in any form or by any means, electronic, mechanical, photocopying, recording or otherwise, without the prior permission in writing of the publishers.

All brand names and product names used in this book are trade names, service marks, trademarks or registered trademarks of their respective owners. The publisher is not associated with any product or vendor mentioned in this book.

Medical knowledge and practice change constantly. This book is designed to provide accurate, authoritative information about the subject matter in question. However, readers are advised to check the most current information available on procedures included and check information from the manufacturer of each product to be administered, to verify the recommended dose, formula, method and duration of administration, adverse effects and contra indications. It is the responsibility of the practitioner to take all appropriate safety precautions. Neither the publisher nor the author(s)/editor(s) assume any liability for any injury and/or damage to persons or property arising from or related to use of material in this book.

This book is sold on the understanding that the publisher is not engaged in providing professional medical services. If such advice or services are required, the services of a competent medical professional should be sought.

Every effort has been made where necessary to contact holders of copyright to obtain permission to reproduce copyright material. If any have been inadvertently overlooked, the publisher will be pleased to make the necessary arrangements at the first opportunity. The **CD/DVD-ROM** (if any) provided in the sealed envelope with this book is complimentary and free of cost. **Not meant for sale.**

Inquiries For Bulk Sales May Be Solicited At: Jaypee@Jaypeebrothers.com

Differential Diagnosis in Computed Tomography

First Edition: 2006
Second Edition: 2012
Third Edition: 2021
ISBN: 978-93-89587-47-0

Contributors

Amit Sahu
Consultant Radiologist
Max Super Speciality Hospital
Saket, New Delhi, India

Anoop Durga Das Agarwal
Consultant Radiologist
Department of Radiology and Imaging
Apollo Hospital
Navi Mumbai, Maharashtra, India

Anupama Tandon
Associate Professor
Department of Radiology and Imaging
University College of Medical Sciences (University of Delhi) and
Guru Teg Bahadur Hospital
New Delhi, India

Anurag Agarwal
Additional Director
National Board of Examinations
New Delhi, India

Atin Kumar
Additional Professor
Department of Radiodiagnosis and Imaging
All India Institute of Medical Sciences
New Delhi, India

Gopesh Mehrotra
Professor
Department of Radiology and Imaging
University College of Medical Sciences (University of Delhi) and
Guru Teg Bahadur Hospital
New Delhi, India

Neema Agarwal
Associate Professor
Government Institute of Medical Sciences
Greater Noida, Uttar Pradesh, India

Nikhil Aggarwal
Former Medical Officer
Department of Radiology and Imaging
University College of Medical Sciences (University of Delhi) and
Guru Teg Bahadur Hospital
New Delhi, India

Pardeep Kumar
Senior Resident
Department of Radiology and Imaging
Maulana Azad Medical College and Associated GB Pant Hospital
New Delhi, India

Rajul Rastogi
Associate Professor
Department of Radiology and Imaging
Teerthanker Mahaveer University
Moradabad, Uttar Pradesh, India

Satish K Bhargava
Former Professor and Head
Department of Radiology and Imaging
School of Medical Sciences and Research, Sharda Hospital
Sharda University, Greater Noida
Uttar Pradesh, India
Former Professor and Head
Department of Radiology and Imaging
University College of Medical Sciences (University of Delhi) and Guru Teg Bahadur Hospital
New Delhi
Former Head
Department of Radiology
JN Medical College
Aligarh Muslim University
Aligarh, Uttar Pradesh, India

Shuchi Bhatt
Head
Department of Radiology and Imaging
University College of Medical Sciences (University of Delhi) and Guru Teg Bahadur Hospital
New Delhi, India

Sumeet Bhargava
Associate Professor
Department of Radiology and Imaging
MS Medical College
Hapur, Uttar Pradesh, India

Swati Gupta
Assistant Professor
Department of Radiology and Imaging
Assistant Professor
Maulana Azad Medical College and Associated LNJP Hospital
New Delhi, India

Usha Thingujam
Associate Professor
Department of Radiodiagnosis
Jawaharlal Nehru Institute of Medical Sciences, Porompat
Imphal, Manipur, India

Vineeta Rathi
Professor
Department of Radiology and Imaging
University College of Medical Sciences (University of Delhi) and Guru Teg Bahadur Hospital
New Delhi, India

Preface to the Third Edition

Due to overwhelming response from the readers, the book has been revised keeping in view the various new requirements. The large number of illustrations have been added to give clear and precise view of the particular disease. We are sure the third edition will be more useful to radiologists and residents in their day-to-day practice and also helpful to the clinicians in patient management.

Sumeet Bhargava
Satish K Bhargava

Preface to the First Edition

Since the discovery of CT scan, this modality has made its visible impact in diagnostic field. Its role is ever increasing in imaging and is an indispensable modality in today's practice. With the emergence of the slip ring technology and then the multidetector configuration made continuous scan acquisition possible in very short time. The isotropic volumetric data acquired can be used for reconstructing images in various planes and displaying them through selective rendering techniques for maximum diagnostic information. This has remarkably improved the image quality and has opened new avenues in the field of diagnosis. All these advances have raised the expectations of the clinicians in acquiring a diagnosis through computed tomography. The plethora of imaging findings are seen and most of which have a list of differential diagnosis. The stress of establishing the closest diagnosis has evoked the need for a book on differential diagnosis based on CT findings.

The book covers the various disease conditions giving similar imaging findings on CT. An attempt has been made to include most of the disease processes/conditions of every organ system which can be diagnosed on CT. The typical CT findings of the conditions have been enumerated with other relevant information. Illustrations have been given wherever necessary to make a visual impact of the imaging finding. A lot of effort has been made to present the information in a vivid manner with the help of tables, so as to segregate the various clinical conditions. The differentiating features have been highlighted in the text. We have purposely avoided repetition of the text related to the various conditions and all have been described at one place or in the system where it is most relevant. We hope the book proves to be of great help for all the radiologists and even the clinicians to have a better understanding of the subject.

Satish K Bhargava

Acknowledgments

We are grateful to our colleagues and friends who gave timely support and stood behind us in our joint endeavor of bringing out this book, which was required keeping in view the fact that no such book is available in an Indian perspective and wide acceptability of this imaging modality for the diagnosis and staging of the disease.

We are especially thankful to Shri Jitendar P Vij (Group Chairman), Mr Ankit Vij (Managing Director), Mr MS Mani (Group President), Ms Chetna Malhotra Vohra (Associate Director—Content Strategy), Ms Pooja Bhandari (Production Head), and Ms Nikita Chauhan (Development Editor) of M/s Jaypee Brothers Medical Publishers (P) Ltd, New Delhi, India, for giving the go-ahead at the very beginning and helping us in every way possible to bring out this book.

Contents

1. **Brain** 1
   - Intracranial Calcification 1
     Sumeet Bhargava, Rajul Rastogi, Shuchi Bhatt
   - Differential Diagnosis of Brain Lesions 12
     *Atin Kumar, Rajul Rastogi, Shuchi Bhatt,
     Satish K Bhargava, Swati Gupta*
     - Supratentorial Midline Tumors 12
     - Supratentorial Midline Cysts 17
     - Supratentorial Paramidline Cysts 17
   - Pseudomasses of Brain 18
   - Intracranial Masses 19
   - Nontumoral Brain Lesions 20
     Rajul Rastogi, Shuchi Bhatt, Anurag Agarwal
   - White and Gray Matter Lesions 21
     - Multifocal White Matter Lesions 22
     - Periventricular Hypodensity 23
     - Brainstem Hypodensity 23
     - Bilateral Focal/Diffuse Hypodensities
       Basal Ganglia 23
     - Bilateral Hyperdense (Calcification)
       Basal Ganglia 25
     - Hyperdense Falx 25
     - Innumerable Small Enhancing Brain Nodules ... 26
     - Gyriform Enhancement 26
     - Pneumonic for Ring Enhancing Lesions
       in Brain 26
     - Multifocal Brain Tumors and Tumor-like
       Lesions 29

- Ventricular Lesions 29
  Rajul Rastogi, Atin Kumar, Satish K Bhargava, Swati Gupta
    - Ventricular Enlargement 29
    - Small Ventricles 29
    - Abnormal Ventricular Configuration 30
    - Hydrocephalus 32
    - Holoprosencephaly 33
    - Hydranencephaly 35
    - Atrophy 35
    - Corpus Callosum Agenesis 35
    - Arnold-Chiari Malformation 36
- Differentiating Features of Brain Lesions 37
  Rajul Rastogi, Shuchi Bhatt, Sumeet Bhargava
- Miscellaneous Lesions of the Brain 69
  Rajul Rastogi, Shuchi Bhatt, Satish K Bhargava
    - Intraparenchymal Hemorrhagic Lesions in Brain 69
    - CT Findings of Hemorrhage 69
    - Aneurysm and Vascular Malformation (AVM, Cavernous Angioma) 70
    - Conditions Primarily Presenting as Cerebral Atrophy 77
    - Conditions Primarily Presenting as Cerebellar Atrophy 77
    - Effaced Basal Cisterns 78
- Differential Diagnosis of Cerebellopontine Angle Masses 81
- Differential Diagnosis of Infratentorial Lesions 84
- Differential Diagnosis of Supratentorial Mass Lesions 88
- Differential Diagnosis of White Matter Diseases 96

2. Spinal Cord 106
- Spinal Cord Lesions 106
  *Sumeet Bhargava, Neema Agarwal,
  Satish K Bhargava, Shuchi Bhatt*
- Lesions Associated with Spinal Stenosis 126
  *Satish K Bhargava, Rajul Rastogi,
  Anoop Durga Das Agarwal*

3. Ear and Temporal Bone 132
Satish K Bhargava, Anurag Agarwal, Rajul Rastogi
- Differential Diagnosis of Ear Lesions 132
- Lesions of the Middle Ear and Mastoid 138
- Infective, Miscellaneous Lesions of the
  Middle Ear and Mastoid 138
- Internal Ear Lesions 146
  - Endolymphatic Sac Lesions 146

4. Orbital Lesions 161
Satish K Bhargava, Rajul Rastogi, Usha Thingujam
- Altered Globe Size 163
  - Microphthalmia 163
  - Macrophthalmia 164
- Orbital Lesions with Bone Involvement 164

5. Nasal or Paranasal Sinus Lesions 183
Sumeet Bhargava, Shuchi Bhatt, Satish K Bhargava
- Hyperdensities on Noncontrast-enhanced
  Computed Tomography in Sinonasal Region 184
- Normal Development of Paranasal Sinuses 209
- Anatomical Variants of Paranasal Sinuses 210

6. Neck 215
- Pharyngeal and Parapharyngeal Lesions 215
  Rajul Rastogi, Satish K Bhargava, Usha Thingujam
  - Pharyngeal Mucosal Space 215
  - Parapharyngeal Space 217

- Neck Space Lesions 220
  Sumeet Bhargava, Satish K Bhargava, Rajul Rastogi
  - Sublingual Space 220
  - Submandibular Space 223
  - Buccal Space 225
  - Masticator Space 225
  - Retropharyngeal Space 227
  - Posterior Cervical Space 228
  - Prevertebral/Perivertebral Space 229
- Parotid Lesions 229
  Rajul Rastogi, Satish K Bhargava, Gopesh Mehrotra
  Parotid Space 229
- Lesions of the Oral Cavity 232
  Nikhil Aggarwal, Shuchi Bhatt, Rajul Rastogi, Sumeet Bhargava
  Lingual Thyroid 233
- Laryngeal or Visceral Space 233
  Satish K Bhargava, Rajul Rastogi
  Other Lesions 238
- Thyroid and Parathyroid Gland Lesions 238
  Satish K Bhargava, Shuchi Bhatt
  Parathyroid Lesions 242
- Lymph Nodes in the Neck 242
  Rajul Rastogi, Satish K Bhargava
  - Superficial 242
  - Deep 242
  - Size Criteria for Lymphadenopathy 243
  - Shape Criteria 244
  - Central Hypodensity in Nodes 244
  - Calcification in Nodes 245
- Differential Diagnosis of Thyroid Diseases 245
- Differential Diagnosis of Parotid Lesions 249

7. Chest 255

- Pulmonary Nodular and Cavitating Lesions........... 255
  Sumeet Bhargava, Shuchi Bhatt, Rajul Rastogi
  Solitary Pulmonary Nodule 255
- Mass within a Cavity 271
- Interstitial Lung Diseases...................................... 272
  Pardeep Kumar, Shuchi Bhatt, Rajul Rastogi
  - Pulmonary Edema 274
  - Lymphangitis Carcinomatosa 274
  - Fibrosing Alveolitis (Idiopathic Pulmonary Fibrosis) 274
  - Sarcoidosis 275
  - Extrinsic Allergic Alveolitis (Hypersensitivity Pneumonitis)... 275
  - Asbestosis 276
  - Langerhans' Cell Histiocytosis......................... 276
  - Lymphangioleiomyomatosis 277
  - Silicosis.. 277
  - Coal Workers' Pneumoconiosis 278
  - *Pneumocystis Carinii* Pneumonia.................... 278
  - Desquamative Interstitial Pneumonia 278
  - Nonspecific Interstitial Pneumonia................... 278
  - Idiopathic Pulmonary Hemorrhage 279
  - Collagen Vascular Disease.............................. 279
  - Tree-in-bud Appearance 280
- Cystic Pulmonary Diseases 281
  Satish K Bhargava, Shuchi Bhatt, Rajul Rastogi
  - CT Angiogram Sign.. 283
  - Differential Diagnosis of Opacity with an Air Bronchogram.. 283
- Mediastinal Masses 285
  Amit Sahu, Shuchi Bhatt, Rajul Rastogi
  - Anterior Mediastinal Masses............................ 286
  - Middle Mediastinal Masses.............................. 293

- ♦ Posterior Mediastinal Masses........................... 298
- ♦ Mediastinal Masses Containing Fat................. 301
- ♦ Mediastinal Cysts.. 302
- Classification of Regional Intrathoracic Lymph Nodes.. 304
  Shuchi Bhatt, Satish K Bhargava, Pardeep Kumar
- Mediastinal Lymphadenopathy 307
- Lesions of Tracheobronchial Tree........................... 312
  Satish K Bhargava, Amit Sahu, Shuchi Bhatt
  - ♦ Congenital Lesions 312
  - ♦ Acquired Lesions 314
- Pleural Lesions 318
  Satish K Bhargava, Amit Sahu, Shuchi Bhatt
  - ♦ Pleural Calcification 318
  - ♦ Local Pleural Masses...................................... 321
  - ♦ Pleural Thickening 326

8. Abdomen..327
- Abdominal Wall Lesions 327
  Shuchi Bhatt, Rajul Rastogi, Vineeta Rathi
- Hernias Through Abdominal Wall 331
  Shuchi Bhatt, Rajul Rastogi
- Hepatobiliary Lesions 335
  Rajul Rastogi, Satish K Bhargava, Sumeet Bhargava
  - ♦ Hepatic Lesions 335
  - ♦ Diffuse Liver Disease...................................... 355
  - ♦ Contour Abnormalities 361
- Gallbladder and Biliary Tract Lesions 362
  - ♦ Biliary Lesions... 362
- Splenic and Pancreatic Lesions.............................. 368
  Satish K Bhargava, Rajul Rastogi
  - ♦ Splenic Lesions... 368
  - ♦ Pancreatic Lesions 372

- Gastrointestinal Lesions 377
  Rajul Rastogi, Satish K Bhargava, Sumeet Bhargava, Anurag Agarwal, Swati Gupta
  - Gastric Lesions 377
  - Small Bowel Lesions 382
  - Colonic Lesions 389
- Peritoneal and Mesenteric/Omental Lesions 396
  - Lipoma 397
  - Liposarcoma 397
  - Enteric Cyst 398
  - Mesenteric/Omental/Mesothelial Cyst 398
  - Lymphangioma 398
  - Pseudomyxoma Peritonei 399
  - Retractile Mesenteritis/Chronic Fibrosing Mesenteritis/Weber Christian Disease/ Mesenteric Panniculitis 399
  - Mesothelioma 401
  - Peritoneal Carcinomatosis 401
  - Splenosis 401
- Retroperitoneal Lesions 403
  - Lymphadenopathy 404
  - Seroma 406
  - Retroperitoneal Mesenchymal Tumors 406
  - Neurogenic Tumors 407
  - Undescended Testis 408
  - Retroperitoneal Fibrosis/Ormond's Disease 408
  - Atherosclerosis of Aorta 409
  - Aortic Aneurysm 409
  - Aortic Dissection 409
  - Thrombosis of the Inferior Vena Cava 409
- Adrenal Lesions 410
  - Causes of Bilateral Adrenal Enlargement 411

- Genitourinary Lesions 414
  - Renal Lesions 414
  - Bladder and Pelvic Lesions 430
- Male Reproductive System Lesions 437
  - Prostatic Lesions 437
  - Seminal Vesicle Lesions 440
  - Testes 441
- Female Reproductive System Lesions 441
  - Vagina and Vulva 441
  - Cervix and Uterus 441
  - Adnexa 442
  - Uterus 443
  - Common Hemorrhagic Lesions of the Ovary ... 447

9. Musculoskeletal System 452
- Bony Lesions 452
  Amit Sahu, Anupama Tandon, Rajul Rastogi
  - Well-defined Lytic Lesions 452
  - Ill-defined Lytic Lesions 453
  - Lytic Lesions with Surrounding Sclerosis 453
  - Bone Sclerosis with a Periosteal Reaction 455
  - Solitary Sclerotic Bone Lesion with a Lucent Center 455
  - Salient Features of Bone Tumors and Tumor-like Lesions 456
- Rib Lesions 488
  Sumeet Bhargava, Shuchi Bhatt, Satish K Bhargava
  - Lytic Lesions 488
  - Sclerotic Lesions 488
  - Lesions Involving Multiple Ribs 489
- Skull and Jaw Lesions 489
  Sumeet Bhargava, Anupama Tandon, Shuchi Bhatt, Rajul Rastogi

- Sclerotic Lesions of the Skull Vault 489
- Hyperdense Skull Base 490
- Lytic Lesion in the Vault of the Skull 490
- Lytic Lesions Involving Base of Skull 492
- Button Sequestrum 492
- Destructive Lesions Affecting the Petrous Pyramid, Middle Ear, and Antrum 493
- Lesions of the Orbit 493
- Lytic Lesions in the Jaw 494
- Sclerotic Lesions of the Jaw 495
- Salient Features of the Jaw Lesions 495

- Bony Spinal Lesions 499

  Sumeet Bhargava, Anupama Tandon
  - Expansile Lesions of the Vertebra 499
  - Lesions Involving Multiple Vertebrae 499
  - Differential Involvement of the Part of Vertebra 500
  - Differential Diagnosis of Selected Craniovertebral Anomalies 500

- Arthritis 505

  Rajul Rastogi, Shuchi Bhatt, Satish K Bhargava
  - Osteopenia 506
  - Joint Effusion 506
  - Joint Space Narrowing 507
  - Erosions, Cysts, Geodes, and Bone Resorption 507
  - Changes in the Ossification Center and the Small Bones 508
  - Subchondral Sclerosis and Osteophytes 509
  - Periosteal New Bone Formation 510
  - Malalignment, Subluxation, and Dislocation 511
  - Disorganization 511
  - Ankylosis 512

- ♦ Distribution and Sequence of Changes 512
- ♦ Soft Tissue Swelling, Atrophy, and Calcification 512
- Spine 513
  - ♦ Differential Diagnosis of Intra-articular Loose Bodies 515
  - ♦ Differentiating Features of Pyogenic and Tubercular Arthritis 516
- Soft Tissue Lesions 516

  Anupama Tandon, Shuchi Bhatt, Rajul Rastogi

  - ♦ Soft Tissue Calcification 516
  - ♦ Differential Diagnosis of Bony and Soft Tissue Lesions 521
  - ♦ Differential Diagnosis of Joint Diseases 526
  - ♦ Differential Diagnosis of Soft Tissue Lesions 530
  - ♦ Differential Diagnosis of Spinal Fractures 535

Index *539*

Chapter 1

Brain

INTRACRANIAL CALCIFICATION

Details of intracranial calcification are given in Tables 1 and 2.

TABLE 1: Causes of intracranial calcification.

Criteria	Physiological	Pathological
Midline	<ul><li>Pineal</li><li>Habenular</li><li>Falcine</li><li>Interclinoid ligament</li><li>Pituitary</li><li>Third and fourth ventricular choroid plexus</li></ul>	<ul><li>Craniopharyngioma</li><li>Pinealoma</li><li>Chordoma/clival chondrosarcoma</li><li>Pituitary adenoma</li><li>Lissencephaly</li></ul>
Off-midline Unilateral		*Neoplasms*<ul><li>Meningioma</li><li>Ependymoma</li><li>Papilloma of choroid plexus</li><li>Dermoid/epidermoid/teratoma</li><li>Metastases</li></ul>

Contd...

Contd...

Criteria	Physiological	Pathological
		Infections • Viral (CMV, herpes, rubella) • Bacterial (TB, *Staphylococcus spp.*) • Fungal (*Coccidioides*)
		Infestations • Cysticercosis • Echinococcosis • Toxoplasmosis • Paragonimiasis • Trichinosis • Torulosis
		Vascular • Atheroma • Glioma • Aneurysm • Angioma • Subdural/intraparenchymal hematoma • Sturge-Weber syndrome
Bilateral • Symmetrical	• Choroid plexus • Basal ganglia • Dentate nucleus • Petroclinoid ligaments • Tentorial	• Lipoma • Hypoparathyroidism • Pseudohypoparathyroidism • Fahr syndrome (Figs. 1A to E) • Neurofibromatosis
• Asymmetrical	• Pacchionian bodies	• Glioblastoma multiforme • Tuberous sclerosis

(CMV: cytomegalovirus)

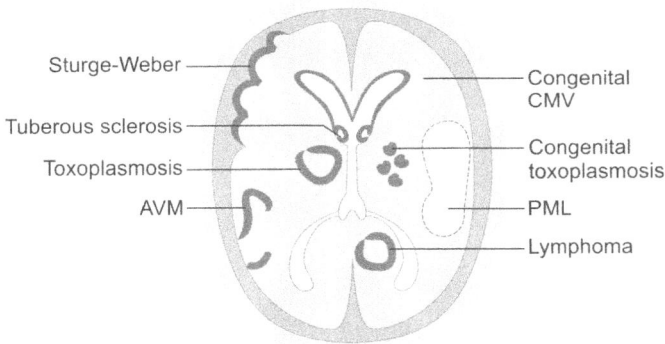

Fig. 1A: Pictorial representation of common causes of intracranial calcification.
(AVM: aneurysm and vascular malformation; CMV: cytomegalovirus; PML: progressive multifocal leukoencephalopathy)

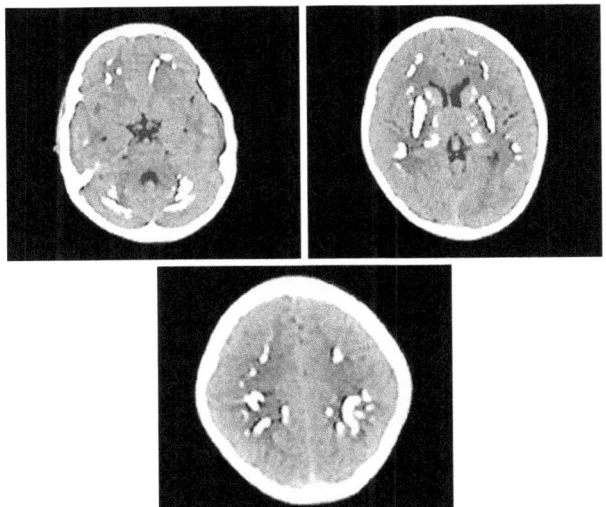

Fig. 1B: Axial computed tomography (CT) images showing extensive intraparenchymal calcification in a case of Fahr's disease.

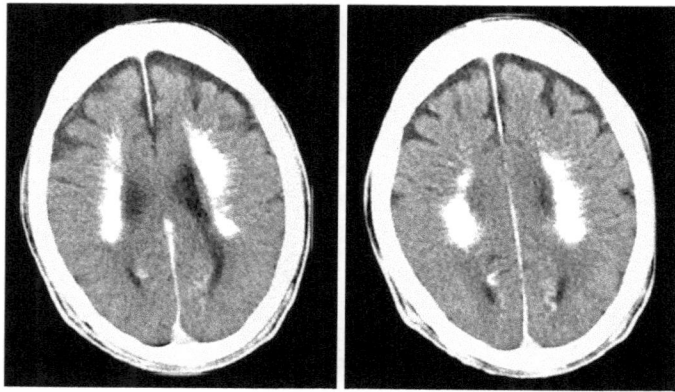

Fig. 1C: Intracranial calcification in hypoparathyroidism.

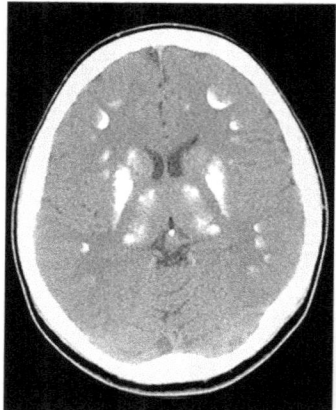

Fig. 1D: Intracranial calcification in pseudohypoparathyroidism.

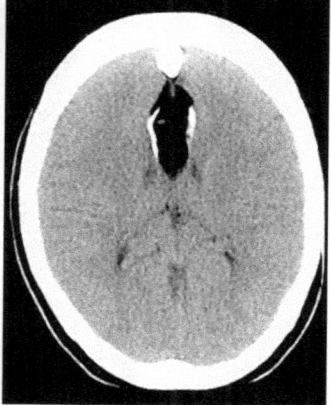

Fig. 1E: Intracranial lipoma with Bracket calcification.

TABLE 2: Differentiating features of various intracranial calcification.

Sites of calcification	Differentiating features	Comments
Pineal gland	It is seen as a punctate or nodular calcific density immediately posterior to the calcific density of habenular commissure	• It is seen in most adults • It may be seen as early as 1 year of life and in 90% cases by 10 years of age
Habenular	• It is usually 3–4 mm in diameter • It is seen as a crescentic, calcific commissure	The concavity of the crescent faces density at the back of the third ventricle posteriorly
Choroid plexus	It varies from punctate to large calcific density measuring up to 1 cm in diameter	Most common in the glomus at the trigone of lateral ventricle
Dural	It is seen as thin linear calcification of falx or sheet-like in cases of tentorium cerebelli	Commonly seen in the elderly
Petroclinoid ligaments	It is seen as a linear calcification extending from the tip of the dorsum sellae to the petrous apex	Commonly seen in the elderly
Interclinoid ligaments	It is seen as a thin linear calcification of ligaments between the clinoid processes	It gives rise to bridging sella extending across the midline appearance
Pacchionian bodies	They are seen as multifocal, punctate or nodular calcific densities usually near the vertex	They are usually bilateral and asymmetric in distribution
Pituitary gland	It is seen as a punctate calcification in the location of the gland in the sella	It is very rare and may be normal variant

Contd...

Contd...

Sites of calcification	Differentiating features	Comments
Basal ganglia and dentate nucleus	It is seen as amorphous calcification in the basal ganglia and dentate nuclei, usually in symmetrical and bilateral pattern	• Globus pallidus is the first to calcify • This can be idiopathic or secondary to metabolic disorders
Glioma	• Any type of glioma can show any pattern of calcification • Oligodendroglioma are the commonest to show calcification (approximately half of the cases)	Slow growing and the less malignant glioma are the most likely to reveal calcification
Craniopharyngioma	• Punctate calcification is seen in three-fourths of the cases in children. • Occasionally, when the tumor is cystic, the calcification is curvilinear in the wall of the cyst with a characteristic location in midline just above the sella	The shape of the sella is changed as the anterior part is pressed downward from above
Meningioma	The calcification may be characteristically ball-like and amorphous in a characteristic parasagittal location and other specific sites	• Hyperostosis in the adjacent calvarium and increased meningeal vascular markings upto the site of the bony lesion are other clues to the diagnosis • Heavily calcified meningiomas: *Brain Rocks!!*
Dermoid	• They may show arcs of calcification • There may be associated central defect in the occipital bone in posterior fossa dermoid	• They are most common in the posterior fossa and the base of the skull • Teratoma can also be seen in the pineal and suprasellar region

Contd...

Contd...

Sites of calcification	Differentiating features	Comments
	• Presence of the dental element confirms the diagnosis of the mature dermoid/teratoma	
Lipoma	They show characteristic marginal calcification giving rise to the bracket configuration in the region of the corpus callosum	Less specific calcification may also be seen
Chordoma	It shows irregular calcification associated with soft tissue mass in the region of the clivus that may present into the nasopharynx after basal erosion	The calcification is, however, seen in minority of cases
Aneurysm	They show characteristic arc-like or circular marginal calcification	The most common site is the circle of Willis
Angioma	Small proportion of these show scattered flecks of calcification along with one or more rings or arc-like calcification	The arc-like calcification is seen in the aneurysmally dilated venous channels
Subdural hematoma	It shows typical marginal calcification of the membrane in concavo-convex configuration	Characteristic location of being adjacent to the calvaria is typical
Atheroma	Linear flecks of calcification in the carotid siphons secondary to atherosclerosis is very characteristic	Similar findings can occasionally be seen in other intracranial vessels

Contd...

Contd...

Sites of calcification	Differentiating features	Comments
Postinfectious/Post-infestation	• Congenital toxoplasmosis typically shows linear streaks in the basal ganglia and multiple scattered calcific specks in the cortex (Figs. 2A and B) • Congenital CMV infection results in widespread periventricular calcification that may take the shape of the dilated ventricle; the calcification is typically stippled, bilateral and symmetric (Fig. 3) • *Paragonimus westermani* lesions are usually seen in the parietal region and often give rise to the extensive *soap bubble* calcification in the cysts that are usually 3–4 cm in diameter	• Treated cases of tuberculoma, cysticerci, and toxoplasma may also result in nodular and punctate calcification at the site of the inactive lesion • Active tuberculoma and cysticercus may also reveal speck of calcification within the lesion

Contd...

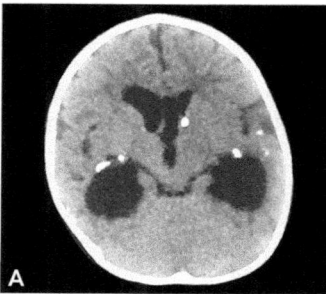 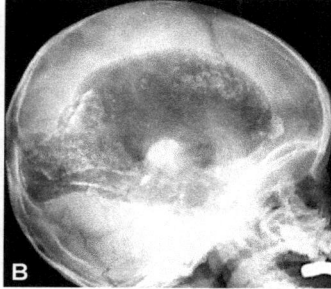

Figs. 2A and B: Axial CT and lateral skull X-ray images in a case of congenital toxoplasmosis shows foci of calcification in left basal ganglia, bilateral periventricular region, and in left temporal lobe.

Brain

Contd...

Sites of calcification	Differentiating features	Comments
Neurofibromatosis	Rare feature of neurofibromatosis is extensive calcification of the choroid plexi of the lateral and third ventricles	
Tuberous sclerosis	• Multiple, nodular, subependymal calcification are seen in this condition (Fig. 4) • Giant cell astrocytoma seen with this condition may also be the cause of calcification	The nodules are usually subcentimeter in size except in the case of the giant cell astrocytoma where larger nodules may be seen
Sturge-Weber syndrome (Figs. 5A to F)	• It is characterized by gyral pattern of calcification typically extensive and bilateral involving the parieto-occipital cortex • The calcification resembles *tram track* configuration	The cortex showing calcification is typically atrophic and may show areas of intense postcontrast enhancement representing angiomas with large choroid plexi
Lissencephaly	Characteristic calcified nodule is seen in the septum pellucidum just behind foramen of Monro	The nodule is typically subcentimeter in size, usually 3–5 mm in diameter

(CMV: cytomegalovirus)

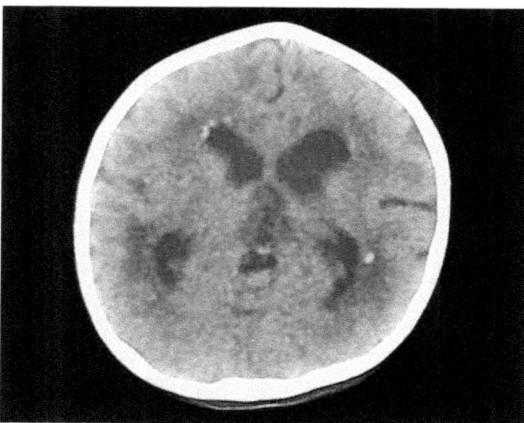

Fig. 3: Axial CT image in a case of congenital cytomegalovirus (CMV) shows bilateral symmetrical periventricular calcification.

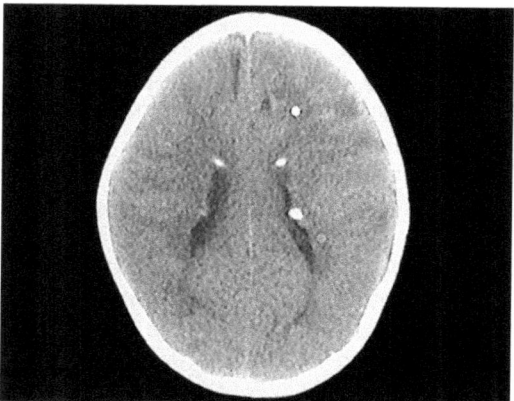

Fig. 4: Axial CT image in a 10-year-old boy with tuberous sclerosis shows bilateral calcified subependymal nodules and a partially calcified tuber in left frontal lobe.

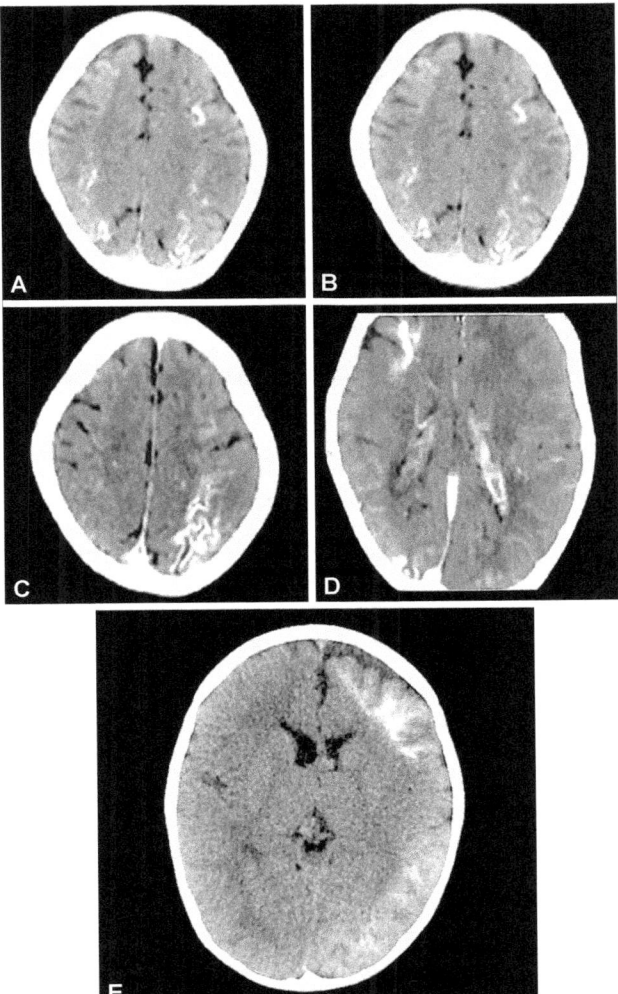

Figs. 5A to E: Axial CT images showing features in a typical case of Sturge-Weber syndrome.

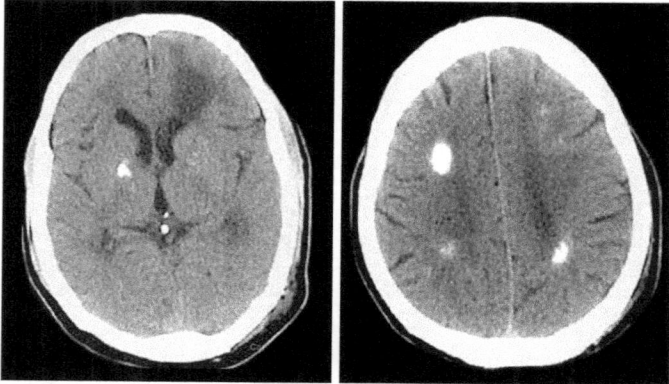

Fig. 5F: Leukoencephalopathy with intracranial calcifications.

DIFFERENTIAL DIAGNOSIS OF BRAIN LESIONS

Details of differential diagnosis of brain lesions are given in Tables 3 and 4.

Supratentorial Midline Tumors

- Optic and hypothalamic glioma
- Craniopharyngioma
- Astrocytoma
- Pineoblastoma
- Germinoma
- Lipoma
- Teratoma
- Pituitary adenoma
- Meningioma
- Choroid plexus papilloma.

TABLE 3: Causes of space occupying lesions of brain.

	Supratentorium	*Infratentorium*
Intra-axial (Table 6)	*Cerebral hemisphere* • Glioma (astrocytoma, oligodendroglioma, ependymoma, glioblastoma multiforme, gliomatosis cerebri) • Lymphoma • Parasitic cysts • Abscesses • Metastases *Pineal region* • Germ cell tumor (germinoma, teratoma) • Pineoblastoma • Pineocytoma • Pineal cyst *Intraventricular* • Astrocytoma • Primitive neuroectodermal tumor (PNET) • Choroid plexus papilloma • Meningioma • Medulloblastoma • Ependymoma, subependymoma • Giant cell astrocytoma • Central neurocytoma • Oligodendroglioma • Metastases • Colloid cyst • Hemangioblastoma *Corpus callosum* • Lipoma • Glioblastoma multiforme • Lymphoma	*Brainstem* • Hematoma • Cavernous angioma • Glioma *Cerebellar hemisphere/ vermis* • Hematoma • Abscesses • Telangiectasia • Glioma • Ganglioglioma • Hemangioblastoma • Medulloblastoma • Pilocytic astrocytoma • Metastases *Fourth ventricle* • Choroid plexus papilloma/carcinoma • Ependymoma/ subependymoma • Medulloblastoma • Pilocytic astrocytoma • Dermoid/epidermoid • Hemangioblastoma • Metastases • Cysticercus *Foramen magnum* • Astrocytoma • Hemangioblastoma

Contd...

Contd...

	Supratentorium	Infratentorium
	Sellar and suprasellar • Pituitary adenoma • Metastases • Craniopharyngioma • Epidermoid, dermoid • Germinoma • Lymphoma • Lipoma • Opticochiasmatic/ hypothalamic • Infundibular glioma • Neurosarcoid • Rathke cyst • Parasitic cyst • Hamartoma of the tuber cinereum • Histiocytosis	

Extra-axial (Table 6)	*Suprasellar*
	• Arachnoid cyst
	• Parasitic cyst
	• Meningioma
	• Osteocartilaginous tumors
	Parasellar
	• Vascular tumors (internal carotid artery aneurysm)
	• Cavernous sinus lesions
	  – Hemangioma Hemangiopericytoma
	  – Meningioma
	  – Lymphoma
	  – Metastases
	  – Neural tumors (Schwannoma, neurofibroma)
	  – Intracranial aneurysm (ICA)
		Cerebellopontine angle
		• Schwannoma (V, VIII) (Fig. 6)
		• Meningioma
		• Epidermoid
		• Metastases
		• Paraganglioma
		• Arachnoid cyst
		• Lipoma
		• Cholesterol granuloma
		• Lymphoma
		• Sarcoidosis
		• Bony tumors from the petrous bone
		Skull base
		• Posterior cranial fossa lesions
		  – Nerve sheath tumor
		  – Paraganglioma
		  – Meningioma
		  – Metastases

Contd...

Brain

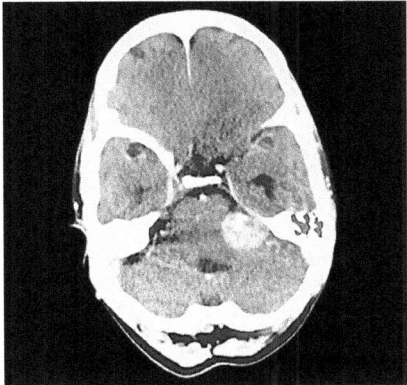

Fig. 6: An intensely enhancing extra-axial mass lesion seen in left cerebellopontine (CP) angle cistern with intracanalicular extension suggestive of acoustic Schwannoma.

Contd...

Supratentorium	*Infratentorium*
Skull base	*Foramen magnum*
• Anterior cranial fossa lesions	• Meningioma
– Invasive polyposis	• Schwannoma
– Inverted papilloma	• Metastases
– Meningioma	• Paraganglioma
– Malignant sinonasal masses	• Epidermoid
– Lymphoma	• Arachnoid cyst
– Esthesioneuroblastoma	• Tumors arising from the clivus and skull base
– Metastases	*Tentorial*
– Mucocele	• Meningioma
– Encephalocele	*Epidural lesions*
– Dermoid cyst	• Hematoma
– Osteoma	• Abscess
– Osteomyelitis secondary to sinusitis	• Soft tissue mass arising from bony lesions the skull vault
• Middle cranial fossa lesions	
– Metastases	
– Malignant naso-pharyngeal lesions	

Contd...

Contd...

Supratentorium	Infratentorium
– Juvenile nasopharyngeal angiofibroma – Osteomyelitis secondary to sinusitis – Granulomatous sinusitis (Wegener's granulomatosis) – Lymphoma – Meningioma – Chordoma – Leprosy – Sarcoidosis – Tuberculosis – Myeloma *Dural/falcine/subdural lesions* • Hematoma • Effusion/empyema • Sarcoidosis and histiocytosis (Rosai-Dorfman disease) • Arteriovenous (AV) malformation • Meningioma (en plaque)/meningiosarcoma • Hemangioma/hemangiopericytoma • Metastases (leukemic and lymphoma deposits) *Epidural lesions* • Hematoma • Abscess • Soft tissue mass arising from the skull vault	

TABLE 4: Causes of brain tumors in the pediatric age group.

Presenting at birth	Presenting at a later age
• Choroid plexus papilloma/carcinoma • Craniopharyngioma • Ependymoma • Hypothalamic astrocytoma • Medulloblastoma • Primitive neuroectodermal tumor (PNET) • Teratoma	• Astrocytoma • Choroid plexus papilloma • Colloid cyst • Craniopharyngioma • Ependymoma/subependymoma • Germinoma • Hamartoma • Medulloblastoma • Meningioma • Metastases • Oligodendroglioma • Optic nerve glioma • Pinealoma • Teratoma

Supratentorial Midline Cysts

- Cavum septum pellucidum (5th ventricle)
- Cavum vergae (6th ventricle)
- Cavum velum interpositum
- Arachnoid cyst in the region of the quadrigeminal plate cistern
- Vascular lesions (aneurysm)
- Cholesterol granuloma
- Pineal cyst
- Rathke's cleft cyst

Supratentorial Paramidline Cysts

- Epidermoid
- Trichilemmal cyst (sebaceous)
- Leptomeningeal cyst
- Arachnoid cyst (middle cranial fossa/convexity)

PSEUDOMASSES OF BRAIN

Pseudomasses of brain are shown in Table 5.

TABLE 5: Causes of pseudomasses of the brain.

	Supratentorium	Infratentorium
Intra-axial	*Pineal region* • Enlarged suprapineal recess • Enlarged cavum velum interpositum *Intraventricular* • Subependymal giant cell tumor • Enlarged calcified choroid plexus *Sellar and suprasellar* • Encephalocele	*Vermis* • Superior vermis *Fourth ventricle* • Prominent choroid plexus
Extra-axial	*Suprasellar* • Empty sella • Congenital ectopic neurohypophysis *Parasellar* • Vascular tumors (caroticocavernous fistula, cavernous thrombosis) *Dural/falcine/subdural lesions* • Thrombosis	*Cerebellopontine angle* • Enlarged flocculonodular lobe of cerebellum • Prominent choroid plexus from foramen of Luschka *Foramen magnum* • Tonsillar herniation *Skull base* • High jugular bulb • Jugular vein thrombosis • Prominent jugular tubercles

Brain

INTRACRANIAL MASSES

Details of intracranial masses are shown in Table 6.

TABLE 6: Differentiating features between intra-axial and extra-axial intracranial masses.

Features	Intra-axial	Extra-axial
Local bony changes	Usually absent until late in the disease	Commonly seen
Dural tail	Absent	May be seen
Cerebrospinal fluid (CSF) cleft	Absent	Present
Effect on adjacent subarachnoid spaces and cisterns	Effaced to variable degree	Enlarged to variable degree
Feeding vessels	Pial source	Dural source (Meningioma has dual blood supply from dural as well as pial arteries)
Buckling of gray/white matter junction	Absent	Present
White matter bucking sign	Absent	Present
Intervening gray matter between mass lesion and white matter	Absent	Present
Rotation of the brainstem in infratentorial lesions	Absent	Present (toward the contralateral side)

NONTUMORAL BRAIN LESIONS

Nontumoral brain lesions are given in Table 7.

TABLE 7: Causes of hypodense, nonenhancing lesions.

Soft tissue	Fluid		Fat	Air
	With mural nodule	Without mural nodule		
• Edema • Infarct • Nonhemorrhagic contusion (Fig. 8) • Encephalitis (including limbic) • Gliosis • Periventricular cerebrospinal fluid (CSF) seepage • Demyelinating diseases • Leukodystrophies • Gliomatosis cerebri	• Neurocysticercosis (granular nodular) • Toxoplasmosis	• Chronic infarcts • Virchow-Robin spaces • Chronic hematoma • Encephalomalacia • Porencephaly • Schizencephaly • Neurocysticercus (vesicular, colloid vesicular) • Hydatid cyst • Arachnoid cyst • Choroid plexus cyst • Choroid fissure cyst • Ependymal cyst • Epidermoid	• Lipoma • Dermoid	• Aeroceles (Fig. 7) • Abscess

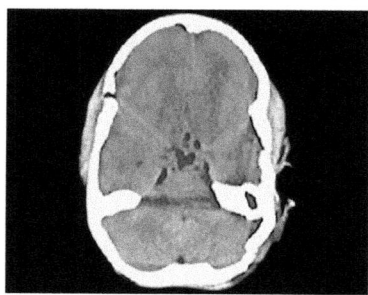

Fig. 7: Axial CT image showing multiple aeroceles in the basal cisterns.

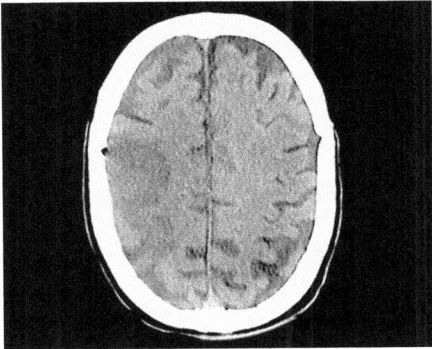

Fig. 8: Contrast-enhanced computed tomography (CECT) axial image of head hypodense area with loss of gray-white matter differentiation in a case of head trauma suggesting nonhemorrhagic contusion.

WHITE AND GRAY MATTER LESIONS

Details of white and gray matter lesions are given in Tables 8 and 9.

TABLE 8: Causes of myelinating/demyelinating lesions.		
White matter (Leukodystrophy)	*Gray matter (Poliodystrophy)*	*Both gray and white matter*
<ul><li>Multiple sclerosis</li><li>Vascular disease</li><li>Diffuse axonal injury</li><li>Postinfectious demyelination</li><li>Toxic demyelination</li><li>Metachromatic leukodystrophy (MLD)</li><li>Krabbe disease</li><li>Adrenoleuko-dystrophy (ALD)</li><li>Pelizaeus-Merzbacher disease (PMD)</li><li>Alexander disease</li><li>Canavan disease</li><li>Aminoaciduria</li></ul>	<ul><li>Lipidoses</li><li>Mucopoly-saccharidoses</li><li>Mucolipidosis</li><li>Fucosidosis</li><li>Glycogen storage diseases</li></ul>	<ul><li>Mitochondrial encephalopathies [myoclonic epilepsy with ragged red fiber (MERRF); mitochondrial encephalopathy with lactic acidosis and stroke-like episodes (MELAS)]</li><li>Peroxisomal disorders</li></ul>

TABLE 9: Characteristic pattern involvement in leukodystrophy/demyelinating diseases.

Characteristic patterns	Diseases involved
Diffuse lobar involvement	• Canavan disease • Pelizaeus-Merzbacher disease • 4H syndrome
Predominantly frontal white matter involvement	Alexander disease
Predominantly occipital white matter involvement	Adrenoleukodystrophy
Associated with enlarged ventricles	• Alexander disease • Canavan disease
Associated with hyperdense basal ganglia	Krabbe disease
Associated with focal hypodensity in basal ganglia	• Alexander disease • Canavan disease • Metachromatic leukodystrophy
Associated with postcontrast enhancement	• Adrenoleukodystrophy • Alexander disease

Multifocal White Matter Lesions

- Virchow-Robin spaces (when bilateral and diffuse, these are called Etate Crible)
- Demyelinating diseases (vascular, postinfectious) (Table 9)
- Multiple sclerosis (MS)
- Diffuse axonal injury
- Cysticerci
- Abscesses
- Leukoencephalopathy
- Neurocutaneous syndromes [tuberous sclerosis, neurofibromatosis-1 (NF-1)]
- Multifocal glioma
- Primary CNS lymphoma
    - Progressive multifocal leukoencephalopathy (PML)
    - Encephalitis
    - Iris

- Gliomatosis cerebri
- Metastases.

Periventricular Hypodensity

- Gliosis
- Encephalomalacia
- Porencephaly
- Resolving hematoma
- Infarct
- Interstitial seepage of cerebrospinal fluid (CSF) in hydrocephalus
- Multiple sclerosis
- Migraine
- Vasculitis
- Encephalitis
- Acute disseminating encephalomyelitis
- Diffuse necrotizing leukoencephalopathy
- Progressive multifocal leukoencephalopathy
- Virchow-Robin space
- Leukodystrophy.

Brainstem Hypodensity

Brainstem hypodensity is given in Table 10.
- Physiological
- Syringobulbia
- Infarction
- Central pontine myelinolysis
- Gliosis
- Glioma
- Metastases
- Granuloma.

Bilateral Focal/Diffuse Hypodensities Basal Ganglia

- Physiological (VR spaces)
- Infection (TB, HIV)/infestation (toxoplasmosis, cryptococcosis)
- Arterial infarct (lacunar infarcts)
- Venous infarct (internal cerebral vein thrombosis)

TABLE 10: Causes of hyperdense brain lesions.

Nonenhancing lesions	Enhancing lesions
- Acute hematoma (Figs. 9 and 10) - Capillary/cavernous angioma - Colloid cyst - Calcified lesions	- Tuberculoma - Neurocysticercus - Lymphoma - Meningioma - Medulloblastoma - Choroid plexus papilloma - Tumors with matrix calcification [oligodendroglioma, glioblastoma, ependymoma, capillary/cavernous angioma, arteriovenous malformation (AVM)] - Metastases [mucinous primary tumor—gastrointestinal tract (GIT), ovary, pancreas, melanotic melanoma osteosarcoma]

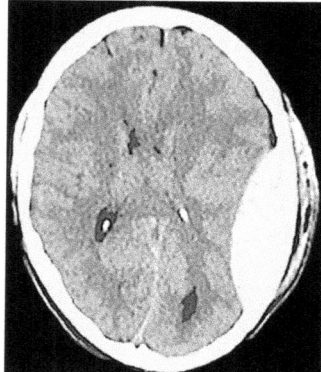 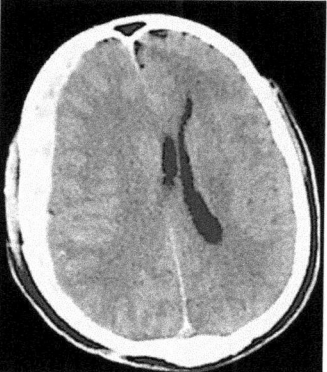

Fig. 9: Axial CT image shows lentiform shaped acute extradural hematoma along the lateral parietal convexity.

Fig. 10: Axial CT image showing acute subdural hematoma along right frontoparietal lateral convexity with a coincidental small hemorrhagic contusion in right parietal lobe.

- Hypoxic—ischemic encephalopathy
- Metabolic encephalopathy (severe hypoglycemia, osmotic myelinolysis)
- Toxic encephalopathy (methyl alcohol, CO, cyanide)
- Inherited disorders (Alexander disease, Canavan disease, Hallervorden Spatz disease, Huntington disease, Leigh disease, metachromatic leukodystrophy, methylmalonic aciduria, Wilson disease)
- Acquired neurodegenerative disorders (MS, Parkinson disease, striatonigral degeneration).

Bilateral Hyperdense (Calcification) Basal Ganglia

- Idiopathic (Globus pallidus is most commonly affected)
- Fahr disease
- *Toxic causes*: CO poisoning, lead poisoning, mineralizing angiopathy.
- Secondary to infection (TB, HIV, TORCH)/infestation (toxoplasmosis, cysticercosis)
- Congenital disorders (Cockayne syndrome, Down syndrome, MELAS/MERRF (mitochondrial encephalopathy with lactic acidosis/myoclonic epilepsy with ragged red fiber) syndrome, methemoglobinopathy, neurofibromatosis, tuberous sclerosis)
- *Metabolic*: Hypoparathyroidism, pseudohypoparathyroidism, pseudopseudohypothyroidism, hyperparathyroidism.
- *Miscellaneous*: Postradiotherapy/chemotherapy.

Hyperdense Falx

- Subarachnoid hemorrhage (associated with sulcal bleed in the parasagittal brain parenchyma)
- Subdural hemorrhage
- Diffuse cerebral edema (there is pseudohyperdensity due to diffusely hypodense brain parenchyma)
- Dural calcification (usually seen in the elderly population)
- Normal variant (usually seen in the children).

Ring Enhancing Lesions Crossing the Corpus Callosum

- *Glioblastoma multiforme (butterfly glioma)*: More heterogeneous with areas of necrosis and hemorrhage
- Astrocytoma
- *Oligodendroglioma*:
    - *Lymphoma*: Primary lymphoma is usually homogeneous and does not show necrosis/hemorrhage. Secondary lymphoma or lymphoma associated with immunocompromised states (AIDS) show necrosis.

Innumerable Small Enhancing Brain Nodules (Table 11)

- *Disseminated infection*: Tuberculosis (TB), neurocysticercosis (NCC), and histoplasmosis
- *Inflammation*: Sarcoidosis, MS
- Primary CNS lymphoma
- Metastases
- *Subacute multifocal infarction*: Hypoperfusion, multiple emboli, cerebral vasculitis, meningitis, cortical vein thrombosis.

Gyriform Enhancement (Table 12)

- Infarct
- Leptomeningitis (Fig. 11)
- Sequelae to subarachnoid hemorrhage

Pneumonic for Ring Enhancing Lesions in Brain

MAGICAL DR

M: Metastasis
A: Abscess
G: Glioblastoma

TABLE 11: Causes of hypodense, enhancing lesions.

Ring enhancement (Fig. 12)

- *Infectious*:
  - Abscess/empyema
  - Granuloma
  - Fungal (cryptococcosis)
- *Parasitic*:
  - Cysticercus
  - Toxoplasmosis
- *Neoplastic*:
  - Primary (anaplastic astrocytoma, CNS lymphoma in AIDS patient)
  - Metastatic
- *Miscellaneous*:
  - Subacute infarct
  - Subacute hematoma
  - Non-neoplastic cysts (Rathke's cleft cyst, colloid cyst)
  - Multiple sclerosis
  - Thrombosed aneurysm/vessel/AVM

Nonring enhancement

- Postictal edema
- Cerebritis
- Brain tumors (majority)

(AIDS: acquired immunodeficiency syndrome; AVM: arteriovenous malformation; CNS: central nervous system)

TABLE 12: Causes of ependymal enhancement (Fig. 11).

Focal

- Prominent subependymal veins (physiological, collateral veins secondary to dural sinus occlusion)
- Subependymal nodules
- Subependymal giant cell astrocytoma
- Nodular heterotopia
- Subependymal cysticercus
- Neoplastic (lymphoma, infiltrating glioma, medulloblastoma, carcinomatosis)

Diffuse

- Infection (pyogenic, CMV, ependymitis granularis)
- Neoplastic (lymphoma, infiltrating glioma, pineal tumors, medulloblastoma, carcinomatosis)
- Postchemotherapy and shunt placement

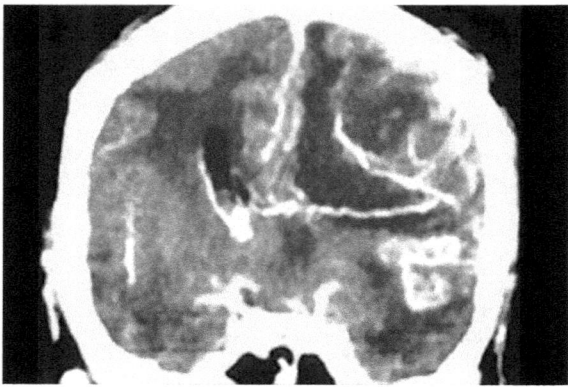

Fig. 11: Coronal MPR CT image with nodular enhancement of the leptomeninges and ependymal enhancement.

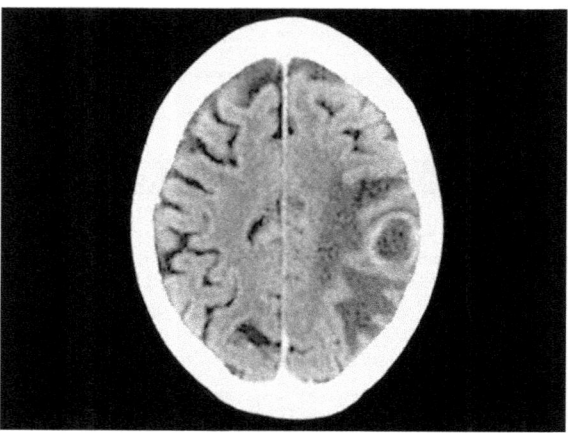

Fig. 12: Axial CT image showing a ring-enhancing lesion with perilesional edema in the left frontoparietal region.

I: Infarct (subacute phase)
C: Contusion
A: AIDS
L: Lymphoma
D: Demyelinating disease
R: Radiation necrosis or resolving hematoma

Multifocal Brain Tumors and Tumor-like Lesions

- Infections and infestations [tuberculoma, toxoplasmosis, NCC, multiple abscesses (pyogenic/fungal)]
- Multiple sclerosis
- Phakomatosis
- Metastases from primary CNS tumor
- *Multicentric CNS lesion*: True multicentric glioma, primary CNS lymphoma
- Multicentric meningioma without neurofibromatosis.

VENTRICULAR LESIONS

Ventricular Enlargement

- Hydrocephalus
- Holoprosencephaly
- Hydranencephaly
- Schizencephaly
- Porencephaly
- Encephalomalacia
- Deep cortical atrophy.

Small Ventricles

- Physiological variation (sulci and cisterns appear normal)
- Chronic ventricular shunt drainage (sulci and cisterns appear normal)
- Increased intracranial pressure (sulci and cisterns appear effaced).

Abnormal Ventricular Configuration

- *Colpocephaly (dilatation of the trigone and occipital horns of the lateral ventricles)*:
  - Corpus callosal agenesis
  - Arnold-Chiari malformation
  - Holoprosencephaly (lobar type).
- *Abnormal frontal horns*:
  - Square or box-like—absence or hypoplasia of septum pellucidum (septo-optic dysplasia, callosal dysgenesis, schizencephaly, holoprosencephaly)
  - Convex or flat lateral wall (caudate lobe atrophy).
- *Miscellaneous*:
  - Schizencephaly (nipple-like elevation along the lateral wall)
  - Porencephaly
  - Corpus callosum dysgenesis (high riding third ventricle with communication with a dorsal interhemispheric cyst)
  - Chiari II malformation (elongated, slit-like fourth ventricle)
  - Dandy-Walker syndrome (communication between the fourth ventricle and the retrocerebellar cyst) (Figs. 13A and B)
  - Dandy-Walker variant (slit-like communication between the fourth ventricle and the cisterna magna with a typical *key-hole appearance*) (Figs. 14A and B)
  - Ventricular diverticulum (CSF-outpouching from the medial atrial wall of the lateral ventricle)
  - Herniation
    - *Subfalcine*: It is characterized by displacement of the lateral and third ventricle under the falx away from the side of mass lesion with dilatation of the contralateral lateral ventricle (Fig. 15).
    - *Transtentorial herniation*: There is change in size and configuration of the fourth ventricle depending upon the ascending or descending transtentorial herniation. Ascending type is associated with compression and displacement of the third ventricle and its aqueduct as well while descending type is characterized by dilatation of the ambient, quadrigeminal, and cerebellopontine cisterns and rotation of the brainstem.

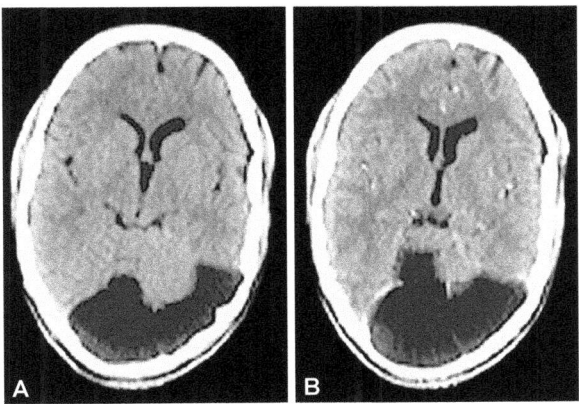

Figs. 13A and B: Axial CT images showing Dandy-Walker syndrome.

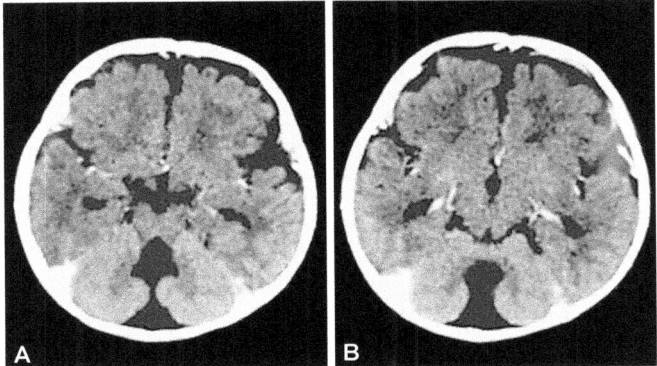

Figs. 14A and B: CECT axial images of head showing hypoplastic vermis and fourth ventricle communicating with cisterna magna in a case of Dandy-Walker variant.

Hydrocephalus

- There is enlargement of part or entire ventricular system with proportionate enlargement of the temporal horns of the lateral ventricles (Fig. 16)
- There is rounding of the frontal horns of the lateral ventricle
- There is effacement of the basal cisterns, fissures, and the sulcal spaces to a varying degree
- There is transependymal seepage of the CSF resulting in periventricular hypodensity in moderate and severe cases
- The dilated ventricles are always surrounded by cortical mantle irrespective of the severity.

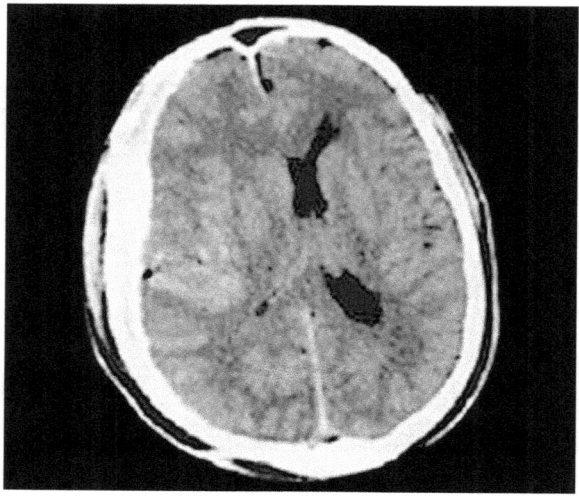

Fig. 15: Axial CT image showing subfalcine herniation of the right lateral ventricle to the left side in a patient with acute SDH on right side with a small aerocele.
(SDH: subdural hematoma)

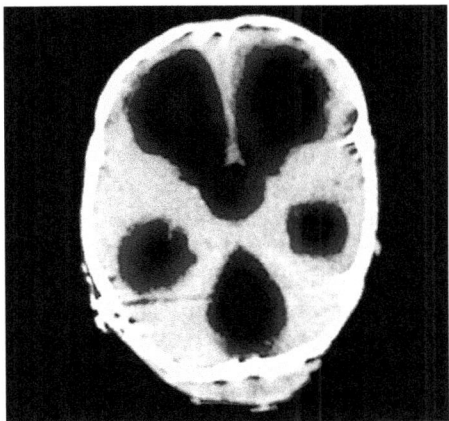

Fig. 16: Axial CT image of the brain showing hydrocephalus with dilatation of all the ventricles.

Holoprosencephaly

The CT appearance varies with the type of the holoprosencephaly.

Alobar Type

It is characterized by:
- Single, large, crescentic ventricle devoid of horns
- Large dorsal cyst with a wide communication with the ventricle
- Grossly distorted supratentorial brain morphology with no hemispheric development and absence of the interhemispheric fissure, falx, and tentorium, septum pellucidum, third ventricle, corpus callosum, Sylvian fissure, straight sinus, vein of Galen, and internal cerebral veins
- Fused thalami and basal ganglia protruding into the ventricle
- Cortical mantle is seen in the posterosuperior part of the cranium and is usually pachygyric

- Midbrain, pons, and cerebellum are morphologically normal
- Associated abnormalities include cyclopia, ethmocephaly, cebocephaly, cleft lip, and palate.

Semilobar Type

It is characterized by:
- Single, large ventricle with rudimentary or poorly developed temporal and occipital horns
- Large dorsal cyst with a wide communication with the ventricle
- Supratentorial brain morphology is distorted with no hemispheric development and rudimentary interhemispheric fissure (separating occipital lobes), falx, and tentorium, third ventricle, but with absence of septum pellucidum and corpus callosum, Sylvian fissure, straight sinus, vein of Galen, and internal cerebral veins
- There is partial separation of the thalami and basal ganglia that are anterior relative to their usual location
- Cortical mantle seen is thicker than in alobar type and is pachygyric
- Midbrain, pons, and cerebellum are morphologically normal
- Associated abnormalities include cleft lip and palate.

Lobar Type

It is characterized by:
- Two distinct, well-formed lateral ventricles with closely apposed bodies
- The ventricles are dilated with relatively greater enlargement of the occipital horns of the lateral ventricle
- The frontal horns are fused due to absence of the septum pellucidum and dysplastic frontal lobes, falx, and interhemispheric fissure
- Sylvian fissures are absent
- Corpus callosum is usually present

- Thalami and basal ganglia may be fused or separated
- Cortical mantle is usually pachygyric and lissencephalic
- Midbrain, pons, and cerebellum are morphologically normal
- Associated abnormalities include cleft lip and palate.

Hydranencephaly

- There is a large CSF—isodense, cystic lesion surrounded by a membrane with no identifiable brain tissue usually involving one half of the cranial cavity
- Hemispheric division is usually maintained
- Except for the atrophic brainstem, rest of the brain appears morphologically normal even on the side of the cyst
- Ventricle with the choroids plexus are usually preserved.

Atrophy

- It is characterized by symmetric enlargement of the ventricular system with proportionate enlargement of the basal cisterns, fissures, sulcal spaces, and the other CSF spaces in the cranial cavity
- It is associated with loss of volume of both gray and white matter with reduction in gray white matter differentiation.

Corpus Callosum Agenesis (Fig. 17)

- It is characterized by absence of corpus callosum, cingulated gyrus, and sulcus with a high riding third ventricle opening into the interhemispheric fissure. A cyst may or may not be present.
- The medial hemispheric surface of the brain shows a radial arrangement of the gyri and sulci in a *spoke-wheel like configuration*.
- Abnormal upward course of the anterior cerebral arteries (ACAs).
- The lateral ventricle are arranged parallel to each other (*Racing car sign*) with pointed frontal horns (*Viking horn sign*) and dilated atria and Brain occipital horns

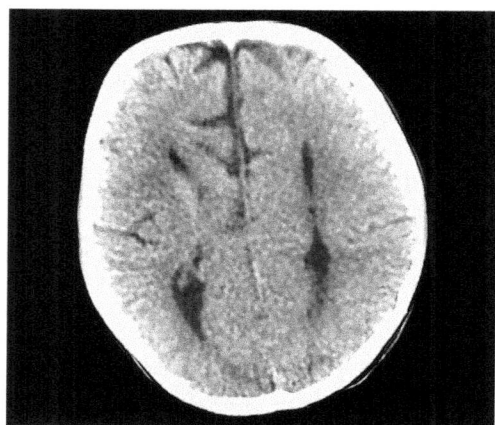

Fig. 17: Axial CT image shows parallel oriented lateral ventricles with colpocephaly with absence of corpus callosum.

- With partial agenesis, rostrum and splenium of the corpus callosum are hypoplastic or absent with varying degrees of development of the body and genu.

Arnold-Chiari Malformation

- *Type II* is the classical type in this group and is commonly associated with colpocephaly
- It is characterized by small posterior fossa, with low lying transverse sinuses and concave clivus and petrous ridges
- There is beaking of tectum, creeping of cerebellum around brainstem with inferiorly displaced vermis and medullary spur and kink
- There is hydrocephalus with tube-like, elongated fourth ventricle
- Meningomyelocele is invariably seen with syringomyelia and diastematomyelia in many cases
- Associated anomalies in the brain include corpus callosum dysgenesis, polymicrogyria, and heterotopias.

DIFFERENTIATING FEATURES OF BRAIN LESIONS

Differentiating features of brain lesions are listed in Table 13.

TABLE 13: Differentiating features of various brain lesions.

Diseases	Differentiating features	Comments
Edema (Fig. 18)	• Ill-defined area of non-enhancing hypodensity involving primarily the white matter • Mass effect is evident in form of flattening of gyri, displacement, and deformation of ventricles and even midline shift	• *Cytotoxic*: Ischemia/anoxia • *Vasogenic*: Commonest, associated with neoplasms, metastases hemorrhagic infarction, and inflammation
Arterial infarct (Fig. 19)	• It is seen as well-defined lesion involving both gray and white matter conforming to an arterial territory that may show ring or gyriform enhancement in subacute stage • Indirect signs include hyperdense clot in MCA; subtle effacement of sulci and fissures; obscuration of gray and white matter interface and hypodensity of insular cortex	Larger infarcts may show hemorrhagic transformation in the form of petechial or frank hemorrhage
Nonhemorrhagic contusion	• It is seen as a hypodense, nonenhancing, ill-defined lesion affecting both gray and white matter • Gyral enhancement can be seen in the resolving stage	History of trauma can be elicited

Contd...

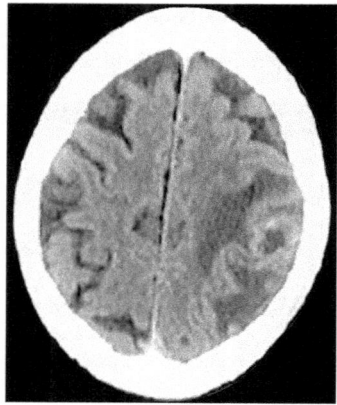
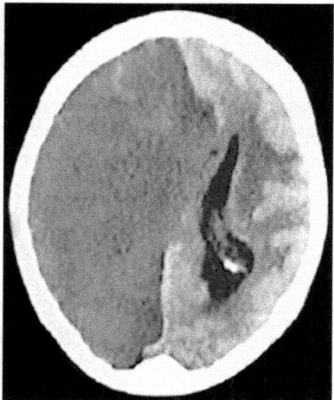

Fig. 18: Axial CT image shows nonenhancing edema around the ring enhancing lesion

Fig. 19: Axial CT image a large right cerebral acute arterial infarct.

Contd...

Diseases	Differentiating features	Comments
Gliosis	It is seen as an ill-defined lesion involving both gray and white matter with signs of volume loss on ipsilateral side with dilatation of the ipsilateral ventricle, fissure, and sulci	It may be due to any type of insult to the brain parenchyma (vascular or inflam- matory or traumatic)
Periventri-cular CSF seepage	It is seen as a marked, white matter hypodensity along the contour of the ventricular system, most prominent at the horns	It is associated with moderate-to-severe hydrocephalus
Lipoma	• It is typically seen as a curvilinear, midline, non-enhancing, fat attenuating mass taking the shape of the corpus callosum, when the latter is normal	Dorsal, pericallosal region is the most common site followed by basal cisterns (Figs. 20A and B)

Contd...

Brain

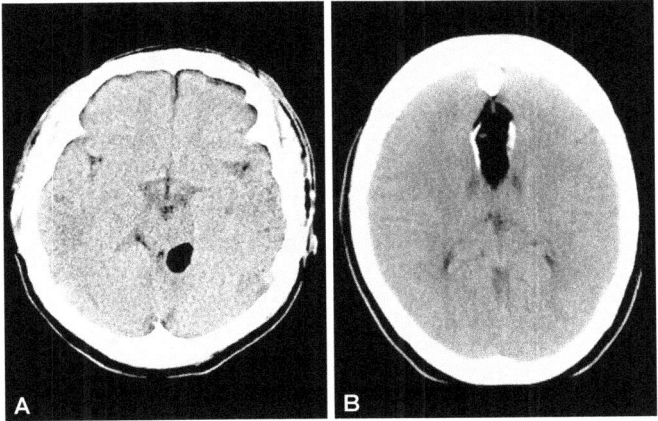

Figs. 20A and B: Axial CT images show a fat density lesion in left ambient cistern suggestive of lipoma.

Contd...

Diseases	Differentiating features	Comments
	• In cases of corpus callosal dysgenesis, the mass is tubulonodular in shape • Calcification may be seen in curvilinear (bracket-shaped) or nodular	
Hemangio-blastoma	It is seen as a sharply marginated mass of CSF density with peripheral, intensely and homogeneously, enhancing mural nodule	• It may be associated with von Hippel-Lindau disease • The size of the tumor and mural nodule is less than pilocytic astrocytoma

Contd...

Contd...

Diseases	Differentiating features	Comments
Neuro-cysticercus (Figs. 21A to C)	• The CT appearance varies with the stage of the disease • In vesicular stage, the lesion is seen as a sub-centimeter cystic focus with imperceptible walls at gray white matter junction or in subpial location. There is no edema or enhancement • In vesicular nodular stage, there is a cystic lesion with usually an eccentric, hyperdense nodule with perilesional edema and variable postcontrast enhancement • Granular nodular stage shows appearance similar to the previous stage but with greater postcontrast enhancement and edema • Nodular calcified stage is characterized by nodular focus of calcification with no postcontrast enhancement or edema • When multiple, the lesions are seen in different stages	When multiple, lesions are seen in different stages (vesicular, colloid vesicular, granular nodular, nodular calcified), with edema around some lesions corresponding to the middle two stages
Toxo-plasmosis	• It is characterized by solitary or multiple, ring-enhancing lesions with edema in immunocompromised patients. Target appearance is characteristic	• It is the most common opportunistic infection in acquired immunodeficiency syndrome (AIDS) patients

Contd...

Brain

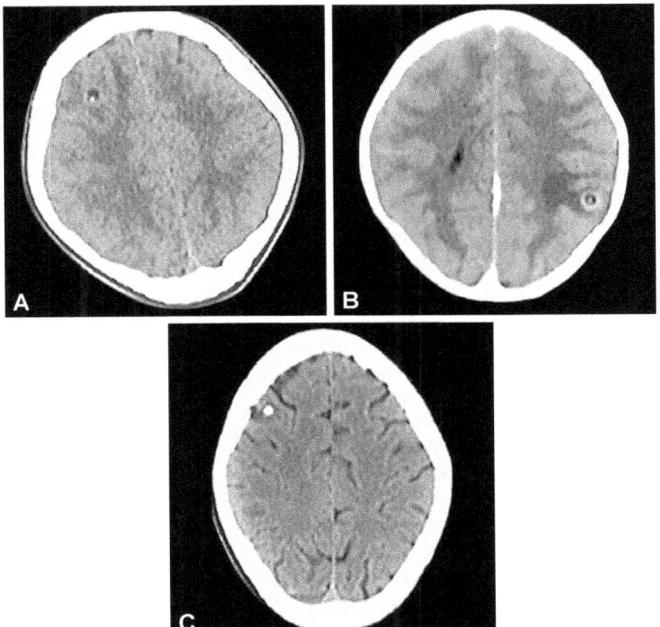

Figs. 21A to C: Axial CT scans showing colloid vesicular and granular nodular and nodular calcified stage of cysticercus.

Contd...

Diseases	Differentiating features	Comments
	• Hemorrhage and calcification is common in treated patients • It is seen as multifocal, calcified lesion in the region of basal ganglia, periventricular white matter, and cortex in cases of congenital infection and is commonly associated with hydrocephalus	• The most common differential diagnosis is AIDS-related lymphoma • Multiplicity of the lesions favor toxoplasmosis • It is the second most common congenital infection after CMV infection

Contd...

Contd...

Diseases	Differentiating features	Comments
Cryptococcosis	• It is seen as multifocal, cystic lesions with variable postcontrast enhancement in the region of basal ganglia and midbrain with absence of edema • The most common differential diagnosis is VR spaces	Diffuse disease in the form of cryptococcomas is common in AIDS patients while meningitis is common in immunocompetent patients
Chronic infarct (Fig. 22)	• It is seen as a well-defined, hypodense to CSF attenuating lesion corresponding to the vascular territory and involving both gray and white matter • No evidence of volume loss is seen	Usually refers to the infarct older than 8 weeks
Virchow-Robin spaces (VR spaces)	• It refers to the CSF attenuating oval lesions with their long axis perpendicular to the body of the ventricle • They are usually multiple	• They are commonly seen in the ganglionic region and periventricular region • Dilated VR spaces are also seen in cryptococcal infection in AIDS patient
Hematoma	• The CT appearance varies with the age of the hematoma • Acute hematoma appears hyperdense • Subacute hematoma appears isodense to the gray matter and may show some ring enhancement on postcontrast images • Chronic hematoma is hypodense and does not show evidence of enhancement	History of trauma or hypertension is suggestive

Contd...

Brain

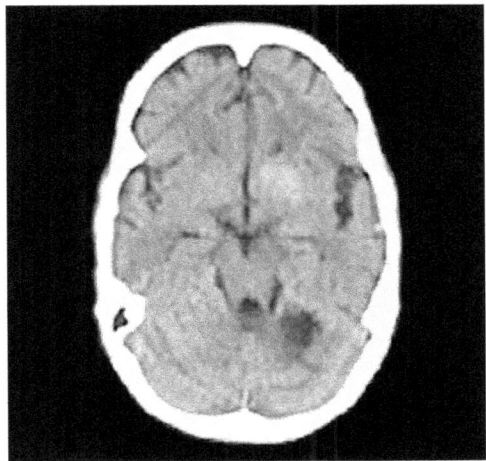

Fig. 22: Axial CT image showing chronic infarct in left cerebellar hemisphere.

Contd...

Diseases	Differentiating features	Comments
Encephalomalacia	Ill- or well-defined CSF attenuating lesion with signs of volume loss	It resembles gliosis in appearance but is lower in attenuation value
Porencephalic cyst (Fig. 23)	• It is a well-defined, intra-axial, CSF attenuating lesion involving both gray and white matter but is surrounded by white matter • It may or may not communicate with the ventricular system	The differentiation is to be made with arachnoid cyst and schizencephaly

Contd...

Contd...

Diseases	Differentiating features	Comments
Schizen-cephaly (Fig. 24)	• It is seen as an extra-axial CSF collection that is communicating with the ventricular system through a gray matter lined cleft in the brain matter • The open lip type shows a clear communication between the collection and ventricular system • In the closed lip type, cleft is often not visualized but the diagnosis is suggested by a nipple-like projection in the lateral wall of the ipsilateral lateral ventricle	• The condition can be bilateral and may be associated with congenital malformation of the brain • Heterotopias are commonly associated

Contd...

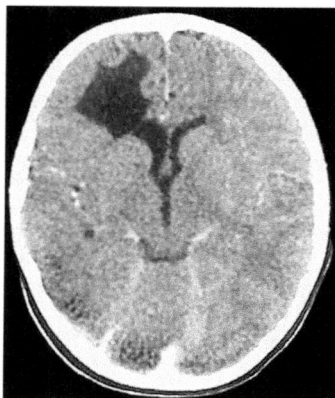 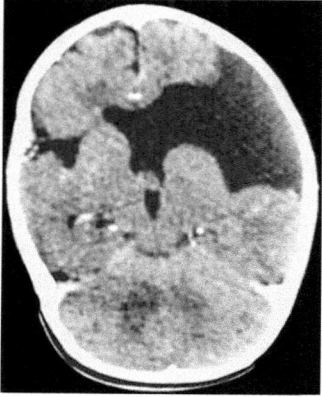

Fig. 23: A cerebrospinal fluid (CSF) containing cavity seen in right frontal lobe communicating with the frontal horn of right lateral ventricle suggestive of porencephalic cyst.

Fig. 24: Bilateral schizencephaly—open lip on left side and closed lip on right side.

Brain

Contd...

Diseases	Differentiating features	Comments
Hydatid cyst	• It is seen as a spherical, intra-axial, CSF attenuating lesion with thin, nonenhancing walls • It may be multiple and gliomatosized	The most common site is the parietal region
Choroid plexus cyst	• It is seen as a CSF attenuating lesion within the choroid plexus of the ventricle • It is usually bilateral	It may be an incidental finding
Choroid fissure cyst	It is seen as a well-defined, CSF attenuating lesion with no postcontrast enhancement in the choroidal fissure. The latter is located between the diencephalon and hippocampus	It is usually discovered incidentally
Ependymal cyst	• It is seen as a well-defined, CSF attenuating, nonenhancing lesion lying within the ventricular system commonly in the atria • The lesion is unrelated to the choroid plexus of the ventricles and is usually unilateral and may just be seen as focal enlargement of the ventricle	Large cyst may present with obstructive hydrocephalus
Arachnoid cyst (Figs. 25A and B)	• It is seen as a well-defined, CSF attenuating, extra-axial lesion with no communication with the ventricular system • There may be mass effect on the adjacent structures as scalloping of the inner table of the skull • There is no edema/enhancement/internal septa	• The most common site is the temporal region in the Sylvian fissure • It may be idiopathic or secondary to meningitis

Contd...

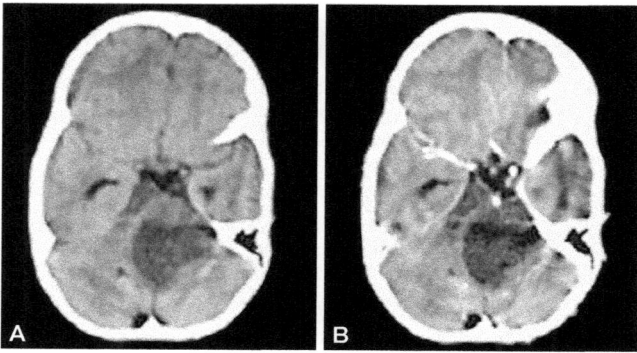

Figs. 25A and B: Axial CT images showing arachnoid cyst in the left cerebellopontine angle.

Contd...

Diseases	Differentiating features	Comments
Epidermoid (Figs. 26A and B)	• It is typically seen as a lobulated, homogeneous, nonenhancing, extra-axial, off-midline mass of CSF or fat density • It engulfs the vessels; cisternal and fissures insinuation is characteristic • It molds itself around the brain surface • Calcification is uncommon and the periphery may show occasional enhancement	The most common site is the basal cisterns especially the cerebellopontine cistern
Dermoid	• It is seen as a rounded, midline, fat attenuating, nonenhancing mass usually seen in the parasellar and basifrontal region • Mural calcification is common but enhancement is almost never seen unless infected • Basifrontal type may be associated with dermal sinus tract	Rupture is commoner than epidermoid

Contd...

Brain

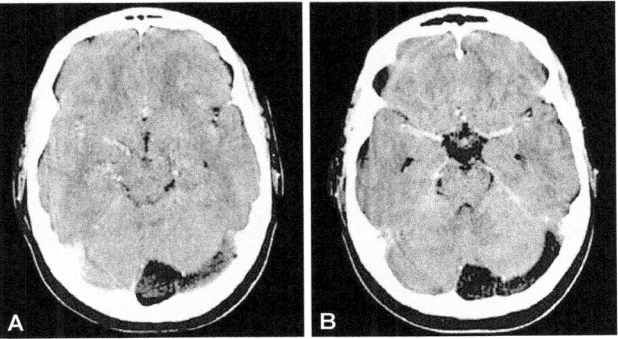

Figs. 26A and B: CECT axial images of head showing fluid density extra-axial lesion on left side of posterior fossa insinuating along the subarachnoid spaces suggestive of epidermoid.
(CECT: contrast-enhanced computed tomography)

Contd...

Diseases	Differentiating features	Comments
Capillary/ cavernous angioma (Figs. 27A to C)	• They are iso- to hyperdense on NECT with variable degree of enhancement in capillary type and absent or minimal in cavernous type • Calcification is common • Edema and mass effect are almost never seen	Capillary type has a predilection for brainstem
Abscess	• It is seen as a ring enhancing lesion on CECT with variable thickness of smooth, regular walls and surrounding edema and mass effect • Granulomatous abscesses have thicker, nodular, and hyperdense walls with lobulated shape • Associated ependymal and meningeal enhancement are commonly seen	• The closest differential diagnosis is necrotic mass where the walls are relatively thicker and irregular and nodular with thicker wall on ependymal side • Abscesses seen in systemic diseases (leukemia, lymphoma) associated with immunosuppression resemble necrotic masses

Contd...

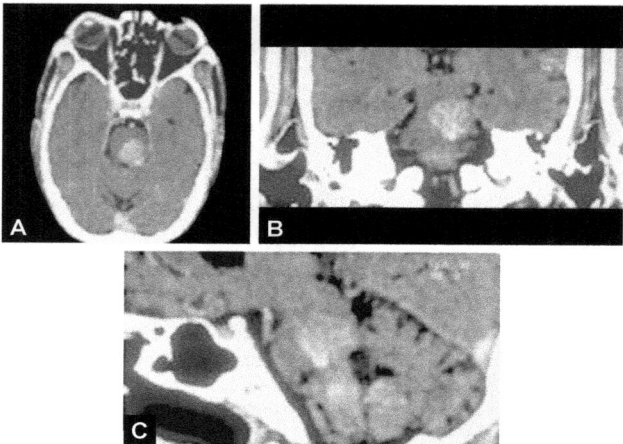

Figs. 27A to C: Axial, coronal, and sagittal CT images showing a cavernous angioma in the pons on left side.

Contd...

Diseases	Differentiating features	Comments
	• The wall on the ependymal side appear thinner than the one toward the cortex • The presence of satellite nodules and air are characteristic • An abscess can be thin-walled with minimal mural enhancement with minimal or no edema in chronic stage or when patient is on steroid therapy	

Contd...

Brain

Contd...

Diseases	Differentiating features	Comments
Empyema	• It is seen as an extra-axial, hypodense collection with enhancing walls and often with edema in the adjacent brain parenchyma • Enhancing septae are sometimes evident • Cerebral convexity and interhemispheric fissure are the common sites	They are commonly associated with meningitis, chronic suppurative otitis media (CSOM), trauma, or post-operative condition
Aeroceles	The CT HU value ranges from –100 to –1,000	The important causes include trauma and neoplasm invading sinus
Colloid cyst	• It is seen as a hyperdense but sometimes as a isodense, round mass at the inferior aspect of the septum pellucidum protruding into the anterior portion of the third ventricle between the columns of the fornix on NECT • CECT shows mild to absent enhancement	It is usually an incidental finding but may present with features of increased intracranial pressure
Rathke cleft cyst	• It is usually seen as hypodense, noncalcified, rim enhancing, intra- and suprasellar lesion • It may be entirely intra- or suprasellar in location	It is commoner in females
Enterogenous cyst	It is seen as a well-defined, lobulated, hypodense, nonenhancing, extra-axial lesion commonly seen in the cerebellopontine angle cistern and anterior to the brainstem	These are very rare lesions; commoner in the spine

Contd...

Contd...

Diseases	Differentiating features	Comments
Tuber-culoma (Figs. 28 and 29)	• It is seen on noncontrast images as an iso- to hyperdense, ring or nodular lesion usually at the gray white matter interface with significant perilesional edema • On postcontrast images, it shows moderate, nodular, or ring enhancement • The lesion is usually larger than 1 cm in diameter with irregular, nodular walls • Mature tuberculoma can appear as target lesions with central or eccentric, punctate calcified, or enhancing hyperdensity • Multiple, conglomerate masses with associated basilar meningitis are highly suggestive of the diagnosis	In pediatric age, these are commonly seen in the infra-tentorium; while in the adult, it is commonly supratentorial
Lymphoma	• It is characterized as multiple, hyperdense, centrally located (deep white matter, basal ganglia, corpus callosum), mild-to-moderately and homogeneously enhancing, nodular lesions • Subependymal spread is common • Hemorrhage and ring enhancement is commonly seen in cases associated with AIDS	• Primary cerebral lymphoma is usually of the non-Hodgkin type • Calcification/necrosis is seen in post-treatment cases

Contd...

Brain

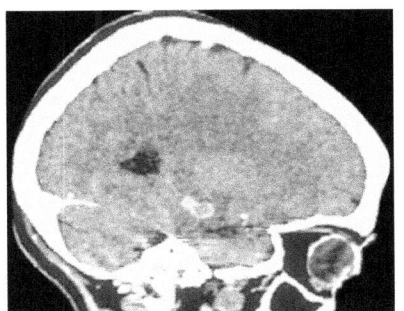

Fig. 28: Axial CT image showing tuberculoma in the temporal lobe.

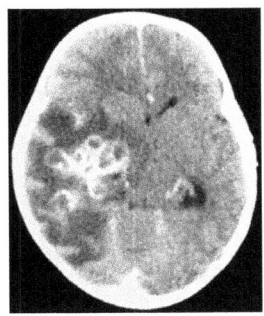

Fig. 29: Axial CECT image shows multiple conglomerate ring enhancing lesions with perilesional edema in the right temporal lobe and basal ganglia suggestive of tuberculomas.

Contd...

Diseases	Differentiating features	Comments
	• Metastatic involvement of the CNS is usually seen as a leptomeningeal involvement or focal, nodular. Enhancing, intra-axial mass • Perineural tumors are also common sites of metastatic lymphoma	
Leukemia	It is seen as an extra-axial, enhancing, lobulated dural-based masses	These are commonly seen in the pediatric age group and the most common leukemia to metastasize to brain is acute myeloblastic leukemia (AML)

Contd...

Contd...

Diseases	Differentiating features	Comments
Meningioma (Figs. 30A and B)	• It is seen as a round, iso- to hyperdense, (Fig. 30) moderate to intensely enhancing, extra-axial mass with dural tail • Edema in the adjacent brain parenchyma is common with larger lesions • Sometimes, it is present as a calcified, minimally enhancing mass or as a small, dural-based, enhancing plaque (focal dural thickening) • Hyperostosis in the adjacent bony calvaria are highly suggestive • Atypical varieties may show ring enhancement and bone erosion	Most common sites are the falx cerebri, cerebral convexities, sphenoidal ridge, and the tentorium
Medulloblastoma	• It is seen as a midline, vermian, predominantly solid mass arising from the roof of the fourth ventricle that is hyperdense on noncontrast images and shows moderate postcontrast enhancement. Calcification is seen in up to 50% cases • CNS dissemination is seen at the time of presentation in up to 50% cases. Therefore, image the entire neuraxis	• It is usually seen before 15 years of age • The features are more atypical if the tumor is seen in adults • If tentorial calcification present, rule out Gorlin-Goltz syndrome.

Contd...

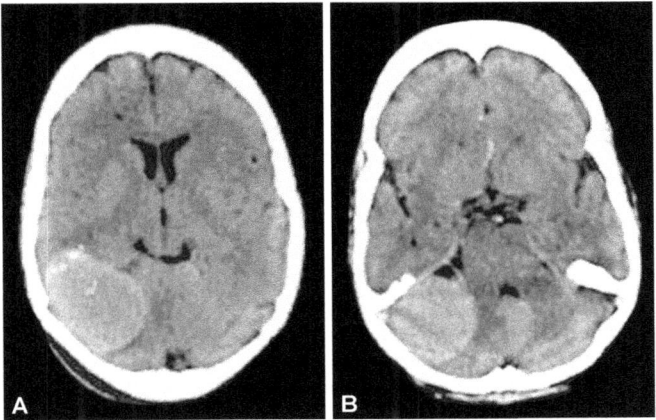

Figs. 30A and B: Axial CT images showing tentorial meningioma on right side.

Contd...

Diseases	Differentiating features	Comments
	• Predominantly cystic mass; no postcontrast enhancement and isoattenuating on NECT may be seen in atypical cases • The tumor can arise in the cerebellum	
Choroid plexus papilloma	• It is seen as a cauliflower like, solid, moderate to intensely but heterogeneously enhancing mass arising in the ventricular system usually associated with hydrocephalus due to CSF over-production • Calcification is seen in up to one-quarter of the cases • CSF dissemination is common	• The most common site is the trigone of the lateral ventricle • In children, it is commoner in the supratentorium and in adults in the infratentorium

Contd...

Contd...

Diseases	Differentiating features	Comments
Choroid plexus carcinoma	• CT findings are similar to choroid plexus papilloma • Parenchymal and CSF dissemination is seen	• The most common age group is under 5 years • Differentiation from papilloma is not possible on imaging
Astrocytoma (Figs. 31A and B)	• *Pilocytic type* is seen as a round, hypo- to isoattenuating, nonenhancing tumor with a heterogeneously enhancing mural nodule • Edema is usually absent • *Low-grade glioma* is seen as focal or diffuse hypodense, non or minimally enhancing mass in the cerebral white matter with or without involvement of the gray matter • Hemorrhage, necrosis, and edema are uncommon but calcification may be seen in up to 20% cases • *Anaplastic glioma* or *glioblastoma multiforme* are seen as ill-defined, inhomogeneous, usually nodular, ring enhancing masses in the cerebral white matter with massive edema and mass effect • Hemorrhage and necrosis are common as opposed to calcification, which is uncommon. • CNS dissemination is common	• *Pilocytic type* is seen usually in childhood • *Common site* is around the third and fourth ventricle • *Low-grade glioma* usually in children and young adults • Presence of the lesion in the corpus callosum and its spread on either of midline is more suggestive of glioblastoma multiforme

Contd...

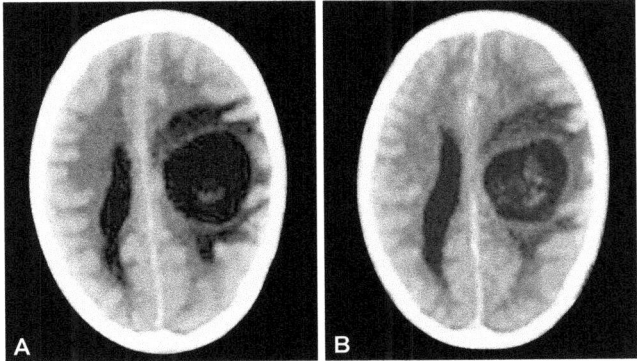

Figs. 31A and B: Axial CT images showing cystic glioma.

Contd...

Diseases	Differentiating features	Comments
Gliomatosis cerebri	It is seen as a diffusely, infiltrating, non-enhancing, white matter lesion causing cerebral enlargement but with preservation of the overall brain morphology	The common sites include optic nerves, corpus callosum, fornices, and cerebral ped-uncles
Brainstem glioma (Fig. 32)	They are usually seen as enlargement of the brainstem due to their infiltrative quality and appear as hypodense on noncontrast images and may show variable enhancement	• It may encase the basilar artery • They are commonly seen in children and may be exophytic
Subependymal giant cell astrocytoma (Fig. 33)	It is seen as a cystic, partially calcified, heterogeneously enhancing mass at the foramen of Monro with features of obstructive hydrocephalus	• It occurs with tuberous sclerosis • Other stigmata of tuberous sclerosis may be suggestive of the diagnosis

Contd...

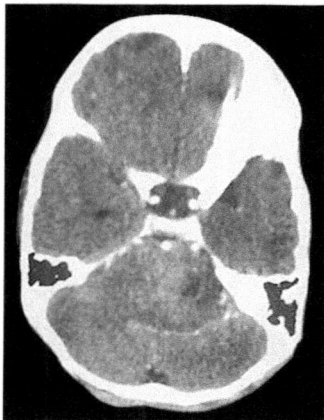

Fig. 32: Axial CECT image in a patient with brainstem glioma shows expansion of the brainstem with encasement of the basilar artery.

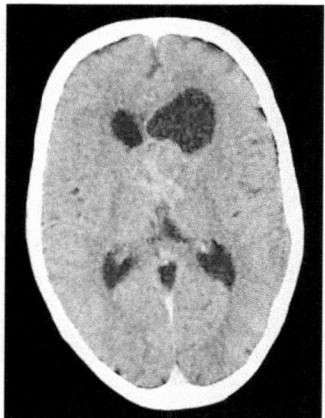

Fig. 33: Subependymal giant cell astrocytoma—heterogeneous enhancing mass lesion seen in the region of foramen of Monro in this patient of tuberous sclerosis.

Contd...

Diseases	Differentiating features	Comments
Oligodendroglioma (Fig. 34)	• It is usually seen as a partially calcified, iso- to hyperdense, mild-to-moderately enhancing mass in the white matter usually of the frontal lobe with extension into the gray matter • Cystic degeneration is common but hemorrhage, necrosis, and edema are uncommon • Overlying skull may show signs of pressure erosions	• It is seen in the middle-aged adults • Allelic deletion of 1p and 19q is favorable for chemotherapy

Contd...

Contd...

Diseases	Differentiating features	Comments
Ependymoma	• It is characterized by heterogeneous, lobulated mass with cyst and calcification with variable postcontrast enhancement • It is most commonly seen arising from the floor of the fourth ventricle • *Plastic growth*: Squeezes out laterally from foramen of Luschka and posteriorly from foramen of Magendie.	It is extraventricular in location when supratentorial while intraventricular in location when infratentorial
Subependymoma	It is seen as a well-defined, homogeneously, iso- to hypodense, nonenhancing or minimally enhancing mass usually in the region of the frontal horns and the inferior aspect of the fourth ventricle	It is a rare tumor seen in the middle-aged and the elderly

Contd...

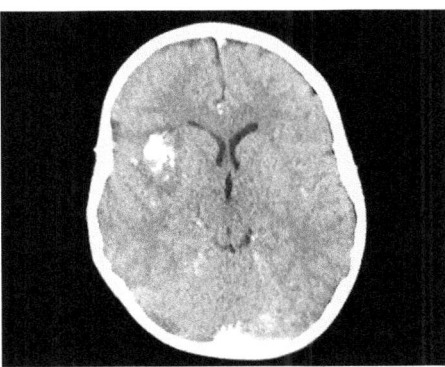

Fig. 34: A partially calcified oligodendroglioma seen in right perisylvian region.

Contd...

Diseases	Differentiating features	Comments
Ganglio-glioma	• It is seen as a well-defined, cystic lesion with iso- to hypodense mural nodule that may often be calcified. Enhancement is variable • They are usually located peripherally and so may be associated with scalloping of the over-lying calvaria	They are commonly seen in pediatric age group and most commonly in the supratentorium in the temporal lobe
Hemangio-pericytoma (Fig. 35)	• They are seen as heterogeneous density lesions with cystic areas on noncontrast images • Postcontrast images show intense heterogeneous enhancement. Vascular channels may be seen within the lesion • Extra-axial signs may be suggestive of the lesion	They have a strong propensity for extraneural meta-stases to bone, both local and distant

Contd...

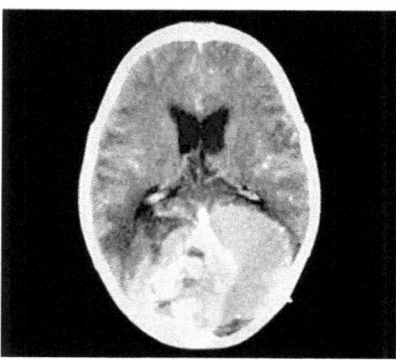

Fig. 35: Intensely enhancing vascular mass lesion seen along posterior falx—hemangiopericytoma.

Brain

Contd...

Diseases	Differentiating features	Comments
Pineal cell tumors	It is seen as a well-defined, hyperdense strongly enhancing mass with presence of calcification in 80% cases. Pineal tumors show blast-type calcification.	They account for two-thirds of the pineal tumors and usually occur in second decade
Germ cell tumors Germinoma, teratoma (Fig. 36)	Synchronous lesions in the suprasellar region are also present. Appears to engulf calcification.	Germinoma are eight times more common in males
Parenchymal cell tumors pineocytoma pineoblastoma	• They appear as heterogeneous masses containing cysts, calcification, and fat and showing minimal enhancement • They appear as a well-defined, partially calcified cystic mass • It may resemble a medulloblastoma on imaging	• Distinction from pineal cyst is not possible on imaging • It is a primitive neuroectodermal tumor (PNET) tumor

Contd...

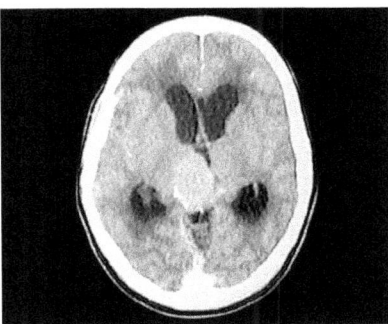

Fig. 36: Well-defined enhancing mass lesion seen arising from the pineal gland.

Contd...

Diseases	Differentiating features	Comments
Neural tumors	• *Schwannoma* is seen as well-defined, homogeneous, Hypo- to isodense lesions with moderate-to-intense homogeneous postcontrast enhancement. Cystic degeneration in the larger lesion is common resulting in heterogeneous postcontrast enhancement. Calcification and hemorrhage are rare • *Neurofibroma* is seen as a poorly delineated, infiltrative mass lesion, isodense with muscle with variable contrast enhancement. Erosion and enlargement of the neural foramina of the affected nerve is common	• *Schwannoma* is seen in middle-aged females and can involve any cranial nerve except Ist and IInd • It commonly involves VIIIth cranial nerve and seen as cerebellopontine angle (CPA) mass. When it involves the V nerve, it has to be differentiated from neurofibroma • Association is seen with neurofibromatosis-2 (NF-2), when they are multifocal and seen at an early age • *Neurofibroma* is associated with NF-1 and is seen at all ages with no sex predilection • It commonly involves the VIth cranial nerve
Pituitary adenoma (Figs. 37A and B)	• Microadenoma may cause slight contour asymmetry of the pituitary gland, and is visualized as a hypodense lesion on CECT due to lesser enhancement relative to the normal parenchyma • Macroadenoma appears as well-defined, isodense sellar mass showing moderate homogeneous enhancement and displacing the part of normal pituitary gland and its infundibulum. It balloons the sella causing pressure erosion of the surrounding bone. Suprasellar extension gives a typical figure-of-eight appearance to the lesion	• Microadenoma measures less than 10 mm in size • It is the most common intrasellar tumor in adults • Though rare in children, most lesions occur in adolescent girls • Cystic adenoma is indistinguishable from other cystic lesions of the sella

Contd...

Brain

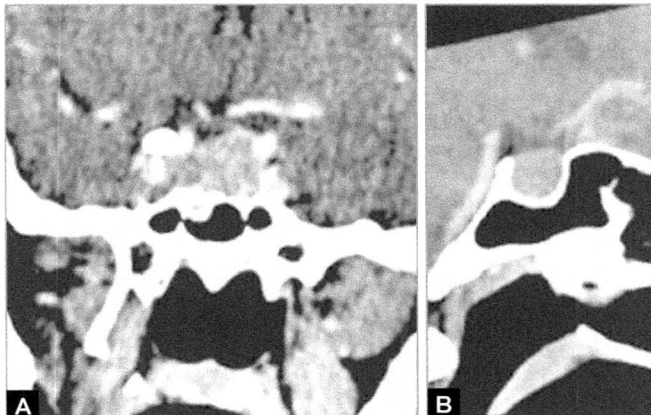

Figs. 37A and B: Coronal and sagittal CT images showing pituitary macroadenoma.

Contd...

Diseases	Differentiating features	Comments
	• Calcification is rare, however, hemorrhage is seen within the lesion which imparts an inhomogeneously hyperdense appearance to the tumor	
Craniopharyngioma (Fig. 38)	• It appears as heterogeneous, lobulated, suprasellar mass showing variable enhancement • Calcification is common in the lesion either ring-like or globular • Erosion of the posterior clinoid process is common	• It commonly occurs in children and middle-aged adults • Most lesions have a sellar component as well

Contd...

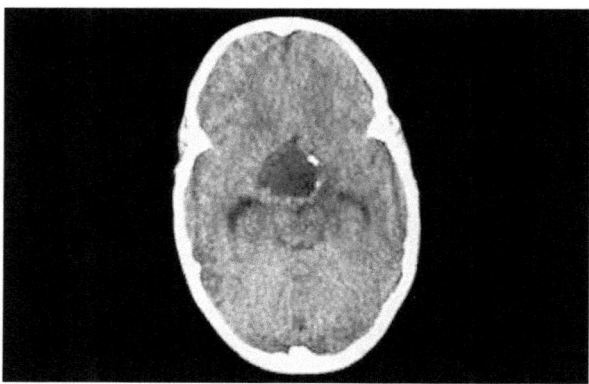

Fig. 38: Craniopharyngioma—a suprasellar cystic mass lesion with calcification.

Contd...

Diseases	Differentiating features	Comments
Metastases	• *Parenchymal* lesions are seen usually at the gray white matter interface as well-defined lesions of variable attenuation and edema that is out of proportion to the size of the lesion. Postcontrast images show variable enhancement including thick, nodular, ring-like appearance • *Leptomeningeal* lesions are seen as focal or diffuse, enhancing, nodular lesions in the sulcal and fissural location • *Dural* metastases as an isolated entity are rare and can be missed on CT	• The common sites of the primary tumor metastasizing to brain include lung, breast, melanoma, gastrointestinal, genitourinary tract (GUT), etc. • Hemorrhage may be seen within the lesions in case of breast, renal cell carcinoma, and choriocarcinoma • Leptomeningeal variety is commonly seen with highly malignant astrocytoma

Contd...

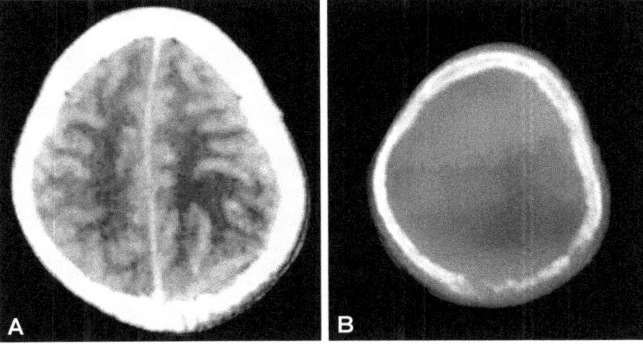

Figs. 39A and B: Axial CT images showing bony lytic metastases with extradural soft tissue mass.

Contd...

Diseases	Differentiating features	Comments
	• *Calvarial* metastases have variable appearance ranging from small lytic areas to large areas of bony destruction associated with enhancing extradural, soft tissue mass (Figs. 39A and B)	
Metachromatic leukodystrophy (MLD)	• Symmetric hypodensity in the deep white matter with relative sparing of the subcortical U-fibers is characteristic • The anterior fibers are first and more severely affected	Cerebellum is often atrophic
Krabbe disease/globoid cell leukodystrophy (GLD)	• Symmetric hypodensity in the deep white matter with relative sparing of the subcortical U-fibers is characteristic • The parieto-occipital lobes are the first to be involved	• The brain is small and atrophic • Cerebellum is relatively spared or less severely affected

Contd...

Contd...

Diseases	Differentiating features	Comments
Adreno-leukodys-trophy (ALD)	• Large, symmetric hypodensity in the parieto-occipital or peritrigonal region with sparing of the subcortical white matter in the early stages is typical • Postcontrast images show rim enhancement at the advancing edge of the demyelination surrounded by peripheral edema in the adjacent brain	• Predominantly unilateral or frontal involvement is seen in atypical cases • Degenerative changes are seen in the internal capsule, brainstem, and cerebellum
Pelizaeus–Merz-bacher disease (PMD)	• It is characterized by patchy hypodensity in the deep white matter with relative sparing of the internal capsule and subcortical fibers • In the less common form, there is nonspecific diffuse hypodensity involving all the white matter • The cortex is intact	• Atrophic changes are seen in the cerebrum and cerebellum • Enlarged ventricular system is usually present
Alexander disease	• There is diffuse, symmetric, hypodensity involving the frontal white matter and the basal ganglia • Postcontrast images may show patchy nodular or discoid enhancement within the hypodensity	There is increased volume of the brain in the affected region with effacement of the sulcal spaces and other subarachnoid spaces
Canavan disease	• Preferential involvement of the subcortical fibers is the hallmark	Thalami and basal ganglia may be involved in severe cases

Contd...

Contd...

Diseases	Differentiating features	Comments
	• But in severe cases, there is diffuse hypodensity of the white matter of the entire brain with sparing of only the internal capsule	
Amino-aciduria including phenyl-ketonuria (PKU)	These are characterized by diffuse, nonenhancing, periventricular hypodensity with relative sparing of the subcortical fibers	
Tay-Sachs disease	• Basal ganglia show symmetrical, homogeneous, hyperdensity • Early stages show enlarged caudate nuclei protruding into the lateral ventricles • Late stages are characterized by severe cortical atrophy	It is a type of lipidosis
Mucopoly-sacchari-doses	The findings that characterize these conditions include thickened dura, perivascular hypodensities, and varying degree of cortical atrophy	The conditions are indistinguishable from each other only on the basis of the brain findings
Mucolipi-dosis, fucosidosis and glycogen storage diseases	These are characterized by thinning of the cortex with nonspecific white matter changes in the form of nonspecific hypodensity, gliosis, and atrophy	It is not possible to distinguish these diseases on CT imaging

Contd...

Contd...

Diseases	Differentiating features	Comments
Leigh disease	• It is characterized by nonenhancing, hypodensity in the periaqueductal, subependymal, and tegmental gray matter • Periventricular white matter also shows similar hypodensity	It is also known as subacute necrotizing encephalopathy
MELAS/ MERRF syndrome	• It is characterized by the nonspecific, gray, and white matter cerebral infarcts affecting any part of the brain but the occipital lobes are the sites of predilection • Multifocal venous occlusion are also associated	It falls into the category of mitochondrial encephalopathy
Zellweger syndrome	It is characterized by heterotopias, pachygyria and polymicrogyria with a generalized reduction in the white matter thickness	It is included in the peroxisomal disorders
Multiple sclerosis	• It is characterized by multiple, iso- to hypodense, ovoid lesions in the periventricular white matter arranged perpendicular to the long axis of the lateral ventricles showing variable degree and patterns (ring or nodular) of postcontrast enhancement • Callososeptal interface is also a common site of involvement with periventricular extension of the lesions into the deep white matter referred to as the Dawson' finger	• The disease is commonly seen in young females • Brainstem and cerebellum involvement is commoner in children than adults

Contd...

Contd...

Diseases	Differentiating features	Comments
Vascular disease (arteriosclerosis, vasculitis, embolism, hypoxic-ischemic encephalopathy)	• It is characterized by a spectrum of white matter changes ranging from nonspecific, nonenhancing hypodensity to frank infarcts with gliosis and encephalomalacia in late stages with variable involvement of the gray matter • The site of involvement depends upon the age • In preterm infants, bilateral periventricular white matter involvement is typical with resultant loss of white matter and atrophy in late stages • In term infants, the cortical and subcortical white matter are the sites of involvement; deep gray matter nuclei are also commonly involved • In children and adults, gray matter is more commonly affected with cortical loss • In the elderly, the periventricular white matter is the usual site of lesions	
Toxic demyelination (alcohol, drugs and chemicals, osmotic demyelination)	• These are characterized by nonspecific white matter hypodensity at variable location depending upon the cause of insult • In osmotic demyelination, the usual site is pons	Common agents associated with such type of lesions include cyclosporine, methotrexate, 5-fluorouracil, hydrocarbons, mercury, lead, etc.

Contd...

Contd...

Diseases	Differentiating features	Comments
	• In alcoholism, pons (osmotic cause) and corpus callosum (Marchiafava-Bignami disease) are the common sites • In chronic alcoholism associated with Wernicke encephalopathy, both white and gray matter are involved. Periventricular region, midbrain, Tectum, and thalami are commonly involved	
Acute disseminated encephalitis (ADEM)	It is characterized by multifocal, bilateral, non-enhancing, hypodense lesions typically involving the subcortical white matter, but deep white matter, diseases, brainstem, and cerebellum may also be involved	• The disease occurs following childhood exanthematous RTI, and vaccination against rabies, DPT, etc. • The lesions usually appear 1–2 weeks after the contact with the inciting agent
Subacute sclerosing panencephalitis	• It is characterized by hypodense, nonenhancing foci in the subcortical and deep white matter progressing to gliosis • Gray matter involvement is common especially the basal ganglia • Generalized atrophy of the brain is common	It occurs several years after the measles infection

MISCELLANEOUS LESIONS OF THE BRAIN

Intraparenchymal Hemorrhagic Lesions in Brain

Hemorrhagic lesions in brain can be broadly categorized into:
- *Nontraumatic*:
    - Hypertension
    - Aneurysm and vascular malformation (AVM, cavernous angioma)
    - Perinatal hemorrhage
    - Hemorrhagic infarction (reperfusion or venous)
    - Neoplastic
    - Miscellaneous:
        - Amyloid angiopathy
        - Coagulopathies and blood dyscrasias
        - Drug abuse
        - Eclampsia
        - Infections (vasculitis, encephalitis, abscess, endocarditis with septic emboli)
- *Traumatic*:
    - Diffuse axonal injury
    - Cortical contusions
    - Deep cerebral and brainstem lesions.

CT Findings of Hemorrhage

- *Acute hemorrhage (0–72 hours)*: It appears hyperdense to human brain. Unretracted semiliquid clot appears hypodense within the hyperdense acute hematoma, giving rise to the so-called *swirl sign*.
- *Subacute hemorrhage (4–14 days)*: Subacute hemorrhage becomes virtually isodense with the adjacent brain parenchyma. It may sometimes show a peripheral postcontrast enhancement.
- *Chronic hemorrhage (>2 weeks)*: It appears hypodense to the adjacent brain. High attenuation within chronic hematomas is usually secondary to the rebleeding. Rim enhancement around a resolving hematoma typically appears within a few days and disappears between 2 and 6 months. A *target sign* on

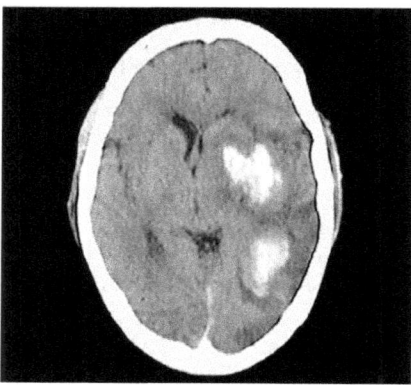

Fig. 40: Axial CT image showing hypertensive acute hematoma in the left cerebral hemisphere.

postcontrast images can be seen if rehemorrhage takes place within an organizing hematoma; if rebleeding occurs outside an organized hematoma, it can resemble a *tumoral hemorrhage*.

Hypertensive ICH

- Hypertensive intracerebral hemorrhages (HICH) are the most common nontraumatic cause in adults (Fig. 40)
- Most are associated with systemic hypertension and in some, ruptured microaneurysms are implicated
- Common location include putamen/external capsule followed by thalamus, pons, cerebellum, and subcortical white matter in the decreasing order of frequency.

Aneurysm and Vascular Malformation (AVM, Cavernous Angioma)

Hypertensive intracerebral hemorrhage (Figs. 41A to C):
- *Ruptured aneurysms* are associated with either intraparenchymal or subarachnoid hemorrhage

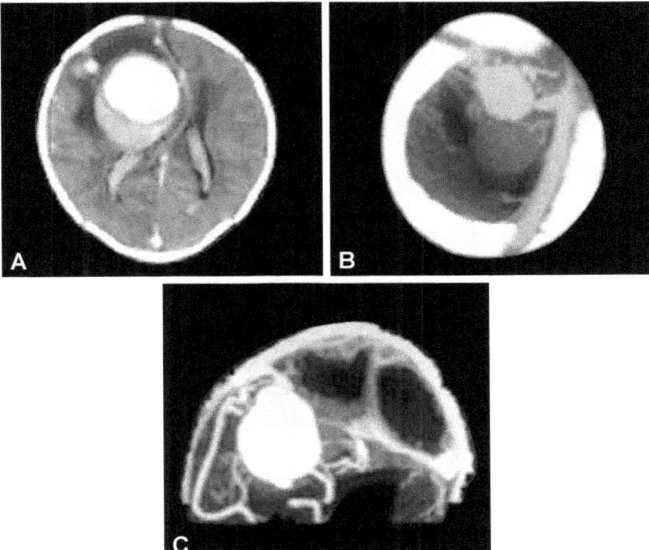

Figs. 41A to C: Axial and sagittal CT images showing a large AV malformation with an aneurysm and hematoma.
(AV: aneurysm and vascular)

- Acute SAH is characterized by hyperdensity in the subarachnoid spaces (basal cisterns, fissures, sulci) (Figs. 42A and B)
- Although SAH tends to be diffuse; more focal cisternal or parenchymal hematomas can be due to ruptured aneurysms and are helpful in localizing the bleeding source
- Blood in the Sylvian fissure—aneurysm on the I/L ICA.
- Focal interhemispheric blood—Anterior com artery aneurysm
- Blood in the fourth ventricle—Posteroinferior cerebellar artery aneurysm
- ICH secondary to *AVM* are usually seen in children or normotensive young adults
- AVM are usually associated with gliotic and encephalomalacic changes

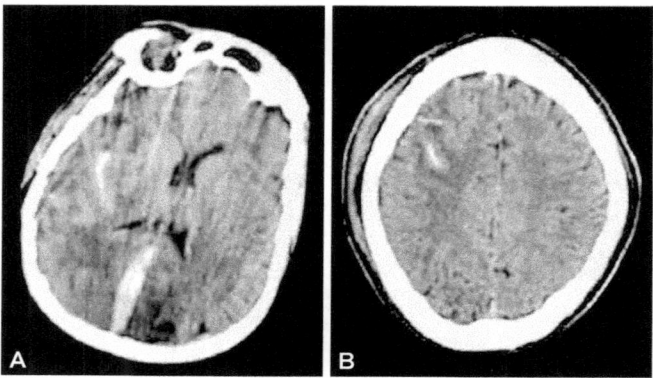

Fig. 42: Axial CT images showing posterior interhemispheric acute SDH and SAH in the right frontal lobe.
(CT: computed tomography; SAH: subarachnoid hemorrhage; SDH: subdural hematoma)

- *Cavernous angiomas* typically have a popcorn-like appearance with calcification and mixed signal foci inside a hemosiderin ring.

Perinatal Hemorrhage

- In *term infants*, it is usually the result of hypoxic-ischemic insult
- Areas of hemorrhage are typically seen in the posterolateral lentiform nuclei and ventral thalamus
- Although the cortex can be involved in profound asphyxia, it is relatively spared compared to the deep gray matter
- In *premature infants*, germinal matrix hemorrhage (GMH) is the most common form of ICH followed by intraventricular and intraparenchymal hemorrhage that are usually secondary to the former.
- Germinal matrix hemorrhage is divided into four grades:
  - *Grade I*: Hemorrhage confined to one or both germinal matrices

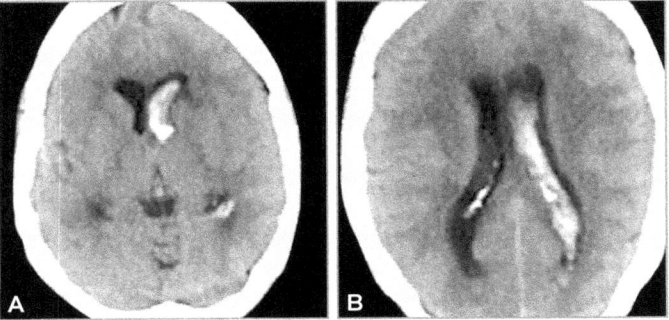

Figs. 43A and B: Axial CT images showing hemorrhage in left lateral ventricle in an adult patient.

- *Grade II*: Hemorrhage ruptured into a normal-sized ventricle
- *Grade III*: Intraventricular hemorrhage with hydrocephalus (Figs. 43A and B)
- *Grade IV*: Hemorrhagic extension into the adjacent hemispheric white matter.

Hemorrhagic Infarction (Reperfusion or Venous)

- Hemorrhagic infarction is usually the result of lysis of embolus/opening of collaterals/restoration of normal blood pressure following hypotension/hypertension/anticoagulation causing extravasation in reperfused ischemic brain
- It is seen in approximately 6% of brain infarcts and is usually at the corticomedullary junction
- CT will show the hyperdensity within a previously imaged hypodense acute ischemic infarct
- *Venous infarctions* are usually hemorrhagic, bilateral, and occur primarily in the white matter and are most often associated with cortical vein and dural sinus thrombosis
- CT demonstrates patchy foci of edema and petechial hemorrhage with or without signs of dural sinus thrombosis.

Neoplastic

- Common brain tumors that are commonly associated with hemorrhage include: pituitary adenomas, high-grade gliomas, PNET, epidermoid and metastases from bronchogenic, and renal, chorio- and melanocarcinoma.
- *Points of benign versus malignant hemorrhage:*
  - There is no absolute criteria
  - Tumors are complex and heterogeneous
  - Benign lesions usually have a complete hemosiderin ring
  - Nonhemorrhagic areas of the tumor enhance on post-contrast images
  - Hemorrhage evolution is disordered or delayed in tumoral lesions in contrast to an orderly evolution seen in benign hemorrhage
  - Edema/mass effect resolve with resolution of hematoma in benign lesions while it will persist with malignant lesions
  - Hemorrhagic metastatic deposits will be multifocal.

Amyloid Angiopathy

- This is probably the most common cause of recurrent bleeding in normotensive elderly and the incidence increases with advancing age
- Hemorrhages are characteristically multiple, spare the basal ganglia and brainstem, and are located at the corticomedullary junction
- Computed tomography findings of multiple peripherally located hemorrhages of different ages in an elderly normotensive patient strongly suggests the cause as amyloid angiopathy.

Inflammatory Disease and Vasculitis

- Hemorrhage in immunocompetent persons is uncommon, but immunocompromised individuals are at increased risk of developing hemorrhage in infectious lesions

- Such lesions include infective endocarditis with septic emboli, fungal vasculitis, and necrotizing lesions as herpes encephalitis
- Aspergillosis and other fungal infections may directly invade the vessel wall and cause thrombosis, Hemorrhage, or cerebral infarction
- Type II herpes simplex encephalitis is the most prone to develop hemorrhage especially in neonatal herpes.

Drug Abuse

- Drugs like cocaine can induce a hypertensive episode in which case the location of ICH is similar to that in hypertensive ICH
- Cocaine also promotes arterial and dural sinus thrombosis producing venous infarction and ischemic infarction with subsequent hemorrhage
- Vasculitis with hemorrhage is seen commonly with amphetamines and phenylpropanolamine and less commonly with cocaine.

Blood Dyscrasias and Coagulopathies

- Common causes of noniatrogenic coagulopathy include vitamin K deficiency, hepatocellular disease, antibodies that react to clotting factors, and disseminated intravascular coagulation (DIC). Iatrogenic causes include mainly anticoagulants as heparin, warfarin, thrombolytic agents as streptokinase, antiplatelet agents as aspirin, etc.
- Imaging findings in most coagulopathies are similar.
- Although bleeding can occur at any location, the most common site is supratentorial and intraparenchymal with multifocal lesions with fluid—fluid levels within the hematomas.

Eclampsia

- Posterior circulation is particularly prone
- Lesions are commonly seen at corticomedullary junction and within external capsule and basal ganglia

- The occipital lobes are a frequent location of cortical and subcortical lesions
- CT scans will reveal multiple hypoattenuating foci or hemorrhages in the subcortical white matter or basal ganglia.

Diffuse Axonal Injury

- Diffuse axonal injury (DAI) is most common form of the intra-axial primary traumatic lesion
- It tends to occur in the lobar white matter, corpus callosum, and dorsolateral aspect of the brainstem
- Nearly two-thirds are seen at the gray white matter junction, most often in the frontotemporal region, splenium and posterior body of the corpus callosum
- Early CT scans may be unremarkable. Delayed scans in acute DAI may reveal petechial hemorrhages in the location mentioned above.

Cortical Contusions

- It is the second most common form of the intra-axial primary traumatic lesion (Figs. 44A and B)
- Majority involve the temporal lobes followed by the frontal lobes and other sites as the cerebellar hemispheres
- Early findings include patchy, ill-defined, frontal or temporal hypodense lesions that may be mixed with smaller hyperdense foci of petechial hemorrhages
- Delayed scans at 24-48 hours may reveal hemorrhages developing in the previously hypodense regions.

Deep Cerebral and Brainstem Lesions

- Computed tomography is often normal in these patients
- Petechial hemorrhages are sometimes seen in the dorsolateral brainstem, periaqueductal region, and deep gray matter nuclei.

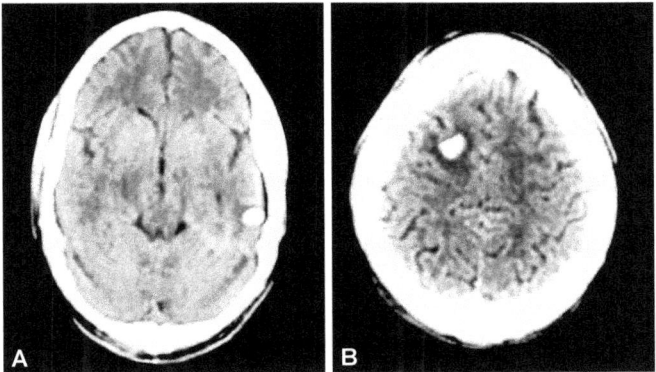

Figs. 44A and B: Axial CT images showing cortical contusions.

Conditions Primarily Presenting as Cerebral Atrophy (Table 14)

- Alzheimer's disease
- Pick's disease
- Vascular dementia
- Extrapyramidal disorders
- Subcortical dementia
- Dyke-Davidoff-Masson syndrome.

Conditions Primarily Presenting as Cerebellar Atrophy (Table 14)

- Diffuse brain atrophy in the elderly
- Secondary to previous infarct/trauma
- Phenytoin toxicity (involves mainly the cerebellar hemispheres)
- Ethanol toxicity (involves mainly the cerebellar vermis)
- Olivopontocerebellar degeneration
- Ataxia-telangiectasia syndrome

- Paraneoplastic cause (secondary to oat cell carcinoma of the lung)
- Postradiotherapy.

Effaced Basal Cisterns

Enhancing:
- Meningitis especially tuberculous
- Leptomeningeal carcinomatosis (usually nodular enhancement)
- Sarcoidosis (thickened leptomeninges).

Nonenhancing:
- Subarachnoid hemorrhage (isodense to hyperdense cisterns)
- Cerebral edema
- Diffuse axonal injury
- Hydrocephalus
- Racemose NCC (cystic, septated appearance of cisterns).

TABLE 14: Differentiating features of common conditions presenting as cerebral and cerebellar atrophy.

Types	Differentiating features	Comments
Alzheimer's disease	• It is characterized by diffusely enlarged ventricles especially the temporal horns • Cortical sulci are also enlarged especially in the anterior temporal lobes and the hippocampal region • Fissures are increased in size especially the choroidal, hippocampal, and Sylvian fissures	• It is the most common acquired neurodegenerative disorder • There is decrease in cortical thickness especially in the temporal lobes

Contd...

Contd...

Types	Differentiating features	Comments
Pick's disease	• It is characterized by asymmetric lobar atrophy involving the frontal and temporal lobes • Parietal and occipital lobes are spared	• There is decrease in cortical thickness in the frontal and temporal lobes • Ventricular system is enlarged
Vascular dementia	Multi-infarct dementia is characterized by multifocal infarcts involving both gray and white matter (cortical and subcortical region), enlarged ventricles, and sulci	It is the second most common acquired neurodegenerative disorder
Dyke-Davidoff-Masson syndrome	• It is characterized by cerebral hemiatrophy with reduced cortical and white matter thickness, enlarged ventricle, and sulci on the side of affection (Table 14) • There is associated thickening of the calvaria, enlargement of the sinuses, and elevation of the petrous bone on the side of affection	It is usually congenital but may be acquired following massive large infarction
Huntington's disease	• It is characterized by cortical and subcortical atrophy • There is striking atrophy of the basal ganglia especially caudate nucleus; cerebellar and brainstem atrophy may also be seen • There is focal dilatation of the frontal horns of lateral ventricle with convex lateral border	It is usually seen in fourth or fifth decade

Contd...

Contd...

Types	Differentiating features	Comments
Fahr's disease	It is characterized by bilateral extensive calcification in the basal ganglia, dentate nuclei, centrum semiovale, and subcortical white matter	It is a hereditary disorder
Wilson's disease	It is characterized by bilateral putaminal, hypodense lesions associated with mild generalized atrophy	It is associated with hepatic cirrhosis and degenerative changes in the brain secondary to deposition of the copper
Ataxia-telangiectasia syndrome	• It is characterized by cortical cerebellar atrophy with dilated fourth ventricle and cerebellar folia • Cerebellar infarct and hemorrhage are frequently associated	This syndrome is characterized by telangiectasia of the skin and eyes; cerebellar ataxia, sinusitis and pulmonary infections; immunodeficiencies; and increased susceptibility to malignancies
Olivopontocerebellar atrophy	• It is characterized by focal or diffuse atrophy of the cerebellum, pons, and inferior olives • The cerebellum is shrunken with dilated fourth ventricle, folia, and cisterns (supracerebellar and cerebellopontine cisterns)	Basal ganglia and spinal cord may be involved

DIFFERENTIAL DIAGNOSIS OF CEREBELLOPONTINE ANGLE MASSES (TABLE 15)

TABLE 15: Differential diagnosis of cerebellopontine angle masses.

Diseases	CT findings	Comments
Acoustic Schwannoma	• Isodense mass over the internal auditory canal forming an acute angle with the temporal bone like an ice cream cone. • Homogeneous enhancement. May contain necrosis, rarely calcified	Most common CPA mass (60–75%), seen in patients between 20–50 years. Arises from the glial—Schwann cell interface of vestibular nerve. Schwannoma bilateral in neurofibromatosis-2.
Meningioma	Isodense or hyperdense, strongly and uniformly enhancing mass. Broad dural base, obtuse angle with the temporal bone. Not centered over the IAC. IAC is not widened. Hyperostosis of the adjacent temporal bone and/or calcification may occur	Second most common CPA mass (10%). Typical age 30–60 years.
Epidermoid (congenital cholesteatoma)	Homogeneously hypodense, irregular, or lobulated nonenhancing CPA mass	4–5% of CPA mass lesions. 20–50 years. Arises from intracranial or intraosseous ectoderm inclusions. Found in the CPA as well as in the petrous temporal bone. Contains cholesterol or keratin debris.

Contd...

Contd...

Diseases	CT findings	Comments
Nonacoustic Schwannoma	Isodense homogeneously enhancing mass associated with one of the cranial nerves, most often 7th cranial nerve	5% of CPA mass lesions.
Paraganglioma (glomus jugulare)	Isodense, strongly enhancing mass with erosion and enlargement of the jugulare foramen	2–10% of CPA masses 40–60 years
Vertebrobasilar dolichoectasia	Tubular, hyperdense, strongly enhancing, often calcified tubular mass	3–5% of CPA masses. An atherosclerotic or degenerative lesion seen in patients over 50 years.
Aneurysm	3–5 mm or larger aneurysms may be seen on CT as oval or round enhancing vascular lesions	1–2% of CPA masses. Seen in between 20 years and 50 years of age. Berry aneurysms originate from the vertebral artery, superior cerebellar artery, or posterior inferior cerebellar artery
Arteriovenous malformation	Serpiginous isointense or hyperintense foci with strong enhancement following administration of contrast material calcification may be present	1% of CPA masses. Typically seen in between 20 years and 40 years of age
Glioma of brainstem or cerebellum	If solid hypodense, often 50% cystic. Solid portions enhance calcification in 20%	More common in cerebellum than brainstem. More common in children than in adults. May be associated with severe hydrocephalus before becoming symptomatic

Contd...

Contd...

Diseases	CT findings	Comments
Metastasis	Extra-axial: destructive mass centered in bone. Intra-axial: enhancing mass in the brainstem with an exophytic component extending into the CPA	Originates in the clivus or temporal bone adjacent to the CPA
Hemangioma	Spherical or nodular sharply delineated hyperdense mass which shows uniform, strong enhancement. Calcification may be present	Rare, less than 1% of CPA lesions. May be difficult to distinguish from meningioma
Lipoma chordoma	• Low-density, non-enhancing lesion • Large isodense or hyperdense destructive clival and skull base mass typically midline. May contain calcification. Minimal enhancement	Rare, less than 1% of CPA lesions 1% of CPA masses, in older adults. Originates from notochordal remnants in the clivus.
Arachnoid cyst	Well-delineated smoothly marginated mass isodense with CSF. May erode adjacent bone	Rare. Split or duplicated arachnoid membranes containing CSF. Dandy-Walker cyst of fourth ventricle can involve the CPA
Inflammatory lesions	Diffuse enhancement of leptomeninges, including both CPA cisterns. Communicating hydrocephalus due to fibrosis of the CPA cisterns	Bacterial meningitis, tuberculosis cause meningeal enhancement. Mass-like effect in cysticercosis, sarcoidosis, and histiocytosis

(CPA: cerebellopontine angle; CSF: cerebrospinal fluid; IAC: internal auditory canal)

DIFFERENTIAL DIAGNOSIS OF INFRATENTORIAL LESIONS (TABLE 16)

TABLE 16: Differential diagnosis of infratentorial lesions.

Diseases	CT findings	Comments
Brainstem glioma	Isodense, hypodense, or mixed with partial contrast enhancement in 50%. Cysts occur in 20%. Encasement of basilar artery seen in 45%	In children, 25% of gliomas occur in brainstem; in adults only 2.5%. Hemorrhage, no enhancement and change from nonenhancing to enhancing tend to indicate aggressive nature of tumor
Astrocytoma of the cerebellum	Hypodense, 50% solid, 50% cystic. Calcification in 20%. Solid lesions enhance well. Obstructive hydrocephalus is common in vermis of fourth ventricle tumors	Common posterior fossa neoplasm in children
Medulloblastoma	Cerebellar vermis; denser than normal cerebellum on unenhanced scans. Enhances well unless necrotic. Hydrocephalus common. Subarachnoid metastatic spread is common as "icing on the cake"	Common posterior fossa tumor in the children
Ependymoma	An inhomogeneous mass in the fourth ventricle. 50% contain small flecks of calcium. Enhances homogeneously or heterogeneously. Hydrocephalus is common	Most often in the first decade. Tendency to hemorrhage.

Contd...

Contd...

Diseases	CT findings	Comments
Choroid plexus papilloma/ carcinoma	Slightly hyperdense fourth ventricular mass, may calcify. Homogeneous contrast enhancement, hydrocephalus common. Carcinomas occur in infancy. Rare but often aggressive, often necrotic, and may invade the brain	More common in the lateral ventricle than in the fourth ventricle
Hemangio- blastoma	• Either solid or cystic with a mural tumor nodule, occasionally multiple. Over 90% located in cerebellar hemispheres. Nearly always in contact with the leptomeninges at some point • Enhancement of the solid component is strong. Calcification is rare	8–12% of posterior fossa tumors. Common in 20–40 years. Rare in children.
Schwan- noma	Most common in the acoustic nerve and located in the cerebellopontine angle. Isodense and well enhancing unless necrotic	Associated with neurofibromatosis-2
Meningioma	Hyperdense (75%) or isodense (25%) in nonenhanced scans. Broad dural surface is common. Calcification seen in 15–20%. Adjacent hyperostosis and edema of the underlying brain are common. Strong enhancement is a rule	5–10% of meningiomas occur in the posterior fossa; either in the cerebellopontine angle clivus or foramen magnum

Contd...

Contd...

Diseases	CT findings	Comments
Epidermoid	Hypodense (0–10 HU), round mass usually in the cerebellopontine angle, no enhancement, no surrounding edema	The most common intracerebral tumor. Hydrocephalus is usually absent
Dermoid	Midline thick-walled hypodense (negative HU) inhomogeneous mass with focal areas of fat. No contrast enhancement or edema	Rare pilosebaceous mass lined with skin appendages, most common in the posterior fossa and in the base of the brain. Hydrocephalus is rare
Teratoma	Contains fat, nonadipose tissue and calcification. No enhancement or edema.	Rare obstructive hydrocephalus, usually absent despite large mass
Lipoma	Fat-density nonenhancing lesion in the CPA or in the cerebellum. May contain ring or central fleck calcification and enhance. No edema	Rare obstructive hydrocephalus usually absent
Metastasis	Appearance is variable, including densely enhancing nodules with surrounded by edema; large inhomogeneously enhancing mass; or ring enhancing tumors with central necrosis	Most common cerebellar tumors in older patients
Lymphoma	Poorly defined solid hyperdense enhancing mass, usually near the fourth ventricle or cerebellar surface. Little or no peritumoral edema	May be multicentric, does not respect normal anatomic boundaries. Seen in immunocompromised patients

Contd...

Contd...

Diseases	CT findings	Comments
Infarct	Low-density lesion appears 12–24 hours after ictus; subacute infarcts may enhance and may simulate a neoplasm	Due to artefacts, CT is poor in detecting cerebellar or brainstem infarcts. PICA infarcts are the most frequent and involve portions of the cerebellar hemispheres and brainstem
Hemorrhage	High attenuating lesion that may compress or obstruct the fourth ventricle and cause hydrocephalus	Hemorrhage into the cisterns may appear as thin hyperdense layers adjacent to the tentorium or cisterns
Arteriovenous malformation	Rapidly and strongly enhancing tortuous structures, variable degree of mass effect may be indistinguishable in precontrast scans	Cyst-like lesions or calcification may represent previous hemorrhage
Multiple sclerosis	Large, fresh cerebellar and brainstem plaque may appear expansile, enhances and mimics a neoplasm	
Gliosis	Single or multiple low-density, nonenhancing lesion in the cerebellar hemisphere	May be seen in neurofibromatosis type 1

DIFFERENTIAL DIAGNOSIS OF SUPRATENTORIAL MASS LESIONS (TABLE 17)

TABLE 17: Differential diagnosis of supratentorial mass lesions.

Diseases	CT findings	Comments
Astrocytoma	• Low-grade astrocytoma: usually well-delineated low-density mass with little or no enhancement. • Some tumors may calcify. Juvenile pilocytic astrocytoma: sharply marginated isodense, hypodense or mixed mass around third/fourth ventricle (optic chiasm, hypothalamus, cerebellar vermis) cysts are frequent and contain an enhancing mural nodule. Anaplastic astrocytoma: less well-defined, often heterogeneous density showing greater mass effect and contrast enhancement	• 25–30% of these are relatively benign, occurs usually between 20 years and 40 years in white matter. May become more malignant. Pilocytic astrocytoma is a subtype of astrocytoma in children and young adults, often associated with neurofibromatosis. Rare in cerebral hemispheres. Most common in temporal lobes • 25–30% of astrocytomas, usually after 40 years of age
Glioblastoma multiforme	Tumor in supratentorial white matter characterized by necrosis, hemorrhage, vasogenic edema, mass effect, heterogeneity, and substantial contrast enhancement	50% of astrocytomas; occurs in 50–70 years of age. Tends to be more malignant in older patients. Tumor cells diffuse widely outside the region of contrast enhancement

Contd...

Contd...

Diseases	CT findings	Comments
Oligoden-droglioma	Typically low-density tumor with little enhancement. Most often in frontal lobe. Usually partly calcified	- 5% of primary brain tumors. - *Peak age*: 35–40 years. 85% supratentorial. Nearly 50% astrocytic elements
Ependy-moma	Often periventricular/parenchymal. Calcified in 50%. Cysts are common, hemorrhage uncommon. May be indistinguishable from astrocytoma. Occurs at all ages	5% of intracranial tumors. 50% occur in children younger than 5 years. Two-thirds are infratentorial from the floor of fourth ventricle and often extend into CP angle or vallecula 15–20% of intracranial tumor
Menin-gioma	Rounded, sharply delineated (hypodense in 75%) in juxtadural location, parasagittal or convexity in 30–40%, sphenoid wing 15–20%. Intense enhancement in 90%. Calcification in 15–20%	- Rare in children and adolescents. Arises from arachnoid lining cells and attached to dura - Hyperostosis is virtually pathognomonic. Histologic type variable
Ganglio-cytoma, ganglio-glioma, ganglio-neuroma	Well-circumscribed, low- or mixed-density lesion in frontal; or temporal, occipital lobe with little mass effect. Cysts are common (50%) calcification in one-third, enhancement is variable. Can erode the inner table of skull	Uncommon, 80% occur under the age of 30, occurs in third or fourth ventricle and cerebellum. Ganglioneuroma consists of preganglionic cells, ganglioglioma contains glial cells. Usually well-differentiated, may be anaplastic

Contd...

Contd...

Diseases	CT findings	Comments
PNET	Grossly well-circumscribed hyperdense cerebral deep white matter mass with variable enhancement; cysts and calcification occur in 50% hemorrhage in 10%. Can be intraventricular	Less than 5% of supratentorial tumors, mostly seen in patients under 5 years of age. Highly malignant. Pathology is controversial.
Primary cerebral neuroblastoma	Periventricular/intraventricular mass with little edema. Inhomogeneous enhancement. Calcification, cyst, and hemorrhage are common. Pattern is highly variable and nonspecific	Uncommon; 80% in patients under 10 years. Can be considered a subset of PNETs
Hemangioblastoma	Solid/cystic mass with strong enhancement. Nearly always in contact with leptomeninges at some point. Rarely calcifies	Uncommon supratentorially. Occurs in young/middle-aged adults. Sporadic or associated with VHL. Over 90% occur in cerebellar hemispheres, medulla, or spinal cord. (10% of posterior fossa tumors)
Lymphoma	Isodense or hyperdense, poorly delineated, strongly enhancing mass, most often involving deep gray matter or corpus callosum; calcification is rare. In AIDS patients, may be necrotic and mimic infection (e.g. toxoplasmosis) with ring enhancement. 50% multiple	Traditionally rare. Incidence is rapidly growing with increase in AIDS patients. Occurs in immunocompromised patients, may be most common tumor in some locations. Primary CNS lymphomas are usually non-Hodgkin's type

Contd...

Contd...

Diseases	CT findings	Comments
Langerhans cell histiocytosis	Focal isodense or hyperdense mass, most often in hypothalamic region. Strong and uniform enhancement	Previously known as histiocytosis X, brain parenchymal involvement is rare. May also involve leptomeninges and cranial nerves
Germinoma	Well-delineated suprasellar mass, may involve the infundibulum, rarely the thalamus, or basal ganglia. Hyperdense/calcified in 80%; strongly enhancing	Pineal gland is most common site (more than 50% of pineal tumors); other locations called "ectopic." The ectopic are histologically identical to testicular seminoma and ovarian dysgerminoma. Striking male preponderance, up to 10:1
Teratoma	Heterogeneous pineal/suprasellar mass that may contain calcification, fat, cystic/solid component; minimal enhancement	Most common in pineal gland, lower incidence than germinomas but same age group (second decade) histology is variable
Pineal cyst	Small nonenhancing cystic lesion associated with pineal gland	Pineal cyst is relatively common but not always recognized on CT
Metastasis	Parenchymal mets are most commonly hypodense and enhance with contrast; most necrotic metastases are thick-walled and are surrounded by vasogenic edema	Metastases of lymphoma, osteosarcoma, melanoma, and choriocarcinoma are often hyperdense

Contd...

Contd...

Diseases	CT findings	Comments
Lipoma	Midline; most often interhemispheric fat density mass. No enhancement but may show curvilinear calcification	Callosal lipomas, often associated with partial/complete agenesis of corpus callosum
Craniopharyngioma	Multilobulated sellar/suprasellar mass with variable enhancement. Contains cysts and calcification in 90%	
Radiation necrosis	Deep focal hypodense mass near the irradiated tumor bed. May show an irregular ring of contrast enhancement.	Develops 9–24 months after radiation therapy. May be impossible to differentiate from residual/recurrent tumor
Cerebral infarction	*From 12 hours to 48 hours*: Poorly circumscribed, low attenuation subtle mass effect (sulcal effacement, ventricular displacement if large infarction). Enhancement uncommon. Hemorrhage in 5–10% as high density components. *From 48 hours to 96 hours*: Increasing mass effect. Focal area of triangular/wedge-shaped hypodensity involving the cortex and the underlying white matter down to ventricular surface	• Early infarcts may become isodense and not detected unless CECT is performed. • Hyperosmolar contrast may be harmful in acute stroke. High-density atherosclerotic thrombus may be seen in the arterial lumen (dense MCA sign); shape of infarct corresponds to distribution of specific vessel and has characteristic peripheral enhancement; onset of symptoms is usually abrupt unlike glioma;

Contd...

Contd...

Diseases	CT findings	Comments
	• *From 4 days to 7 days*: Gyral contrast enhancement appears and may persist up to 8 weeks, hypodense infarct surrounded by low-density edema. • *From 2 weeks to 8 weeks*: Mass effect resolves, contrast enhancement may persist. • *Old infarct*: Well-delineated low-attenuation area, enlargement of adjacent sulci and ventricle. Calcification is rare	most clinically detectable stroke is embolic and occur in MCA distribution. Thrombotic strokes are small and most often spare the cortex. • Post-traumatic infarctions occur due to vascular compression secondary to mass effect and are most often in PCA distribution
Pyogenic brain absces	Sequence from early and late cerebritis stage with focal enhancement. Central hypodense zone represents pus/necrotic tissue. Isodense uniformly enhancing ring represents fibrous capsule also, a peripheral low-density rim of white matter occurs representing reactive edema	C/F: Fever, leukocytosis, obstruction, extracranial infection, previous operation. Ring enhancement of gliomas may be irregular in thickness and may be impossible to differentiate from malignant gliomas
Hydatid cyst	Round, sharply marginated, smooth-walled hypodense mass.	Rare. Cysts in parenchyma tend to be large, multiple, thin-walled with no reactive edema or contrast enhancement

Contd...

Contd...

Diseases	CT findings	Comments
Cerebritis	Irregular, poorly marginated hypodense edematous area in white matter/basal ganglia which may behave as a mass and result in effacement of sulci or ventricles. No enhancing capsule on unenhanced scans, but ring-like enhancement occurs	Usually bacterial/fungal infection. May progress to abscess in 10–14 days
Intracerebral hemorrhage (ICH)	*Acute*: Homogeneously dense well-defined lesion with round or oval configuration and moderate mass effect. *Resolving (3–6 weeks)*: Hypodense region with thin uniform ring of enhancing tissue. May mimic a neoplasm	*Causes*: Head trauma, surgery, hypertension, rupture of vascular aneurysm, or malformation. Acute hemorrhage may be isodense in patients with anemia/coagulopathy
Epidural hematoma (EDH)	Biconvex high density extra-axial mass displacing adjacent interface between gray-white matter. Usually temporoparietal, less commonly frontal or occipital	Caused by traumatic laceration of meningeal arteries or disruption of dural sinuses/veins (especially in children); look for contralateral lesion of brain, subfalcine, or descending trans-tentorial herniation and signs of increased intracranial pressure, which are common associated findings

Contd...

Contd...

Diseases	CT findings	Comments
Subdural hematoma (SDH)	*Acute SDH*: Crescentic high-density extra-axial hyperdense fluid collection. Typically frontoparietal, may extend into interhemispheric fissure and along falx displacement of adjacent interface between gray and white matter. Small subtemporal, subfrontal, and tentorial SDH are seen best on coronal scans. Subacute SDH (from few days to 3 weeks old): Isodense mass effect on adjacent interface between gray and white matter, underlying veins may be displaced as evident on contrast-enhanced scans. Underlying membrane may enhance chronic SDH (over 3 weeks old): Well-defined hypodense crescentic mass adjacent to inner table of skull. Thin marginal enhancement	Often associated with underlying brain injury (contusion, focal brain hematoma) commonly bilateral in infants. Interhemispheric SDH in child without SDH elsewhere should raise suspicion of nonaccidental trauma. Bilaterally symmetrical SDH may be difficult to detect when isodense with cerebral cortex. Look for indirect signs of mass effect using contrast enhancement. Repeat hemorrhage in previous chronic SDH may give a mixed-density lesion; contrast material may seep into hematoma and give fluid-fluid level (Fig. 45)

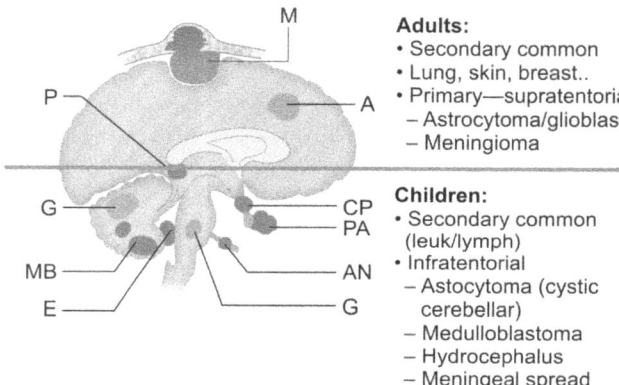

Fig. 45: Central nervous system tumors—summary.
(P: pinealoblastoma; G: glioma; M: meningioma; A: astrocytoma; MB: medulloblastoma; E: ependymoma; CP: choroid plexus papilloma; PA: pilocytic astrocytoma; AN: anaplastic ependymoma)

DIFFERENTIAL DIAGNOSIS OF WHITE MATTER DISEASES (TABLE 18)

TABLE 18: Differential diagnosis of white matter diseases.

Diseases	CT findings	Comments
Congenital demyelinating disorders		
Alexander's disease (fibrinoid leukodystrophy)	Symmetric well-demarcated low-attenuation areas in deep white matter. Frontal lobes involved with extensive posterior extension. May enhance in caudate nuclei, fornices, forceps minor, optic radiation, and periventricular white matter	Rare, unknown biochemical defect, manifests within 1st year with macrocephaly and developmental retardation progresses through spastic quadriparesis and intellectual deterioration to death usually within 5 years. Diagnosis requires brain biopsy

Contd...

Contd...

Diseases	CT findings	Comments
Canavan-van Bogaert disease (spongiform leukodystrophy)	Diffuse symmetric low-density changes throughout white matter, later ventriculomegaly and cerebral atrophy	Aspartoacylase deficiency, mitochondrial disorder that affects the CNS and skeletal muscle. AR, especially in Ashkenazi Jews. Onset before 10 months with neurological deterioration, blindness and death before 5 years
Krabbe's disease	Initially symmetric; hyperdense areas in the (thalami, caudate nuclei, cerebellum, and corona leukodystrophy). Later patchy periventricular; low-attenuation areas and diffuse white matter atrophy	Beta-galactosidase deficiency; autosomal recessive (AR) lysosomal disorder. Onset between 2 months and 6 months as retarded development, irritability, spasticity. Progresses through dementia, blindness, and quadriplegia to death within 1–3 years. Diagnosis is made through lymphocyte or skin fibroblast assay.
Pelizaeus-Merzbacher disease	CT may be normal. Later nonspecific white matter atrophy. Subtle periventricular white matter lucencies reported	X-linked recessive with lack of proteolipid apoprotein in white matter which leads to lack of myelination. Onset within the first few months of life. Nystagmus, abnormal eye movements, optic atrophy, slowly progressive pyramidal, dystonic, and cerebellar signs.

Contd...

Contd...

Diseases	CT findings	Comments
Metachromatic leukodystrophy	Low-attenuation changes in periventricular white matter and centrum semiovale. No contrast-enhancement in brain atrophy	Automatic recessive lysosomal disorder with deficiency of arylsulfatase. A symptomatic, most common before the age of 3 but may present in juvenile, infant, or adult. In adults, mimics Alzheimer's disease, Pick's disease, and schizophrenia
Childhood adrenoleukodystrophy (ALD), most common ALD	Symmetric low-attenuation changes in parieto-occipital white matter, which often show prominent rim enhancement, are characteristic. Changes progress from posterior to anterior and cause brain atrophy. Calcifications and mass effect may occur.	X-linked recessive, fatal peroxisomal disorder with accumulation of saturated very long chain fatty acids. Presents between 4 years and 8 years with behavioral changes, intellectual deterioration, and visual complaints

Disorders of AA metabolism

Propionic acidemia, methylmalonic aciduria ornithine transcarbamylase deficiency	Nonenhancing foci of low-attenuation in white matter/diffuse low-density, white matter. Changes may reverse on effective treatment	Rare. AR. Delayed myelination and degeneration of white matter are characteristic and better seen on magnetic resonance imaging (MRI)

Contd...

Contd...

Diseases	CT findings	Comments
Homocysteinuria	Low-density lesions, which correspond to lacunar infarcts	Defect in cystathione synthetase leads to build up of homocysteine in plasma, urine, and CSF. Homocysteine is thrombogenic and may lead to multiple cerebral infarcts
Leucinosis (maple syrup urine disease)	Edema and later decreased attenuation of cerebral white matter, brainstem, cerebral peduncles, and dorsal parts of internal capsule	Disturbance of valine, leucine, and isoleucine metabolism. The patient's urine has characteristic smell. Deficiency of enzyme necessary for oxidative decarboxylation of ketoacids

Other congenital metabolic disorders

Diseases	CT findings	Comments
Leigh disease (subacute necrotizing encephalopathy)	Symmetric nonenhancing low-attenuation lesions. Similar lesions may be seen in globus pallidus, thalamus, hypothalamus, midbrain, periventricular white matter, centrum semiovale and cortical white matter. Brain atrophy may be seen	AR. Feeding difficulties and psychomotor retardation during first 2 years. Death occurs within 4 years
Wilson's disease (hepatolenticular degeneration)	CT usually negative. Low-density lesions representing gliosis may be seen in basal ganglia, cerebral white matter, brainstem, and cerebellum	AR. Increased absorption of copper from intestine

Contd...

Contd...

Diseases	CT findings	Comments
Hallervorden-Spatz disease	CT usually negative. Focal variation in density of globus pallidus, thalami, red nuclei, and substantia nigra	Rare AR with onset during second decade. Characteristic finding is abnormal iron accumulation in basal ganglia with variable degrees of neuronal loss

Infections and inflammations

Diseases	CT findings	Comments
Congenital herpes simplex encephalitis (type 2)	*Early CT*: Normal. Then bilateral symmetric low attenuation foci due to white matter edema, gray matter highly attenuating. Brain atrophy and gyriform calcifications are late findings	*Incidence*: 1 in 2,000–5,000 live births. Brain involvement in 30%. Basal ganglia, thalami, and posterior-fossa relatively spared. May also cause visceral disease
Herpes encephalitis (type 1)	CT normal until 4 days. Later areas of hypodensity without enhancement, usually in bilateral temporal lobes, 20–50% bilateral. Hemorrhages in 50%. Late gyral enhancement may be seen	Fulminant, necrotizing meningoencephalitis, 70% cases adults, mortality of 70%
Acquired toxoplasmosis	Multiple bilateral low-density lesions with ring enhancement	Often progressive and fatal in immuno-suppressed
SSPE	Only early finding edema, intermediate stage shows multifocal low-density areas in periventricular and subcortical white matter and parts of basal ganglia followed by generalized atrophy in advanced cases	Probably caused by reactivated measles virus in children and adolescents. Affects both gray and white matter. Cause progressive dementia and disorders of movement

Contd...

Contd...

Diseases	CT findings	Comments
ADEM	CT may be normal. Bilateral confluent low attenuation changes in subcortical white matter.	Probably autoimmune reaction to previous infection/vaccination. Mortality 10–25%. Recovery complete
Brain abscesses	<ul><li>*Early cerebritis stage (0–3 days)*: Low-attenuation mass effect with or without patchy or gyriform enhancement.</li><li>*Late cerebritis stage (4–9 days)*: Low-density ring enhancing lesion with mass effect and edema.</li><li>*Early capsule stage (10–13 days)*: Low- density ring enhancing lesion, smooth well-defined lesion.</li><li>*Late capsule stage (days 14 and later)*: Abscess wall thickens and edema decreases with time</li></ul>	Usually focal, can be multifocal. Usually expands directly from temporal bone/frontal sinuses or arrives through trauma. Can be hematogenous. *Differential diagnosis*: Epidural abscess, subdural empyema, glioma, metastasis, chronic intracerebral hematoma, postoperative granulation tissue, multiple sclerosis, Lyme disease
Meningitis	CT normal in early cases; basal cisterns and sulci poorly visualized. Focal cerebral edema may be seen as low-density lesion. Parenchymal and leptomeningeal enhancement seen; complications like ventriculitis, communicating hydrocephalus, subdural effusion, cortical vein thrombosis, and later atrophy and encephalomalacia	Most often hemato-genous. Follows course from meningeal congestion, through possible thrombosis, cortical infarction, cerebritis, or nidus abscess to exudate in basal cistern and sulci with thickened meninges

Contd...

Contd...

Diseases	CT findings	Comments
AIDS	• *Low-attenuation lesion in white matter*: HIV encephalitis as symmetric nonenhancing diffuse decrease of white matter attenuation. Progressive multifocal leukoencephalopathy less common, usually asymmetric decrease of attenuation in parieto-occipital areas. • *Diffuse cerebral atrophy CNS lymphoma*: 6–7% patients as enhancing periventricular/basal ganglia solid/ring lesion. Necrosis++ • *Infection*: Multiple solid/ring enhancing lesion with edema around in basal ganglia characteristic of toxoplasmosis. Cryptococcosis characterized by small bilateral lesions possibly meningitis. CMV primarily seen in ependymal and sub-ependymal areas and cause ventriculitis	CNS involvement cause of initial complaint in 10%. Neurological s/s in one-third; most are opportunistic infections. HIV encephalitis causes white matter demyelination. PML caused by JC papovavirus is late finding with death within 3 months

Contd...

Brain

Contd...

Diseases	CT findings	Comments
Cysticercosis	Can involve parenchyma, ventricles, and meninges cosis. *Acute stage*: Multifocal edema. Lesions may homogeneously enhance. *Chronic stage*: Single or multiple 4–20 mm fluid-filled cysts without enhancement. Cysts contain a mural soft tissue nodule; they later calcify in 70% and develops hydrocephalus in 70%	Caused by larval stage of pork tapeworm, Taenia solium. Presents as seizures and increased cranial pressure
TB	• *TB leptomeningitis*: On unenhanced scans, parasellar, perimesencephalic, and Sylvian cisterns obliterated by abnormal isodense soft tissue. Basal infarctions and communicating hydrocephalus. Granulomas may appear as solid/ring enhancing lesions • *Tuberculoma*: Hypodense parenchymal lesion with irregular contour. Nodular/ring enhancement	• Diffuse leptomeningitis most common presentation of intracranial TB. CSF monocytosis, low sugar content, and high protein content • Tuberculomas may be indistinguishable from gliomas
Lyme disease (borreliosis)	Bilateral focal low-attenuation enhancing lesions due to demyelination and periventricular inflammation in deep cerebral white matter commonly frontal lobes	Tick borne multisystem disease caused by spirochete *Borrelia burgdorferi*. CNS affected in 10–15%: neuritis, meningitis, encephalitis, myelitis

Contd...

Contd...

Diseases	CT findings	Comments
Neoplastic disease		
Metastases	Commonly hypodense and enhance with contrast. Most necrotic mets are thick-walled and surrounded by vasogenic edema	15–30% intracranial tumors on CT are mets; initial clinical presentation in 30% of lung cancers. Mets of melanoma, choriocarcinoma, lymphoma, and osteosarcoma are hyperdense
Degenerative/vascular diseases		
Normal aging brain	Mild-to-moderate enlargement of CSF spaces. Periventricular hypodensities	Atrophy progresses faster after 70 years of age, changes subtle on CT, obvious on MRI
Alzheimer's disease	Cerebral atrophy in anterior temporal lobes and hippocampus. Loss of distinction between gray and white matter. Decreased density in medial temporal lobes	Most common disorder causing dementia. Pathology: Neurofibrillary degeneration, senile plaques, nonspecific neuronal loss with reactive gliosis
Binswanger's encephalopathy	High ventricular and supraventricular non-enhancing white matter lucencies. Volume loss, lacunar infarcts in basal ganglia. Mild ventricular dilatation and sulcal widening, changes which overlap with normal aging and Alzheimer's disease	10% of dementia. Wide spectrum of changes including infarcts, myelin pallor, demyelination, hyaline arteriolar sclerosis, and gliosis

Contd...

Contd...

Diseases	CT findings	Comments
Multiple sclerosis	CT usually negative. Isodense/hypodense white matter foci, which in active demyelination phase may show contrast enhancement. Can mimic neoplasm by having mass appearance with ring enhancement	Most common demyelinating disease. Most common in periventricular white matter, more common in females. CT insensitive in detecting lesions
Schilder's disease	Confluent hypodensities represent areas of demyelination which may show contrast enhancement	May be virulent childhood form of multiple sclerosis. d/d: Childhood adrenoleukodystrophy
Marchiafava-Bignami disease	Well-defined lucency in genu of corpus callosum	Rare selective myelinolysis in corpus callosum, less often in deep white matter. Occurs mainly in alcoholic, malnourished persons
Central Pontine myelinolysis	CT normal, nonenhancing low-density lesions in pons without mass effect may occur. Other areas (basal ganglia and thalami) may be involved	In alcoholic malnourished persons and in those treated with electrolyte and acid-base abnormalities. d/d: Multiple sclerosis, infarct, encephalitis, neoplasm. Thought to be associated with rapid rise in serum sodium concentration: greater than 20 mEq/L in 1–3 days

(ADEM: acute disseminated encephalitis; SSPE: subacute sclerosing panencephalitis)

Chapter 2

SPINAL CORD

SPINAL CORD LESIONS

Spinal cord lesions are shown in Tables 1 and 2.

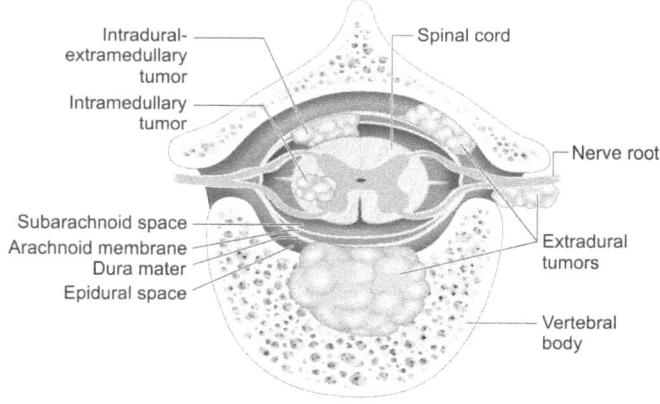

TABLE 1: Causes of spinal cord lesions.

Intramedullary			Extramedullary	
With cord expansion	With cord atrophy		Intradural	Extradural
Neoplasm	• Syringohydro-	*Cystic*	• Dorsal meningocele	• Abscess
• Astrocytoma	myelia		• Sacral meningocele	• Chronic hematoma
• Ependymoma	• Cord		• Neurenteric cyst	• Synovial cyst
• Ganglioglioma	contusion		• Arachnoid cyst	• Dural ectasia
• Paraganglioma	• Chronic injury		• Epidermoid cyst	• Arachnoid cyst
• Lipoma	• Radiation	*Fatty*	• Dorsal dermal sinus	• Lipoma
• Dermoid/	myelopathy		• Tethered filum terminale	• Lipomatosis
epidermoid/			• Lipomyelomeningocele	• Tarlov cyst
teratoma			• Dermoid	
• Hemangioblastoma			• Lipoma	
• Metastases			• Fibrolipoma	
Inflammatory		*Soft tissue*	• Subdural hematoma	• Hematoma
• Abscess			• AV malformation	• Disk bulge/herniated nucleus pulposus/sequestered disk
• Acute transverse myelopathy			• Myelocele/myelo-cystocele/meningo-myelocele	• Postoperative scar/granulation tissue
• Multiple sclerosis				

Contd...

Contd...

Intramedullary		Extramedullary	
With cord expansion	With cord atrophy	Intradural	Extradural

• Granulomata (tuberculosis, sarcoidosis)
Miscellaneous
• Syringohydromyelia
• Cord contusion
• Arteriovenous malformation
• Diastematomyelia
		• Arachnoiditis
		• Neurofibroma
		• Schwannoma
		• Meningioma
		• Ependymoma
		• Paraganglioma
		• Hemangioblastoma
		• Myeloblastoma/chloroma
		• Leptomeningeal carcinomatosis
		• Metastases
			• Ligamentum flavum hypertrophy
			• Neurofibroma
			• Schwannoma
			• Meningioma
			• Vertebral/paravertebral tumors with epidural extension
			• Metastases
			• *Bony lesion*
			  – Osteochondroma
			  – Osteoblastoma
			  – Aneurysmal bone cyst (ABC)/giant cell tumor (GCT)
			  – Hemangioma

Spinal Cord

TABLE 2: Common spinal cord lesions with relevant CT findings.

Diseases	NECT/CECT findings	CT myelography	Comments
Myelomeningocele/ myelocystocele/ myelocele and neural	• Bony defect in the neural arches of the vertebrae with deformity or failure of fusion of lamina • Absence of spinous process • Spinal canal is often widened	• The meningeal sac fills with the contrast medium and outlines the contents of the sac including the cord elements • In the myelocystocele, the cystic sac fills with the contrast medium in delayed phase	• Meningeal contains variable amount of cerebrospinal fluid (CSF) tissue herniating through a defect in the posterior/anterior elements of spine • In myelocystocele, the cystic sac corresponds to the dilated and herniated central canal of the cord
Diastematomyelia/split cord (Figs. 1A and B)	• Bony or fibrous septa in the spinal canal dividing the cord into two complete halves each with its own thecal sac usually between T9 and S1 • Sagittal division of cord into two hemicords lying within one thecal sac without a bony or fibrous septa • Spinal canal usually widened	• It shows one or two separate thecal sacs that fill with contrast medium. In the latter case, the two sacs fuse below the level of the bony or fibrous septa • The fibrous or bony septum are seen as filling defects	• Vertebral anomalies like hemivertebra, block, or butterfly vertebra are commonly associated • Fusion and thickening of adjacent lamina • Spina bifida is seen at multiple levels

Contd...

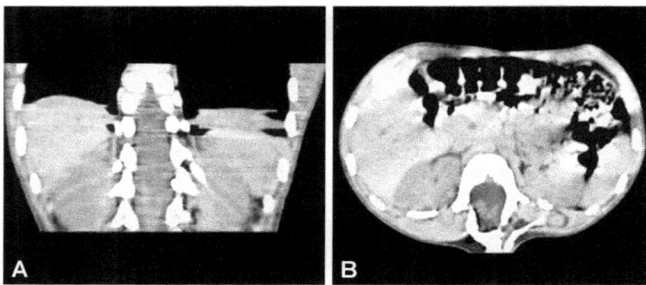

Figs. 1A and B: Coronal and axial CT images of spine showing two hemicords with hypoplastic left lamina and bony outgrowth in a case of diastematomyelia.

Contd...

Diseases	NECT/CECT findings	CT myelography	Comments
Hydromyelia/ syringomyelia/ syringohydro- myelia	• It is seen as a distinct area of fluid attenuation within spinal cord (central— hydromyelia; paracentral— syringomyelia) • The spinal cord may be expanded/ normal sized/ atrophic • There is increase in transverse diameter of the cord with flattened posterior border of the corresponding vertebra	Filling of cavity with contrast is seen early in cases where there is direct communication with subarachnoid space and delayed in other cases	• These can communicate with 4th ventricle with associated hydrocephalus • These may even com- municate with the subarachnoid spaces
Acute transverse myelopathy Radiation myelopathy	• Finding may be normal • There is long segment atrophy of the spinal cord corresponding to the radiation field	• The cord may be swollen • The cord is atrophic with enlarged thecal sac	• The radiation dose should exceed 4,000 rads • The latent period is between 3 months and 40 months

Contd...

Spinal Cord

Contd...

Diseases	NECT/CECT findings	CT myelography	Comments
Spinal cord abscess	• There is a hypodense cavity with extensive edema in the adjacent parenchyma with variable intravenous contrast enhancement • In tuberculosis and sarcoidosis, there is cord expansion with leptomeningeal enhancement		Rare complications of adjacent infections
Astrocytoma (m/c in children)	• Homogeneously hypodense tumor with expansion involving long segment of the spinal cord • The tumor is located eccentrically • It may be cystic with variable degree and pattern of contrast enhancement • Dilated, tortuous veins are seen on surface of the cord	The cord appears widened	• Common in thoracic and cervical spine often extending into lower brainstem • Most common intramedullary mass of childhood
Ependymoma (m/c in adults)	• Heterogeneous attenuation mass with areas of cystic degeneration • Hemorrhages, and calcification with moderate-to-intense contrast enhancement	• The cord widened • When cystic, diffusion of contrast may occur into the cyst in delayed phase	Common in the filum terminale and conus medullaris

Contd...

Contd...

Diseases	NECT/CECT findings	CT myelography	Comments
	• There is focal or diffuse expansion of cord • Syringomyelia may be present • Leptomeningeal enhancement and nodularity may be seen due to metastases		
Hemangio-blastoma	• Spinal cord is expanded by a predominantly cystic, soft tissue mass • Tumor shows a densely enhancing tumor nodule within the cystic component • Large draining veins may be visualized • Syringomyelia is frequently associated	Expanded cord	It may be associated with von Hippel-Lindau disease
Metastases intramedullary	• Nonspecific, enhancing mass lesions are seen with or without cord (usually thoracic segments) expansion	Cord expansion may be seen	Most common primary tumors metastasizing to spinal cord are melanoma, choriocarcinoma, renal cell carcinoma (RCC), lung, breast, lymphoma, and colon

Contd...

Contd...

Diseases	NECT/CECT findings	CT myelography	Comments
Extramedullary, intradural (leptomeningeal carcinomatosis)	• Multiple nodules in cauda equina cord surface • Nerve roots may be matted together • Meninges are thickened and intensely enhancing	• Multiple, nodular filling defects • Expanded, irregular cord • Irregular, nodular spinal cord or matted nerve roots may be seen • Partial intradural block	Drop metastasis of intracranial neoplasms like medulloblastoma, ependymoma, primitive neuroectodermal tumor (PNET), gliomas (anaplastic), usually seen in pediatric age group
Extradural	Abscess	• Thecal sac indentation • Extradural block	• Sclerotic or lytic vertebral body/pedicle lesions • Vertebral collapse, with preserved intervertebral disc (IVD) • Associated soft tissue
Cord contusion/ transection	• Normal or diffusely or focally swollen cord may be visualized • Atrophic cord is seen as a late complication • Associated epidural hematoma. Density varies depending upon its age	• Post-traumatic root avulsions and meningeal injuries can be evaluated • Extradural block may be long segment	• Usually associated with bony spinal fractures and herniated disks • Seen at site of fracture
Chronic injury	Thin atrophic cord with or without syrinx is seen usually in the cervical region	Thin cord is evident with demonstration of syrinx in some cases	History of old trauma is important

Contd...

Contd...

Diseases	NECT/CECT findings	CT myelography	Comments
Dorsal meningocele	• Congenital form is relatively rare and is characterized by dorsal protrusion of meninges and CSF sac with no neural contents. Skin covers the defect externally • Acquired form is the relatively common complication of laminectomy	The sac fills with the contrast medium	Lumbosacral position is the most common site (below L2)
Anterior sacral meningocele	• CSF-filled sac protruding through widened sacral foramina • Dural in sacral area may be absent	The sac fills with the contrast medium	It may occur as an isolated defect or as a part of caudal regression syndrome, neurofibromatosis type 1 (NF-1), and Marfan syndrome
Occult intrasacral meningocele	• Expansile smoothly marginated CSF-filled cyst within the sacral bone • Cysts may or may not communicate freely with subarachnoid space	The cysts that communicate with subarachnoid space may fill up with contrast; and those that do not produce a smooth extradural impression on the contrast column	• Herniation of arachnoid through a dural defect in sacrum • It may be associated with lipoma and neurofibromatosis
Dorsal dermal sinus	• NECT shows a relatively hyperdense sinus tract through the subcutaneous fat and dysplastic lamina into the spinal canal • Associated dermoid (intramedullary or extramedullary) may be seen	• Dorsal tenting of dura and arachnoid mater • Sinus is outlined and may terminate in conus medullaris, filum terminale, nerve	More than half occur in lumbar spine, followed by the occipital region

Contd...

Contd...

Diseases	NECT/CECT findings	CT myelography	Comments
	• Hypoplastic spinous process • Multilevel spina bifida is common	root, fibrous nodule on dorsal aspect of cord, dermoid or epidermoid • Displacement or compression of cord by extramedullary tumors • Expansion of cord by intramedullary tumor • Clumping of nerve roots secondary to adhesive arachnoiditis	
Tight filum terminale (tethered cord)	Lumbar spina bifida occulta with interpedicular widening and scoliosis	• Diameter of filum terminale more than 2 mm at L5-S1 level • Posteriorly located tethered conus medullaris and filum terminale • Conus medullaris below the level of L2 by age 12 years • Abnormal lateral course of nerve roots • Widened triangular thecal sac tented posteriorly	It may be associated with lipoma, diastematomyelia and myelomeningocele

Contd...

Contd...

Diseases	NECT/CECT findings	CT myelography	Comments
Lipomyelo-meningocele	• Dorsal protrusion of meninges, CSF, neural contents, and fat through a focal spina bifida with widened spinal canal • The spinal cord is low lying and is dorsally located in the spinal canal • The lipoma itself lies outside the dura and is contiguous with subcutaneous fat • Lipoma may enter central canal and extend rostrally (intramedullary lipoma) • Lipoma may extend upward within spinal canal external to dura as well (epidural lipoma)	• The sac fills up with contrast medium and shows the complete tract • Lipoma can be suggested as a smooth indentation over the contrast column	• It is analogous to myelo-meningocele that has superimposed lipoma and intact skin • It may be associated with syringomyelia
Fibrolipoma of the filum terminale	There is a small fat density lesion in the filum terminale itself or at a lower level attached to the dura	• It can be seen as thickened filum terminale • The conus medullaris is at a normal position	Usually go undetected on CT but are incidental findings on MR examination
Neurenteric cyst	• Well-delineated lobulated intradural low-density mass characteristically in midline, anterior to spinal cord usually in the thoracic or cervical spine	When intradural may present as a smooth extrinsic impression on the contrast column	• Seen in patients under 40 years of age • Vertebral anomalies and associated clefts are common

Contd...

Contd...

Diseases	NECT/CECT findings	CT myelography	Comments
	• May present as a posterior mediastinal mass, with spinal dysraphism at the same level with defect in the center to accommodate the stalk • May have air-fluid levels if communicating to GI tract		
Intradural lipoma	• There is a spinal cord defect in the midline posteriorly with a fatty mass filling the defect • Fat density mass within the thecal sac that does not enhance on contrast administration • Exophytic component at upper or lower pole of lipoma • Narrow spina bifida	Focal enlargement of cord with enlargement of adjacent neural foramina	• Most common location is dorsal aspect of thoracic cord • Subpial juxtamedullary mass totally enclosed in intact dural sac
Meningioma	• Most common in dorsal aspect of thoracic cord • Cervical meningiomas are usually ventral • Solid smoothly marginated intradural mass isodense, hyperdense to skeletal muscles	• Intradural lesion is seen as a filling defect in the expanded contrast column displacing the cord and nerve roots • Extradural component indents the opacified subarachnoid space	• 25% of primary spinal neoplasm 4:1 female preponderance

Contd...

Contd...

Diseases	NECT/CECT findings	CT myelography	Comments
	• Dumbbell (5%) or extradural (5%) lesion may be seen • Moderate to marked enhancement • May calcify • Enlarged neural foramina in dumbbell lesions		
Neurofibroma (Figs. 2A and B)	• Well-defined mass with dumbbell configuration (extradural component extends through neural foramen) • Widening of neural foramen with erosions of pedicle • Scalloping of vertebral bodies • Hypodense (characteristic) approaching characteristics of water, isodense to skeletal muscles • Usually no contrast enhancement • Dural ectasia cause multilevel posterior vertebral scalloping and lateral meningocele	• Well-defined soft tissue mass is seen as an intradural filling defect with/without an extradural indentation • Widened subarachnoid space having undulating margins or meningoceles may be seen	• When associated with neurofibromatosis • Lesions are multiple • Scoliosis, patulous dural sac, and meningoceles are characteristic
Schwannoma	• Contrast-enhancing soft tissue mass at the lateral aspect of spinal cord • Placed eccentrically along the course of dorsal sensory nerve root	• Intradural lesion is demonstrated well • Extradural component, if present, indents the contrast column	Common in patients with NF-2

Contd...

Spinal Cord

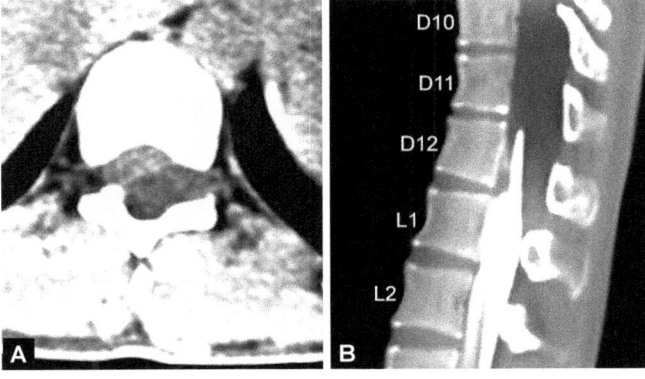

Figs. 2A and B: Noncontrast axial and sagittal CT myelogram showing dumbbell-shaped neurofibroma.

Contd...

Diseases	NECT/CECT findings	CT myelography	Comments
	• Bone erosion may be present • The lesion is almost always solitary		
Ependymoma	• Well-demarcated or diffusely infiltrating tumor • Occupies whole width of spinal cord • Focal mass with areas of extensive cystic degeneration, hemorrhage and calcification • Erosion of vertebral body is common • Enhances extensively	• Widened cord • Contrast block or contrast meniscus	• Common locations are lower spinal cord, conus medullaris, and filum terminale
Paraganglioma	• Strongly and inhomogeneously enhancing intradural, extramedullary mass	• An intradural filling defect is present	Spinal lesions are rare

Contd...

Contd...

Diseases	NECT/CECT findings	CT myelography	Comments
	• Common in cauda equina and filum terminale • Hemorrhage is common in this lesion	• Adjacent dilated vessels are seen as serpiginous filling defects within the contrast column	
Granulocytic sarcoma (chloroma, myeloblas- toma)	Solitary or multiple intradural and/or extradural masses in a patient with myelogenous leukemia	Clearly delineates the location and extent of the mass	Focal masses of leukemic cells associated with myelogenous leukemia
Epidural lipomatosis	There is excessive deposition of the fat in the epidural space with compression of the thecal sac	It reveals long segment narrowing of the thecal sac with crowding of the normal sac contents	It can be idiopathic or secondary to drugs, obesity, and Cushing's syndrome
Arachnoid cyst	• Intradural/extra- dural water density, oval, sharply demarcated lesion, most commonly located posterior to thoracic cord • Thoracic cord displaced anteriorly	• Seen as an intradural filling defect or an extradural indentation on the contrast column • Cyst occasionally opacifies (early/delayed) by intrathecal contrast media	Intradural are congenital or acquired secondary to adhesions due to trauma or infections
Epidermoid cyst	• Intradural soft tissue mass in the lumbar region • Isodense to CSF • No contrast enhancement	• Facilitates detection, almost always presents as complete block • Displacement of spinal cord and nerve roots	Acquired epidermoid is considered as a rare late complication of lumbar puncture

Contd...

Spinal Cord

Contd...

Diseases	NECT/CECT findings	CT myelography	Comments

Arachnoiditis	• Fusion or clumping of nerve roots
	• Featureless empty looking sac with roots adherent to wall
		• Streaking and clumping of contrast
		• Blunting of nerve root sleeves
		• *Three broad patterns recognized*:
		  1. Matted nerve roots located centrally in thecal sac
		  2. Nerve roots adherent peripherally to dura
		  3. Abnormal soft tissue filling the irregularly shaped thecal sac
			Adhesions between nerve roots and dura are common in patients after spinal surgery, and prior infection or intrathecal hemorrhage

Spinal hematoma (subdural and epidural)	• In acute cases, an area of increased density is seen in the spinal canal, most commonly at the thoracolumbar junction and in the thoracic spine • In subacute and chronic cases, it may simulate cord expansion	It is seen as an indentation of different shape and size over the contrast column corresponding to the configuration of the hematoma	• Commonly seen in patients with bleeding diathesis and/or after lumbar puncture • Epidural hematoma is usually associated with vertebral fracture

Contd...

Contd...

Diseases	NECT/CECT findings	CT myelography	Comments
Spinal arteriovenous malformation	• It is seen as multiple, dilated, vascular channels with large arteries and draining veins seen on CECT • Half of the cases are associated with hematoma in the meningeal space • Associated calcification may be seen	• Multilevel, serpiginous, filling defects are seen that may show variation in size with Valsalva maneuver or increased intra-abdominal pressure • Signs of cord atrophy and hematoma may be seen	• It is the most common vascular spinal anomaly • Dorsolumbar region is the most common
Discal disease (bulge, herniation and sequestration)	• Loss of normal posterior disk concavity is seen in bulge with protrusion of disk material beyond the adjacent vertebral endplate • Bulge is usually broad-based and symmetrical • Herniation is seen as a focal nonenhancing soft tissue mass bulging into the spinal canal or neural foramen and is contiguous with the intervertebral disk • Associated spinal canal stenosis is seen • Displacement of the contiguous nerve root is also evident	It is seen as a smooth indentation over the contrast column	• It is commonly associated with degenerative disease of the spine • Most frequent site is L4-L5 and L5-S1 • The herniation is confined to the level of the disk, is subligamental herniation, and is sharply marginated • Transligamental herniation appears at a sharp angle to the contour of the disk

Contd...

Contd...

Diseases	NECT/CECT findings	CT myelography	Comments
	• Sequestration of a herniated disk appears as a soft tissue mass discontinuous parent disk • It appears hyperdense to the adjacent nerve root		• Associated findings are Schmorl's nodes (lucencies in the vertebral endplate surrounded by sclerosis), osteophytes (bony spurs) and endplate sclerosis
Spondylitis, spondylodiscitis	• Bone destruction with large paraspinous abscesses • Hypodensity of disk is the first indicator of disk involvement • Decreased intervertebral disk space with irregularity of the contiguous vertebral endplates is evident • Spinal epidural abscess collection may be present	• An extrinsic impression on contrast column or displacement of thecal sac away from the bony canal with partial or complete block is evident • Encroachment on the nerve roots is also seen clearly	Tuberculosis is by far the most common in India
Spinal epidural abscess	• Extradural soft tissue or fluid attenuation mass involving a larger segment than involved vertebra • It may show homogeneous, heterogeneous, or ring enhancement depending on the stage of abscess	Extradural blockage is seen at the involved level	Isolated abscess is rare, usually associated with spondylitis

Contd...

Contd...

Diseases	NECT/CECT findings	CT myelography	Comments
Spondylolisthesis	• Local narrowing of the spinal canal associated with a symmetrical defect in pars interarticularis • Adjacent sclerosis is evident with the wavy/irregular defect • Anterior dislocation of the affected vertebral body relative to the inferior vertebra	Complete or partial extradural compression	• Common finding at L5-S1 level and trauma is an important cause • When osteoarthritis or dysplasia is the cause, it is referred to as pseudospondylolisthesis
Primary vertebral neoplasm	• Bone destruction or expansion of the vertebra may be evident • Soft tissue mass may be associated and it may also encroach upon the spinal canal	Complete or partial extradural compression	Osteosarcoma, chondrosarcoma, chordoma, giant cell tumor, and aneurysmal bone cyst are the common tumors associated with spinal canal encroachment
Metastases	• Involvement of the pedicle supports the diagnosis • These may form an extradural soft tissue mass that may enhance on CECT	Complete or partial extradural compression	It is the most common destructive bone lesion in patients over age 50 years, followed by myeloma
Degenerative disease of the spine (spondylosis, spondyloarthrosis, ligamentum flavum hypertrophy)	• Schmorl's nodes, osteophytes, and endplate sclerosis are the hallmark for spondylosis • Disk bulge is often associated	Complete or partial extradural compression	

Contd...

Contd...

Diseases	NECT/CECT findings	CT myelography	Comments
	• Dorsal osteophytes may narrow the spinal canal, especially in the cervical spine • Osteophytes arising from the articular surfaces of the facet joints may narrow the spinal canal or lateral recess • Vacuum phenomenon and protrusions of the articular capsule (synovial cyst) may be seen on soft tissue windows • Synovial cyst is seen as a cystic mass adjacent to a degenerating facet joint posterolateral to the thecal sac with enhancement of walls on post-contrast images • Thickness of ligamentum flavum of 5 mm or more is termed as hypertrophy		
Postoperative scar	• Fibrotic soft tissue replaces epidural fat to a variable degree • The thecal sac is often displaced or asymmetric	Complete or partial extradural compression	The degree of contrast enhancement of the postoperative scar tissue diminishes with time

Contd...

Contd...

Diseases	NECT/CECT findings	CT myelography	Comments
	• Fibrotic tissue enhances homogeneously after a high dose of contrast media and the encased nerve root can be seen as a sharply marginated hypodense structure		
Postoperative disk herniation	On CECT, herniation appears as a hypodense zone within contrast-enhanced scar tissue	Complete or partial extradural compression	NECT images are nonspecific

(CECT: contrast-enhanced computed tomography; NECT: noncontrast-enhanced computed tomography; GI: gastrointestinal; m/c: most common)

LESIONS ASSOCIATED WITH SPINAL STENOSIS

These are shown in Tables 3 and 4.

TABLE 3: Common causes associated with spinal stenosis.

Congenital	Acquired

• *Congenital short pedicles*
  – Idiopathic
  – *Syndromes*: Achondroplasia, hypochondroplasia, Morquio syndrome, Down syndrome
• Diastrophic dysplasia
• Klippel-Feil syndrome
• Os odontoideum
• Hemivertebra
	• Degenerative disease of the spine (disk disease, spondylosis, spondylolisthesis, facet joint hypertrophy, ligamentum flavum)
	• Ossification of posterior longitudinal ligament
	• Hydroxyapatite crystal deposition disease
	• Vertebral tumors (benign—aneurysmal bone cyst, osteochondroma; malignant—osteoblastoma, metastases)
	• Fracture vertebra (burst, retropulsed fragment)
	• *Miscellaneous*: Paget's disease, acromegaly

Spinal Cord

TABLE 4: Relevant CT findings of lesions associated with spinal stenosis.

Diseases	NECT/CECT findings	Comments
Achondroplasia, hypochondroplasia	<ul><li>The posterior concavity of the vertebra is exaggerated</li><li>The pedicles of the vertebra are short</li><li>Superimposed spondylosis may further narrow the spinal canal</li><li>The foramen magnum may be stenotic and the spinal cord consequently flattened</li><li>In hypochondroplasia, the foramen magnum and the L1-L5 interpedicular distance may both be narrow</li></ul>	Achondroplasia is most common form of rhizomelic dwarfism throughout the spine
Diastrophic dysplasia	<ul><li>Narrow interpedicular distance are seen especially in the lumbar region</li><li>Hyper- or hypoplasia of odontoid process is common</li><li>Cervical kyphosis with cord compression is common finding</li></ul>	It is as autosomal recessive achondroplasia
Klippel-Feil syndrome	Spinal stenosis may occur in association with block cervical or cervicothoracic vertebra	Associated features include genitourinary abnormalities, atlantoaxial instability, spinal cord compression, and syringomyelia

Contd...

Contd...

Diseases	NECT/CECT findings	Comments
Os odontoideum	• It is seen as a rounded, well-corticated bone superior to dens that has not fused with the body of the C2 vertebra • Atlantoaxial instability may be evident on flexion/extension scans	It is a congenital condition occurring due to nonfusion of ossification centers should not be confused with type 2 os fracture
Hemivertebra	• It produces acute angle scoliosis at the site of affected level compromising the lateral foramen and causing nerve compression • Posterior hemivertebra may cause direct impingement of the spinal canal	
Hydroxyapatite deposition disease (HADD)	• There is excessive deposition of calcified crystals centered at synovial articulations with formation of lobulated, periarticular calcified masses compromising the spinal canal • Erosive changes can be seen in the adjacent bone	Most common in patients with end-stage renal disease

Contd...

Spinal Cord

Contd...

Diseases	NECT/CECT findings	Comments
Ossification of posterior longitudinal ligament (OPLL)	• Longitudinal, multi-segmental linear calcification is seen along the posterior aspect of vertebral bodies • It is seen most commonly in the cervical spine	Often associated with DISH (diffuse idiopathic skeletal hyperostosis)
Ossification of ligamentum flavum (Figs. 3A and B)	• There is enchondral ossification of the hypertrophied ligamentum flavum • The site of predilection is thoracolumbar region	The condition is to be differentiated from calcification of ligamentum flavum seen in calcium pyrophosphate dihydrate deposition disease (CPPD)
Metastases	• Destruction of the vertebral body with involvement of pedicle is suggestive • Associated soft tissue mass may encase or compress the spinal cord or nerve root and may show postcontrast enhancement	It is the most common malignant tumor of the spine
Aneurysmal bone cyst (ABC)	• It is seen as a lobulated, lytic, and expansile lesion that typically involves posterior elements of the vertebra causing stenosis of the vertebral canal • Fluid levels are characteristic, when present • It may extend into the neighboring vertebra or ribs	It is usually seen in patients before 20 years of age

Contd...

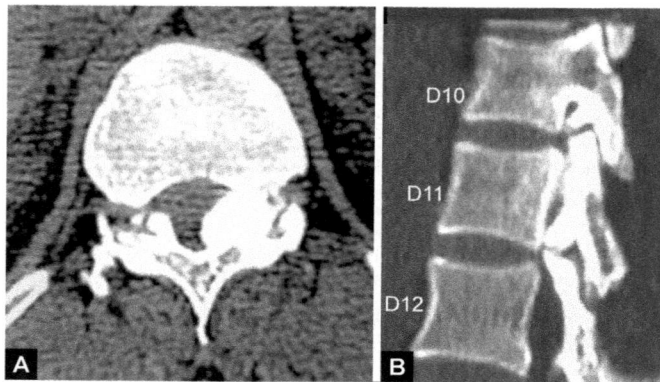

Figs. 3A and B: Axial and sagittal CT images showing spinal canal stenosis due to ligamentum flavum hypertrophy.

Contd...

Diseases	NECT/CECT findings	Comments
Osteochondroma (Figs. 4A and B)	It is characterized by a dense, ossified, sessile, or pedunculated lesion usually in the posterior elements of the cervical spine that may cause narrowing of the canal	
Osteoblastoma	• It is seen as an expansile, lytic lesion with thin sclerotic margins with occasional calcification • Involvement of posterior elements of the vertebra is characteristic	• Usually under 30 years of age • Close differential is aneurysmal bone cyst
Paget's disease (Osteitis deformans)	• Extradural soft tissue mass may displace or compress the spinal cord or thecal sac. Soft tissue mass may contain extramedullary hematopoiesis	• The spine is involved in about a third of cases • Elderly age group • Premalignant condition → overall survival (OS)

Contd...

Spinal Cord

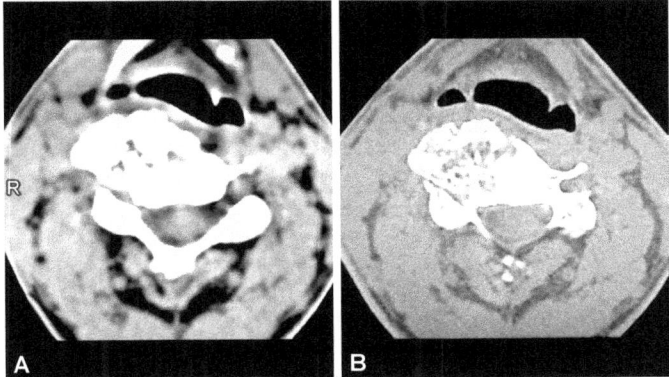

Figs. 4A and B: Axial CT images of spine showing soft tissue mass with flocculent calcification arising from C5 vertebral body suggesting osteochondroma.

Contd...

Diseases	NECT/CECT findings	Comments
	• Associated changes are seen in the vertebral bodies—thickened cortex, bone overgrowth, and heterogeneous increased attenuation	
Acromegaly	• Features include widening of the atlanto-axial joint, enlargement of the vertebrae, abundant osteophytosis with resultant spinal stenosis	

(CECT: contrast-enhanced computed tomography; NECT: noncontrast-enhanced computed tomography)

Chapter 3

Ear and Temporal Bone

DIFFERENTIAL DIAGNOSIS OF EAR LESIONS

Tables 1 and 2 show the differential diagnosis of ear lesions.

TABLE 1: Causes of soft tissue and bony lesions of external ear.

Soft tissue lesions	Bony lesions
• *With osseous destruction*: – Cholesteatoma – Carcinoma – Melanoma – Giant cell tumor – Metastases – Malignant otitis externa • *With no osseous involvement*: – Wax – Keratosis obturans – Fibrous malformation	• Bony malformation • Exostoses • Osteoma • Fibrous dysplasia

TABLE 2: Differentiating features of common external ear lesions.

Diseases	Differentiating features	Comments
Malformation (Fig. 1)	Canal is superiorly angulated instead of extending inferolaterally to superomedially	• Associated with ossicular abnormalities (*viz.* absence or dysplasia of malleus and incus,

Contd...

Contd...

Diseases	Differentiating features	Comments
		fusion of malleus and incus to the attic wall), aplasia of tympanic or mastoid part of the temporal bone, anomalous facial nerve canal course, absent oval or round window, hypoplastic cochlea, hypoplasia or enlargement of the lateral semicircular canal (SCC) and/or enlargement of the vestibule • There is increased incidence of congenital or acquired cholesteatoma
Fibrous type	Soft tissue plug is seen at the site of normal tympanic membrane	Tympanic membrane is absent
Bony type	Bony plate is seen at the site where the normal tympanic membrane	Tympanic membrane is absent
Keratosis obturans	• It is characterized by soft tissue plug which obliterates the medialt portion of external auditory canal (EAC)	• The condition is usually a bilateral • It is common below 40 years of age with history of sinusitis/ bronchiectasis

Contd...

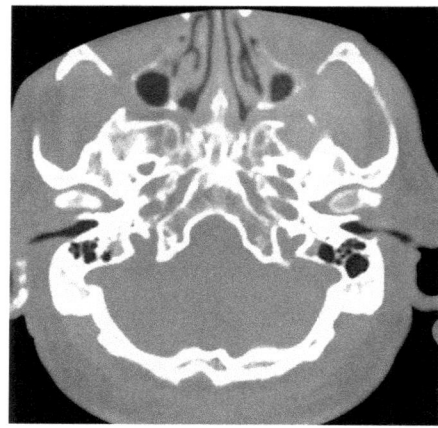

Fig. 1: Axial CT image showing bilateral external acoustic canal stenoses.

Contd...

Diseases	Differentiating features	Comments
	associated with mild diffuse thinning of the cortex with resultant widening of the canal • Tympanic membrane is displaced medially	• Middle ear is normal
Cholesteatoma	• It is seen as a well-defined soft tissue mass causing localized erosion of the inferior canal wall lateral to the isthmus • Sequestration of bone with sinus tract formation may be seen as a complication	• It may be congenital • It may be seen in persons >40 years of age • It is chronic unilateral condition associated with otorrhea

Contd...

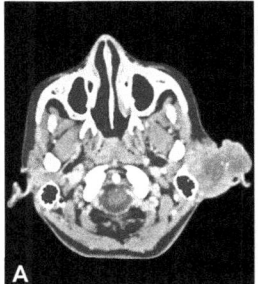
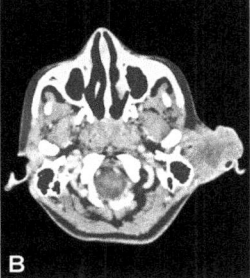

Figs. 2A and B: Contrast-enhanced computed tomography (CECT) axial images of base of skull showing peripherally enhancing lesion arising from left pinna in a case of hemangioma.

Contd...

Diseases	Differentiating features	Comments
Hemangioma (Figs. 2A and B)	• It is seen as lobulated, intensely enhancing soft tissue mass • Smooth pressure erosion may be seen	
Malignant otitis externa (Fig. 3)	• It is seen as a soft tissue thickening or mass of the EAC with clouding of middle ear and the mastoid air cells • Postcontrast images show widespread enhancement with multifocal abscesses with bone destruction	• It is a rapidly progressive infectious condition • Commonly seen in elderly diabetics and in immunocompromised patients
Squamous cell carcinoma	• It is characterized by moderately enhancing, soft tissue mass often with calcific densities • Erosion of the adjacent bone with middle ear extension is common	Temporomandibular joint may be involved

Contd...

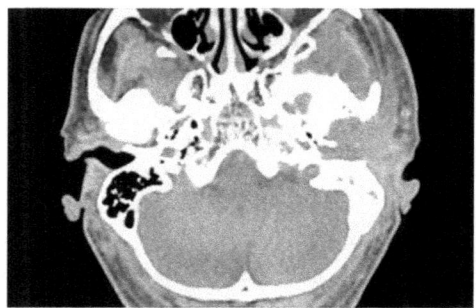

Fig. 3: *Malignant otitis externa*: Noncontrast-enhanced computed tomography (NECT) axial at the level of external auditory canal (EAC) shows a soft tissue mass in the EAC causing bony erosions.

Contd...

Diseases	Differentiating features	Comments
Ceruminoma/ adenocarcinoma	• Computed tomography (CT) features are similar to the squamous cell carcinoma • Regional lymphadenopathy is common with central necrosis and peripheral rim enhancement	
Basal cell carcinoma	• It is characterized by soft tissue mass filling the EAC with extensive bony destruction and expansion, and extension into middle ear with destruction • No nodal or distant metastasis	It is a locally malignant tumor
Malignant melanoma	• It is seen as a soft tissue mass showing intense postcontrast enhancement • Local bony destruction is common	

Contd...

Ear and Temporal Bone

Contd...

Diseases	Differentiating features	Comments
Giant cell tumor	• It is a primary bone tumor with lytic expansile nature with intact cortex and honeycomb pattern • Enhancing soft tissue component may be seen into the adjacent external ear canal simulating a mass	The epicenter of the tumor is bone
Metastases	• Osteoblastic or osteoclastic metastatic lesions can be seen involving the bony external acoustic meatus • Soft tissue component is not a feature	If the primary known, it will help in the diagnosis
Exostoses	These are seen as bony excrescences arising from the anterior and the posterior wall of the tympanic bone deep in the EAC near the tympanic membrane with resulting narrowing of the meatus	The condition usually presents after first decade due to secondary pain, infection and loss of hearing
Osteoma	They are seen as pedunculated growth of the cancellous bone	These are located typically in the outer portion of the bony meatus at the tympanomastoid or the tympanosquamous sutures
Fibrous dysplasia	The affected bones show dense sclerosis and thickening with ground-glass appearance with intact cortex occluding the tympanic cavity	Mostly arise from the mastoids

LESIONS OF THE MIDDLE EAR AND MASTOID

Soft tissue lesions of the middle ear and mastoid are shown in Table 3.

TABLE 3: Common causes of middle ear and mastoid lesions.

Soft tissue lesions		Opacification of air cells and cavity
Enhancing	*Nonenhancing*	
• Granulation tissue • Adenoma • Carcinoma • Neuroma of facial nerve • Glomus tumors (jugulare/tympanicum) • Hemangioma • Eosinophilic granuloma • Rhabdomyosarcoma • Metastases	• Cholesteatoma • Cholesterol granuloma • Tympanosclerosis	• Acute and chronic suppurative otitis media with mastoiditis • Chronic granulomatous otitis media • Adhesive otitis media • Coalescent mastoiditis

INFECTIVE, MISCELLANEOUS LESIONS OF THE MIDDLE EAR AND MASTOID

These lesions are shown in Table 4.

TABLE 4: Causes of infective, miscellaneous lesions of middle ear and mastoid.

Diseases	Differentiating features	Comments
Otitis media with mastoiditis (Figs. 4 and 5)	• Opacified air cells and the fluid levels are identified in the middle ear and the mastoid • Integrity of the mastoid septa, ossicular chain and the external and internal mastoid cortices is preserved	Fluid levels persisting for greater than 3 months suggest chronic infection

Contd...

Ear and Temporal Bone

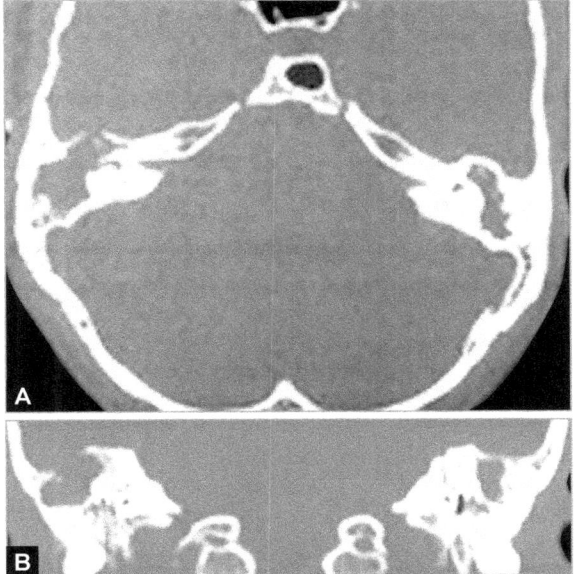

Figs. 4A and B: Axial and coronal CT images showing bilateral CSOM and mastoiditis with destruction of the tegmen tympani on right side.

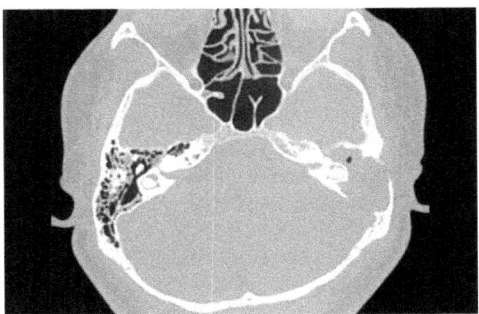

Fig. 5: Axial CT image showing chronic suppurative otitis media (CSOM) with destruction of the tegmen tympani on left side.

Differential Diagnosis in Computed Tomography

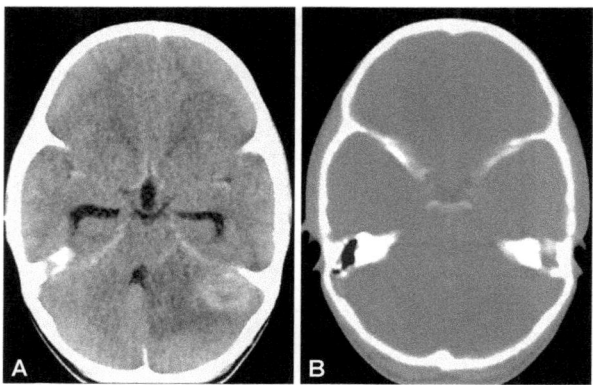

Figs. 6A and B: Transaxial CT images show cerebellar abscess following chronic suppurative otitis media (CSOM) on left side.

Contd...

Diseases	Differentiating features	Comments
Chronic suppurative otitis media (CSOM) and mastoiditis	Residual part is usually thickened and middle ear cavity is partially/completely opacified. Complications like cerebellar abscess may occur (Figs. 6A and B)	
Chronic adhesive otitis media	The thickened tympanic membrane is retracted to the promontory and middle ear cavity is contracted	
Chronic granulomatous otitis media	In addition to the findings of chronic suppurative otitis media polyps, granulation tissue, abscesses and multiple perforations in tympanic membrane are seen	

Contd...

Ear and Temporal Bone

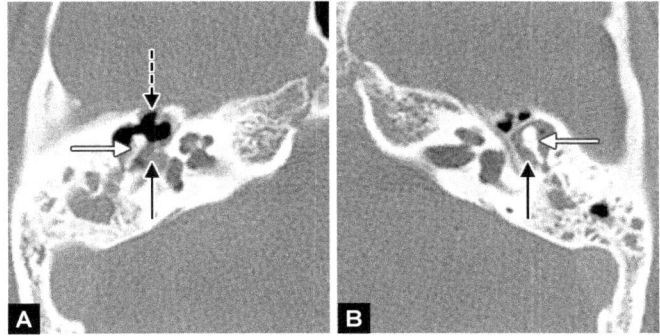

Figs. 7A and B: Axial high-resolution computed tomography (HRCT) of patient with cholesteatoma on right and chronic otitis media without cholesteatoma on left. (A) Mass lesion (black arrow) in tympanic cavity with erosion of ossicles (white arrow) and erosion of epitympanum (dashed arrow); (B) Mass lesion (black arrow) in epitympanum without bony erosion (white arrow).

Contd...

Diseases	Differentiating features	Comments
Coalescent mastoiditis	• Debris in the mastoid cavity with resulting poor definition and destruction of the mastoid septa • Destruction of the external cortex may be seen with perimastoid cellulitis	
Cholesteatoma		
Acquired	• Nonenhancing soft tissue mass is seen in the middle ear with focal or diffuse bone destruction—lateral epitympanic wall, posterosuperior canal wall and ossicles (Figs. 7A and B)	

Contd...

Contd...

Diseases	Differentiating features	Comments
	• Extension into the aditus antrum and mastoid occurs with erosion of these structures and destruction of Korner's septum • Erosion of facial canal, tegmen and bony labyrinth is found as a late complication of the disease	
Primary acquired (pars flaccida)	• Tympanic cavity is contracted • Tympanic membrane is retracted and thickened • Lateral epitympanic wall and anterior tympanic spine is eroded by mass present in epitympanum lateral to the ossicles • The mass expands into the antrum and the mesotympanum with medial displacement of the ossicles away from the Prussak's space	
Secondary acquired (pars tensa)	• The mass lies in the tympanic cavity and extends to epitympanum medial to the ossicles and displaces the head of malleus and incus laterally • Long process of incus is eroded	
Congenital cholesteatoma (epidermoid)	• It is seen as a well-defined soft tissue mass in the middle ear cavity with erosion of the medial wall of the epitympanum	Usually no history of chronic inflammatory ear disease is present

Contd...

Ear and Temporal Bone

Contd...

Diseases	Differentiating features	Comments
	• Associated serous otitis media makes the middle ear cavity cloudy • Tympanic membrane is displaced laterally, however, pure serous otitis media without cholesteatoma causes medial retraction of the tympanic membrane	
Cholesterol granuloma	• It is seen as a well-defined soft tissue mass in an aerated middle ear • Ossicles are eroded, but bony contours are intact	It is formed in a chronic inflammatory setting
Granulation tissue	• It is seen as a soft tissue mass with no ossicular displacement or bone erosion • It usually shows post-contrast enhancement	It is the most common cause of debris in the middle ear
Squamous cell carcinoma	• It is usually seen as a medial extension of external acoustic meatus lesion • An enhancing soft tissue mass with no history of previous cholesteatoma • Bony erosion is also present	Primary tumor is rare
Neuroma of facial nerve	• An expanded bony facial canal is seen in early stage • Later tumor may extend into the middle ear and present as a well-defined enhancing soft tissue mass with associated fusiform • Expansion or erosion of nerve canal	

Contd...

Contd...

Diseases	Differentiating features	Comments
Adenoma	It usually presents as soft tissue mass beginning in posterior tympanum	It is a rare tumor arising from ectopic salivary tissue
Embryonal rhabdomyosarcoma	• It is seen as a middle ear, heterogeneously enhancing, soft tissue mass with bone destruction • It may spread along the eustachian tube	It is seen in children
Eosinophilic granuloma	An enhancing, soft tissue mass with sharply marginated destruction of adjacent bone is seen in middle ear	Mastoid is the most common site of involvement
Glomus tympanicum	• It is seen as an intensely enhancing, soft tissue mass adjacent to the cochlear promontory without bony destruction • Displacement and erosion of ossicles occurs early while floor of hypotympanum is preserved till late	
Glomus jugulare (Fig. 8)	• It is seen as an intensely enhancing, soft tissue mass in middle ear with bony destructive distortion separation of the jugular fossa (jugular spine) and floor of hypotympanum • Mottled appearance of intralabyrinthine compartment is evident	

Contd...

Ear and Temporal Bone

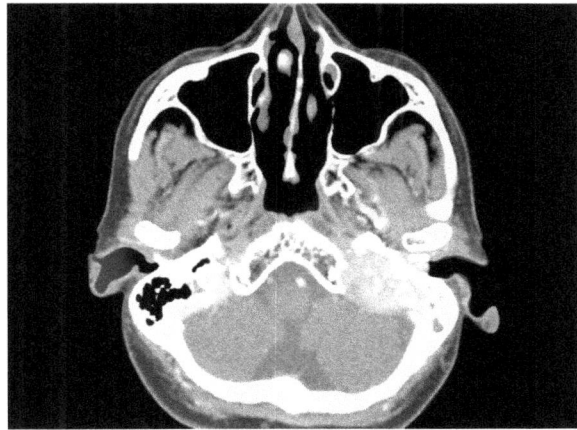

Fig. 8: *Glomus jugulare*: Axial contrast CECT image showing an intensely enhancing soft tissue lesion in the jugular foramen causing expansion of the foramen.

Contd...

Diseases	Differentiating features	Comments
Hemangioma	• An ill-defined, lobulated, enhancing soft tissue mass is seen in the middle ear cavity • Associated bony destruction may be seen	
Tympanosclerosis	Multiple punctuate or web-like calcific densities are seen in the middle ear meatus	It represents dystrophic calcification on due to healed chronic otitis media

INTERNAL EAR LESIONS (TABLES 5 TO 13)

Endolymphatic Sac Lesions

Contrast-enhanced Computed Tomography (CECT)

- Transient enhancement (may be secondary to viral infection).
- Persistent enhancement—causes include:
  - Suppurative infections (may be associated with both destruction and mass effect)
  - Sarcoidosis
  - Metastases
  - Lymphoma
  - Eosinophilic granuloma
  - Autoimmune labyrinthitis
  - Endolymphatic sac tumors.
- It causes local destruction in the retrolabyrinthine petrous bone and may extend into the medial mastoid to invade the facial nerve or transdurally into the posterior cranial fossa.
- On CT, the bony margins are irregular, and intratumoral bony spicules are commonly present.

TABLE 5: Differentiating features of various common lesions associated with demineralization of the cochlea.

Diseases	Differentiating features	Comments
Otosyphilis	It is characterized by a permeative/moth-eaten demineralization	Other associated lesions of syphilis will be seen elsewhere
Otosclerosis	• Crescentic hypodense region parallels the margins of the basal turns of cochlea, entire cochlea or otic capsule (cochlear/retrofenestral type)	

Contd...

Ear and Temporal Bone

Contd...

Diseases	Differentiating features	Comments
	• Lesion may be seen involving the oval window and the stapes footplate (stapedial/fenestral type) • CT shows hypodensity, typically seen when the demineralization is progressing	
Paget's disease	Areas with mixed appearance of bone thickening and sclerosis may be seen	Usually bilateral
Osteogenesis imperfecta	• CT shows proliferation of undermineralized, thickened bone around the otic capsule • As the disease progresses, it may cause middle ear cavity narrowing and oval window obstruction • In the inner ear, CT findings are similar to cochlear type of otosclerosis but is much more extensive and may show a *"double ring sign"* (double lucency due to enchondral band of demineralization)	

TABLE 6: Differentiating features of various common sclerotic lesions in the inner ear/temporal bone.

Diseases	Differentiating features	Comments
Fibrous dysplasia (Fig. 9)	• There is extensive bony overgrowth with diffuse sclerosis and thickening and loss of trabecular pattern of the temporal bone • There may be varying degrees of obliteration of the mastoid air cells • Tympanic cavity may be compressed; external acoustic meatus may be severely narrowed	Secondary cholesteatoma may be seen in the external auditory canal (EAC)
Ossifying fibroma	CT findings are similar to the FD, but it tends to be more localized appearing more as a mass lesion	
Hyperparathyroidism	• It is characterized by ground glass, sclerotic bone • Skeletal manifestations are symmetrically evident throughout the skeletal system	There is associated systemic hypercalcemia
Sclerostenosis (endosteal hyperostosis)	• There is sclerosis and overgrowth of the skull, vertebrae, and mandible, with gigantism and syndactyly • Associated narrowing of the external and internal acoustic canal and the eustachian tube is seen	
Chondroblastoma	• It presents as an expansile soft tissue mass with bone erosion	• It is rare in temporal bone

Contd...

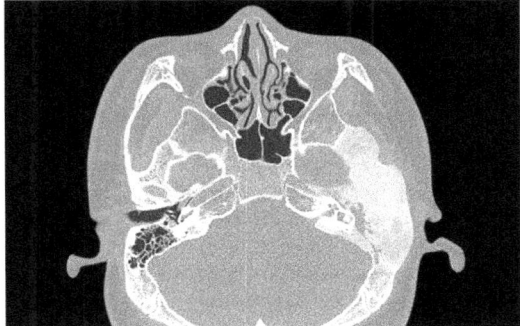

Fig. 9: Fibrous dysplasia: Extensive expansile sclerosis with ground-glass appearance of the left zygoma, sphenoid, and petrous temporal bone.

Contd...

Diseases	Differentiating features	Comments
	• Spotty calcification may be seen and the lesion enhances with contrast administration	• It may simulate fibrous dysplasia
Paget's disease	It is characterized by bilateral lesions exhibiting osteopenia with a small number of sclerotic foci	Patients are usually older as compared to those with fibrous dysplasia
Progressive diaphyseal dysplasia	• CT shows mild-to-moderate thickening of the skull base with hyperostosis and sclerosis • Middle ear may be completely encased by the sclerotic bone, with associated widespread narrowing of the cranial foramina	It is also known as Camurati-Engelmann-Ribbing syndrome

TABLE 7: Differentiating features of common soft tissue masses of inner ear/internal acoustic canal.

Diseases	Differentiating features	Comments
Acoustic schwannoma	There is mushroom-shaped; iso-, hypo- or hyperdense, moderately to markedly enhancing soft tissue mass epicentered at the internal auditory canal	If mass is not seen, asymmetry at the internal auditory canal (greater than 2 mm difference in the internal diameter on both sides) suggests the presence of mass
Meningioma	• Mass may be isodense or slightly hyperdense sometimes calcified • It shows marked homogeneous enhancement after contrast administration	It is rarely seen in the internal acoustic canal arising in the posterior petrous wall
Facial nerve schwannoma	• CT findings similar to acoustic schwannoma • There is erosion of the anteroposterior portion of the internal acoustic canal and the geniculate ganglion • Tumors of facial nerve canal cause enlargement and erosion of the canal • Geniculate ganglion involvement cause enlargement of the geniculate fossa • Extracanalicular type is seen as an eccentric mass beyond the facial nerve canal in the supralabyrinthine area	Geniculate ganglion is the most common site of facial nerve schwannoma

Contd...

Contd...

Diseases	Differentiating features	Comments
Epidermoid cyst	• It is occasionally seen extending into the internal acoustic canal from the cerebellopontine cistern • It is seen as a lobulated, hypodense, nonenhancing mass usually arising in the cerebellopontine cistern	

TABLE 8: Differentiating features of common lesion of the petrous apex lesion.

Diseases	Differentiating features	Comments
Effusion	Fluid level at the petrous apex	Secondary-to-middle ear infections
Acute petrositis	• Debris are seen within petrous apex air cells • Lysis of the bony septa and the disruption of the adjacent bony cortex may also occur	Rarely, it may present as effusion without destruction
Cholesterol granuloma (cyst)	• It appears as cystic, lobulated, sharply, and smoothly marginated • It is ovoid in configuration and expands the petrous apex, especially posteriorly, where the overlying bone is often paper thin or absent • Where the bone is present, the internal margin of the lesion is often sclerotic	

Contd...

Contd...

Diseases	Differentiating features	Comments
	• A lesion is isodense to brain, homogeneous and free of calcium • No contrast enhancement except peripheral rim due to a capsule or the overlying dura	
Epidermoid cyst (primary cholesteatoma)	It is seen as a homogeneous, nonenhancing, sharply defined, ovoid expansile lesion like cholesterol cysts; hypodense to isodense to the brain	Indistinguishable from cholesterol cysts when isodense to the brain
Mucocele carotid artery aneurysm	• It appears similar to the cholesterol cysts • It is seen as an expanding ovoid mass • Mural thrombus is isodense and nonenhancing, the patent lumen shows rapid rise in enhancement	It is rare but important in the differential diagnosis of the petrous lesions
Chondrosarcoma	• It is seen as mass lesion causing bone destruction • It enhances mild-to-moderate on CT and may contain calcification	
Chondroblastoma		Uncommon benign tumor may be indistinguishable from a chondrosarcoma
Apical meningocele	It is characterized by CSF-filled space in the petrous apex	• It may communicate with the middle ear, resulting in the CSF leak • It may mimic cholesterol cyst on CT

Contd...

Contd...

Diseases	Differentiating features	Comments
Petrous apicitis	It is seen as a soft tissue mass with osseous destruction at the petrous apex with enhancement of adjacent dura	

TABLE 9: Differentiating features of various congenital malformations of inner ear (Figs. 10A to D): Dysplasia.

Diseases	Differentiating features	Comments
Bing-Siebenmann dysplasia	Cochlear and vestibular anomalies	
Scheibe dysplasia	In this there is temporal bone dysplasia	• Most common dysplasia • There is profound sensorineural hearing loss
Mondini dysplasia	• It is characterized by normal basilar turns of cochlea with decreased number of upper turns with mediolar hypoplasia • Upper turns are seen as sac-like remnants	
Alexander dysplasia	There is underdevelopment of the basilar turn	
Michel dysplasia	There is complete absence of labyrinth including absence of sensorineural structures of the inner ear	

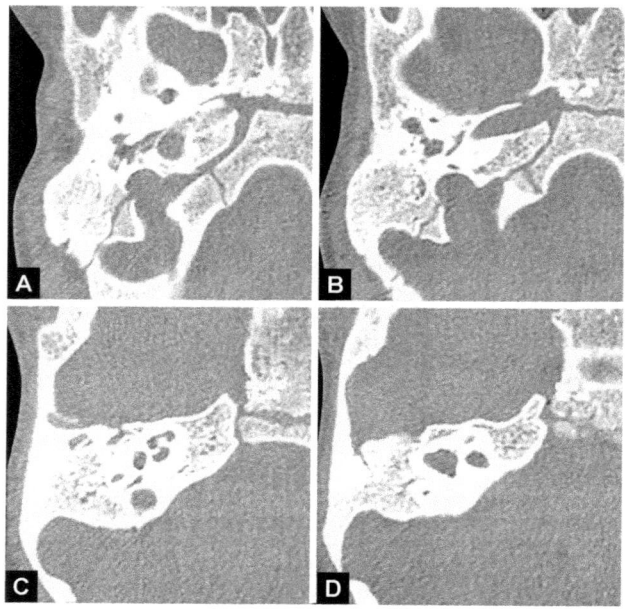

Figs. 10A to D: Axial CT images showing multiple dysplasia involving external, middle, and inner ear.

TABLE 10: Differentiating features of various membranous and bony labyrinthine anomalies.

Diseases	Differentiating features	Comments
Lateral semicircular duct—vestibular dysplasia or a common semicircular duct cavity	There is a common utriculosaccular-lateral semicircular duct or a short wide semicircular ducts or narrowing of the semicircular ducts	It may be bilateral with other associated inner ear anomalies

Contd...

Ear and Temporal Bone

Contd...

Diseases	Differentiating features	Comments
CHARGE syndrome	There is absence of all the semicircular ducts.	Other features of the syndrome are noted
Waardenburg and Alagille syndrome	There is isolated aplasia of the posterior semicircular duct	Other features of the respective syndrome are noted
Complete labyrinthine aplasia (Michel deformity)	No inner ear development is seen instead there is a small, single cystic cavity or several cystic cavities	It is a very rare entity
Common cavity of inner ear	• A large cystic cavity with no internal architecture is seen at the site of inner ear • Semicircular canal may be normal or malformed	
Cochlear aplasia	• There is failure of cochlear formation. • Rest of the inner ear may be normal or malformed	
Cochlear hypoplasia	A small rudimentary cochlea is seen	
Incomplete partition and dilatational defects (including the classic Mondini's dysplasia)	• There is a small cochlea with an incomplete partition or absent of interscalar septum • There is a basilar turn with a common cavity where the normal middle and the apical turns would normally occur • Mondini's dysplasia is classically described as a flat cochlea with one and a half turn	

Contd...

Contd...

Diseases	Differentiating features	Comments
X-linked congenital mixed hearing loss	• There is dilatation of the lateral part of the internal acoustic canal • There is absence or severe hypoplasia of the bony modiolus with normal number of cochlear turns and hypoplasia of the cochlear base with or without widening of the labyrinthine segment of the facial nerve canal and dilatational of the vestibular aqueduct	
Dwarf cochlea	• The cochlea appears relatively normal with normal number of turns • The diameter of the turns of the cochlea is diminished	

TABLE 11: Differentiating features of common facial nerve anomalies.

Diseases	Differentiating features	Comments
Congenital facial nerve hypoplasia or aplasia	This can occur alone or in association with Mobius syndrome (also known as congenital facial diplegia or congenital abducens—facial paralysis)	
Duplication of facial nerve (bifid facial nerve)	• Most commonly the nerve bifurcates along the proximal segment of the tympanic segment inferior to the lateral semicircular canal into a large lateral branch and a small medial branch	

Contd...

Contd...

Diseases	Differentiating features	Comments
	• These two usually reunite at the stylomastoid foramen • Rarely it bifurcates proximal to the geniculate ganglion, in which, there may be also duplication of the internal acoustic canal	
Anterior migration of facial nerve	The nerve attempt to take a more direct course to the pterygopalatine fossa and the ganglion	• It is associated with certain cochlear malformations • In association with cochlear hypoplasia, common cavity malformations, and the dwarf cochlea, lack of a significant cochlear mass results in anterior migration of the proximal or labyrinthine segment of the facial nerve

TABLE 12: Differentiating features of various vascular anomalies.

Diseases	Differentiating features	Comments
Partial absence and aberrant lateral course of internal carotid artery (ICA)	• There is absence of normal vertical petrous portion that is replaced by the more laterally coursing ICA with enlarged inferior tympanic and caroticotympanic arteries • CT shows an enhancing soft tissue mass in the hypotympanum extending toward the oval window, indenting the promontory and displacing the tympanic membrane laterally	

Contd...

Contd...

Diseases	Differentiating features	Comments
	• Grooving of the apical, middle, and the basilar turns of the cochlea by the artery may also be seen • The lateral bony wall of the carotid canal is dehiscent	
Persistent stapedial artery	• It may be found with or without aberrant ICA • It continues to supply middle meningeal artery • Foramen spinosum is absent	
Protruding/ dehiscent jugular bulb	• It is seen as the jugular bulb lying at the level of the basal turns of cochlea • The jugular bulb may be thin or dehiscent	• This renders it vulnerable to trauma • It is more common on right side
Jugular diverticulum (JD)	A smooth outpouching of the jugular bulb that extends superiorly, medially, and posteriorly in the temporal bone. CT demonstrates the jugular diverticulum in the continuity with the jugular bulb, extending superiorly into the petrous pyramid. Bony margins are smooth, due to slow remodeling without permeative destruction. Differentiated from high jugular bulb by its more medial and posterior location in the petrous bone, does not protrude into the middle ear (hence not visible on inspection and not exposed to trauma during surgery), more common on left side and more common in females.	
Jugular foramen agenesis and stenosis	• There is expansion of the occipital bone in the region of the torcular herophili, with a defect through which an enlarged emissary vein passes • This results in an aberrant venous drainage	Extremely rare conditions

Ear and Temporal Bone

TABLE 13: Relevant differentiating features of common malformations of petrous bone associated with meningitis.

Diseases	Differentiating features	Comments
Dehiscence of tegmen tympani	It is characterized by incomplete development of tegmen tympani with or without associated meningocele or meningoencephalocele bulging into the middle ear	It is a perilabyrinthine CSF fistula
Hyrtl's fissure	It is seen as a perilabyrinthine fistula that opens inferior to the round window niche	It is an embryonic remnant, that may persist in adult life
Giant apical air cell	• There is dehiscence in the medial wall of the middle ear anterior to the cochlea • Large air cell at the petrous apex have a thin bony septum separating it from the CSF	This can perforate allowing CSF leak and then CSF ottorhea resulting in a perilabyrinthine fistula
Apical meningocele	• It is a CSF-filled space seen at the apex of the petrous bone • It may communicate with the middle ear, resulting in the CSF leak (perilabyrinthine fistula)	It may mimic cholesterol cyst
Translabyrinthine fistula	• It is characterized by a defect in the lamina cribrosa, a thin, bony layer separating the apex of the internal auditory canal (IAC) from the vestibule • This defect allows communication of the CSF with perilymph of the vestibule or cochlea, causing increase in hydrostatic pressure in the inner ear	• It is also known as *perilymphatic hydrops* • This may cause spontaneous or postsurgical perforation of the stapes foot plate resulting in an acute outpouring of the fluid known as *stapes gusher*

Noncontrast-enhanced Computed Tomography (NECT)

- Ill-defined haziness of membranous labyrinth is seen in stage 2, fibrous type of labyrinthitis ossificans.
- Sclerotic lesion membranous labyrinth is seen in stage 3, bony type of labyrinthitis ossificans.
- Severe type of labyrinthitis ossificans results in total "white out" of the membranous labyrinth.
- Air density in the labyrinth with fluid collection in the middle ear is seen in perilymph fistula with abnormal connection between the inner ear and the middle ear. Unexplained dependent middle ear or mastoid or mastoid fluid collections emanating from the oval window should be viewed with suspicion, and a pneumolabyrinth is very highly suggestive in the context.

Chapter 4

Orbital Lesions

The anatomy and major components of the orbit, and orbital apex are shown in Figures 1 to 3. Common causes of orbital lesions are described in Tables 1 to 4.

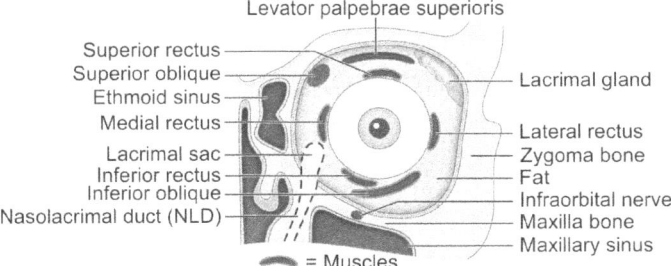

Fig. 1: Coronal anatomy of the left orbit.
Source: 2004 Jane Olver.

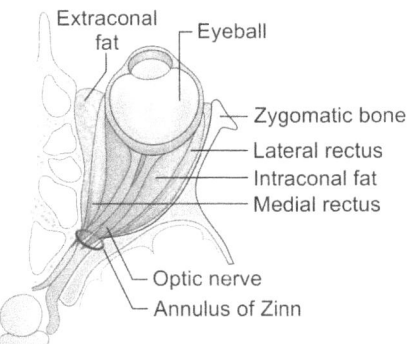

Fig. 2: *Major anatomic components of the orbit*: (1) Globe, (2) Optic nerve and sheath, (3) Conal-intraconal area, and (4) Extraconal area.
Source: Wichmann and Muller-Forell, Eur J Radiol; 2004.

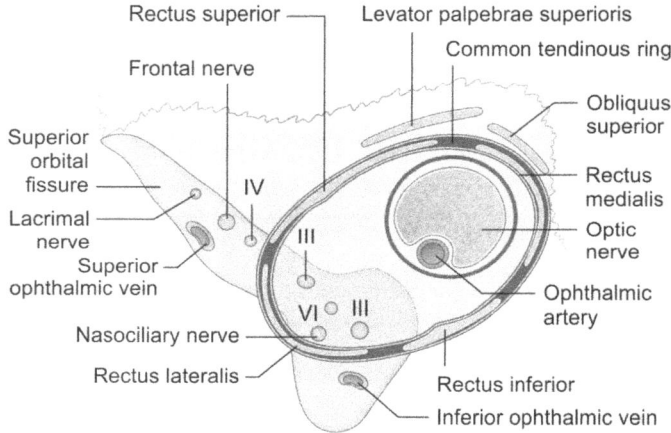

Fig. 3: *Orbital apex*: Common tendinous ring (annulus of Zinn).

TABLE 1: Common causes of orbital lesions.			
		Extraocular lesions	
Diseases	*Ocular lesions*	*Intraconal*	*Extraconal*
Cystic	• Choroidal cyst • Coloboma	Lymphangioma	• Abscess • Hematoma • Dilated lacrimal sac • Dermoid • Lymphangioma

Solid	• Melanoma
	• Metastases
	• Hemangioma
		• Optic nerve lesions
		  – Glioma
		  – Meningioma
		  – Neuritis/ perineuritis
		• Pseudotumor
		• Wegener's granulomatosis
		• Thyroid ophthalmopathy
			• Lacrimal gland lesions
			• Capillary hemangioma
			• Meningioma
			• Rhabdomyosarcoma
			• Lymphoma

Contd...

Orbital Lesions

Contd...

		Extraocular lesions	
Diseases	Ocular lesions	Intraconal	Extraconal
		• Hemangioma • Orbital varix • Thrombosed superior ophthalmic vein • Hemangio-endothelioma/hemangiopericytoma • Nerve sheath tumors (schwannoma, neurofibroma • Rhabdomyosarcoma • Lymphoma • Metastases	• Metastases (rare) • AV malformation
Calcified	• Retinoblastoma • Retinal astrocytoma	• Meningioma	• Cysticercus • Cavernous hemangioma • Dermoid • Meningioma

ALTERED GLOBE SIZE

Microphthalmia

- *Congenital*:
    - Coloboma
    - Rubella
    - Norrie's disease
    - Lowe's syndrome
    - Oculocerebrorenal syndrome
    - Retrolental fibroplasia
    - Persistent hyperplastic primary vitreous.
- *Acquired*: Phthisis bulbi.

Macrophthalmia

- Unilateral
- Congenital bilateral (buphthalmos).

ORBITAL LESIONS WITH BONE INVOLVEMENT

- Optic nerve tumor (causes optic canal enlargement)
- Osteomyelitis
- Wegener's granulomatosis
- Malignant vascular tumors (hemangiopericytoma)
- Dermoid
- Malignant lacrimal gland lesions
- Meningioma
- Rhabdomyosarcoma
- Metastases
- Neurofibromatosis (Figs. 4A and B).

TABLE 2: Common causes of hyperdense vitreous.

On NECT	*Extraconal*

• Hemorrhage:
  – Coats' disease
  – Norrie's disease
  – Warburg disease
  – Retrolental hyperplasia
  – Posterior hyaloid detachment
• Foreign body
• Infective exudates
• *Soft tissue density*:
  – Toxocariasis
  – Retinal detachment
  – Choroidal detachment
• *Calcified lesions*:
  – Retinoblastoma
  – Retinal astrocytoma (astrocytic hamartoma)
  – Drusen
  – Choroidal osteoma
	• Persistent hyperplastic primary vitreous
	• Melanoma
	• Choroidal hemangioma

(CECT: contrast-enhanced computed tomography; NECT: noncontrast-enhanced computed tomography)

Orbital Lesions

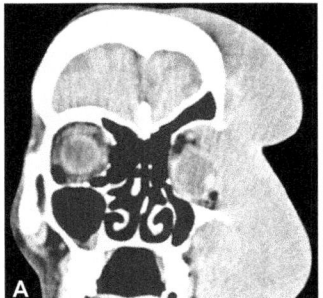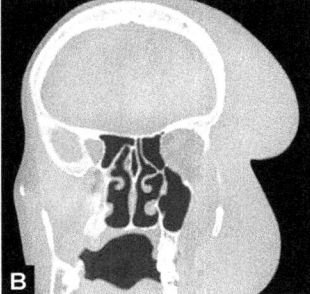

Figs. 4A and B: CT coronal images of orbit showing large soft tissue mass lesion causing right side proptosis and deformed right orbit in a case of plexiform neurofibroma (neurofibromatosis).

TABLE 3: Common causes of thickened coats of eye with enhancement.

- Scleritis
- Endophthalmitis (toxocariasis, infectious)
- Choroidal melanoma
- Ocular metastases
- Choroidal hemangioma
- Macular degeneration

TABLE 4: Common causes and their differentiating features of intraconal lesions.

Diseases	Differentiating features	Comments
Optic nerve glioma (Fig. 5)	• Tubular/fusiform/eccentric, well-circumscribed enlargement of optic nerve • Isodense to optic nerve with little or no contrast enhancement • Posterior extension along optic tracts is seen in 60–70% cases • Ipsilateral optic canal enlargement >3 mm or 1 mm difference compared to contralateral side	• Most common cause of optic nerve enlargement • Peak age group around 5 years • Neurofibromatosis is seen in 10–50% of cases in which the tumors may be bilateral • Calcification may be seen in post-radiotherapy stage

Contd...

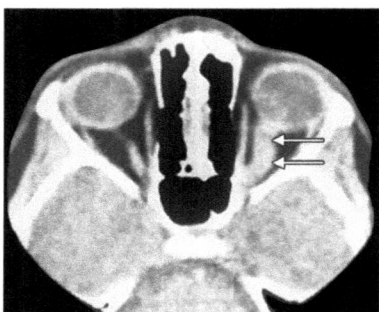
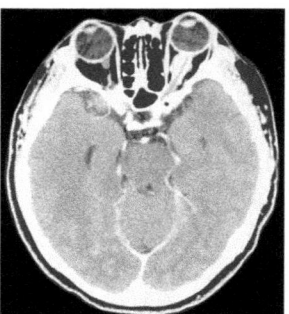

Fig. 5: Axial NECT image shows diffuse enlargement of the left optic nerve (arrows)—optic nerve glioma.

Fig. 6: Axial CECT image shows a brightly enhancing mass encasing the left optic nerve. It has a slightly lobulated contour, and the nerve appears compressed—optic nerve meningioma.

Contd...

Diseases	Differentiating features	Comments
Sheath meningioma (Fig. 6)	• Tubular (most commonly)/ fusiform/eccentric thickening of optic nerve • Hyperostosis of the adjacent bone may be seen • Calcification may be seen within the mass • Contrast enhancement reveals dense linear bands on either side on axial view known as tram-track or ring-like appearance on coronal views around nonenhancing optic nerve	Common in middle-aged females

Contd...

Contd...

Diseases	Differentiating features	Comments
Optic neuritis	Normal to mildly enlarged optic nerve and chiasm with minimal to mild contrast enhancement	Multiple sclerosis is the most common underlying etiology
Optic perineuritis	• Ragged edematous enlargement of the optic nerve • CECT scans show *tram-track* appearance due to edematous, nonenhancing optic nerve with enhancing perineural tissue	It is a localized form of orbital pseudotumor
Elevated intracranial pressure	• Bilateral, tortuous, and thickened optic nerves sheath complex • Dilated, enlarged subarachnoid CSF space is evident around a normal optic nerve	
Metastases	• Enhancing, nodular masses may be seen unilaterally or bilaterally along the nerve sheath complex • Involvement is usually from tumors of adjacent structures such as malignant tumors of the globe, adjacent paranasal sinuses, nose, bony orbit, and intracranial. They have distinctive features related to organ of origin	• Common primary tumors are retinoblastoma and uveal melanoma • Lymphoma and leukemia

Contd...

Contd...

Diseases	Differentiating features	Comments
Cavernous hemangioma	• Sharply demarcated round to oval intraconal mass that often spares the orbital apex • Small phleboliths are characteristic • Expansion without destruction of the orbit and displacement without infiltration of the nerve occurs • Marked uniform or inhomogeneous when thrombosed contrast enhancement is characteristic	Tumor of adulthood common in 20–40 years age group F>M
Orbital varix	• Usually involves superior or inferior orbital veins • Phleboliths are rare • Enlargement of mass after Valsalva or jugular vein compression • Well-defined markedly enhancing intraconal mass • Spontaneous thrombosis is common	• *Congenital*: Venous malformation/ venous wall weakness • *Acquired*: Intraorbital/ intracranial
Arteriovenous malformation	• Irregularly shaped intensely enhancing mass of enlarged vessels • Associated with dilated superior/inferior ophthalmic veins	Least common orbital vascular malformation
Lymphangioma	• Poorly defined, multiseptated, inhomogeneous lesion	Mean age of presentation is 6 years

Contd...

Contd...

Diseases	Differentiating features	Comments
	• Mild-to-moderate enlargement of the orbit • There is only minimal or no displacement/ compression of adjacent structures	
Schwannoma	• Sharply marginated oval or fusiform lesion • Moderate to marked contrast enhancement • Optic nerve is usually displaced	Arises from cranial nerves other than optic nerve in the orbit (cranial nerves III, IV, and VI)
Wegener's granulomatosis	• Diffuse retrobulbar infiltration • Bilateral involvement and bony destruction is common	• Ocular manifestations are also present • Sinonasal involvement is highly suggestive
Capillary hemangioma (Figs. 7A and B)	Ill-defined, enhancing lesion spanning the intraconal and extraconal space	• Most common vascular tumor of orbit in children • 95% in less than 6 months of age • May regresses spontaneously
Pseudotumor (Figs. 8A to C)	• Tumefactive type is seen as discrete poorly defined intra/extraconal mass with intense postcontrast enhancement	• Most commonly in young females

Contd...

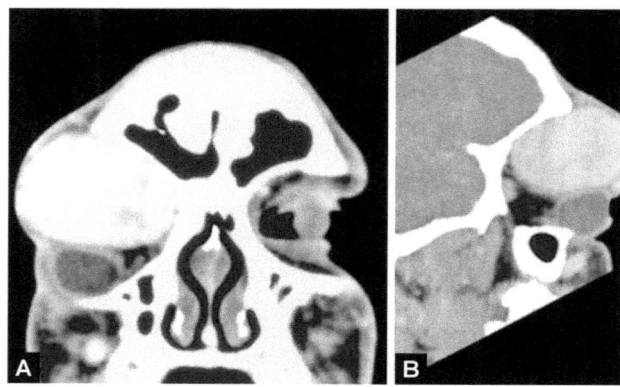

Figs. 7A and B: Hemangioma of the orbit (extraconal compartment).

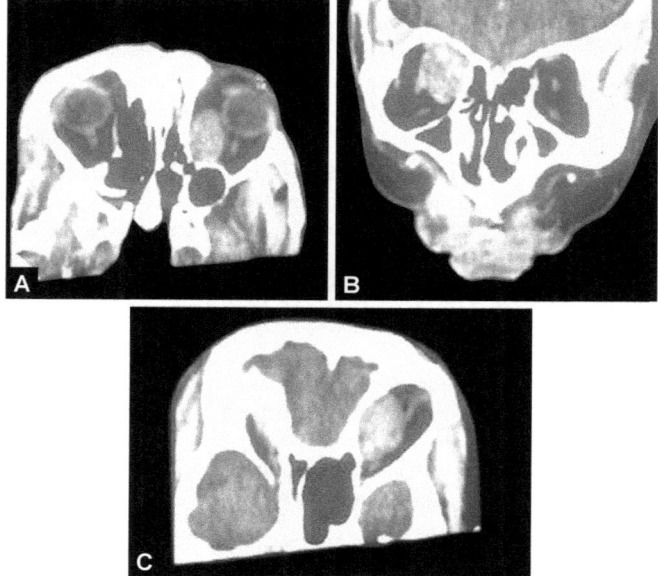

Figs. 8A to C: Axial and coronal CT images showing a pseudomass in the left orbit.

Contd...

Diseases	Differentiating features	Comments
	• Myositic type is rare and involves the extra-ocular muscles with their tendinous insertions • No bony involvement is seen thus differentiating it from aggressive neoplasm • Thickening and enhancement of sclera near Tenon's capsule with enlargement of lacrimal gland is supportive	• Most common cause of intra-orbital mass lesion in adults • It may be idiopathic but may also be associated with Wegener's associated with granulomatosis, sarcoidosis, retroperitoneal fibrosis, thyroiditis, cholangitis, vasculitis and lymphoma, IgG4-related condition
Dermoid cyst (Figs. 9A and B)	• Well-defined cystic mass with or without fat with thick surrounding capsule • It may contain calcifications or teeth	• Most common benign orbital tumor of childhood • Commonly seen in the anterior extraconal orbit
Lymphoma (Figs. 10A and B)	• Well-defined high density mass near or within lacrimal glands • It may cause diffuse infiltration of orbital structures without significant displacements and bony erosions • Mild to moderate enhancement is common	• It may involve the nerve sheath complex • Evidence of systemic disease may be absent • Usually NHL
Rhabdomyo-sarcoma	• *It is seen as a large soft tissue density mass with ill-defined margins*	• Most common primary malignant orbital tumor in childhood

Contd...

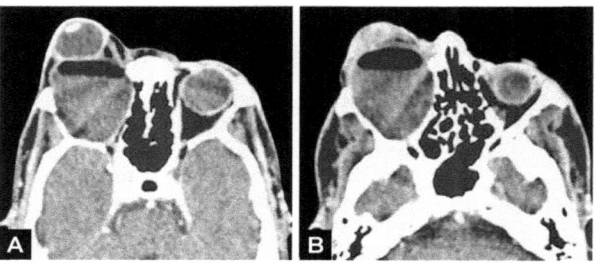

Figs. 9A and B: Transaxial contrast-enhanced computed tomography images of orbit right side intraconal well-marginated retro-ocular lesion with fat-fluid level suggestive of dermoid.

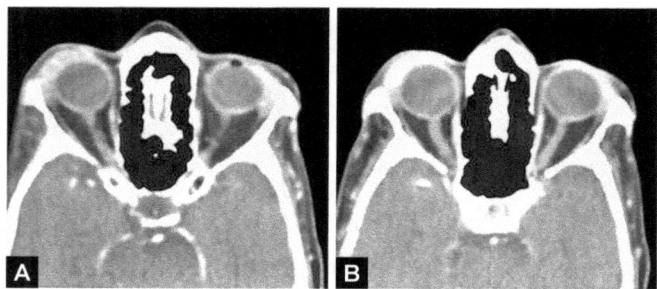

Figs. 10A and B: Transaxial contrast-enhanced computed tomography images of orbit showing bilateral homogeneously enhancing enlarged lacrimal glands due to lymphomatous involvement.

Contd...

Diseases	Differentiating features	Comments
	• Extension into preseptal space, adjacent sinus, nasal cavity, and intracranial cavity is common with adjacent bone destruction • Moderate enhancement is seen on postcontrast images	• Most commonly retrobulbar in location

Contd...

Orbital Lesions

Contd...

Diseases	Differentiating features	Comments
Lacrimal gland tumor	• Round or oblong extraconal mass is seen in the superolateral aspect of the orbit • May or may not be associated with destruction or erosion of adjacent bone • Benign tumors have smooth well-defined outline while malignant tumors may have irregular margins	Pleomorphic adenoma and adenoid cystic carcinoma are common and they cannot be differentiated on imaging
Orbital infection/cellulitis (Figs. 11A and B)	• Imaging features depend on the stage of infection • Inflammatory edema is seen as presents as thickening of eyelids and septum, scleral thickening, enlargement, and displacement of extraocular muscles (medial rectus) with increased attenuation of retroorbital fat with obliteration of fat planes and intense postcontrast enhancement • Abscess appears as subperiosteal or intraorbital space-occupying central necrotic lesions with rim enhancement of the walls • Ophthalmic vein and cavernous sinus thrombosis are the frequent complications	• Orbital infections commonly occur secondary to the spread from adjacent sinuses • However, mycotic infections are common in diabetics and immunocompromised individuals show aggressive course with early and marked bone destruction

Contd...

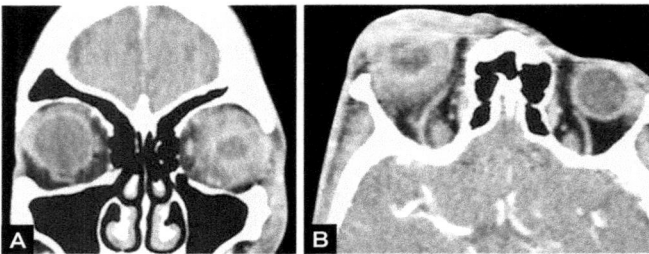

Figs. 11A and B: Contrast-enhanced computed tomography coronal and axial images of orbit showing soft tissue enhancing lesion involving walls of globe, extraocular muscles, and right eyelid in a case of orbital cellulitis.

Contd...

Diseases	Differentiating features	Comments
Sarcoidosis	Unilateral lacrimal gland and optic nerve sheath complex enlargement may occur	It may simulate primary neoplasm of the structures involved
Thyroid ophthalmopathy (Graves' disease of orbit)	• Enlargement of extraocular muscles with typical sparing of tendentious insertions to the globe is characteristic • Disease may be limited to a single-muscle belly or several muscles • Proptosis and increase in retrobulbar fat are common • Slight uveal scleral thickening • Dilatation of superior ophthalmic vein is common	• Bilateral involvement may also occur • Most common cause of unilateral or bilateral exophthalmos in adults • Other causes of extraocular muscle enlargement include acromegaly, myositis, and hematoma

Contd...

Contd...

Diseases	Differentiating features	Comments
	• Increase in diameter of retrobulbar optic nerve sheath • Hyperattenuating of orbital fat	
Dacryoadeno-cystitis	• Diffuse enlargement of lacrimal gland often with marked contrast enhancement • In acute phase scleritis and lateral rectus muscle myositis may be associated	• Acute cases have viral or bacterial etiology • Chronic occurs in Sjögren's syndrome, rheumatoid arthritis, etc.
Superior ophthalmic vein thrombosis	• Enlarged superior ophthalmic vein with enhancing wall and a low-density clot • Ipsilateral cavernous thrombosis is usually present	
Microphthalmia	• Congenital type is associated with small hypoplastic orbits • In the acquired type the orbits may be of normal size	Congenital type is usually bilateral and associated with cataracts
Macrophthalmia	• Enlarged globes • Orbit size may be enlarged	Associated with glaucoma and high-grade myopia
Buphthalmos	Uniformly enlarged globes assuming a round to oval shape	Usually associated with juvenile onset glaucoma

Contd...

Contd...

Diseases	Differentiating features	Comments
Coats' disease (congenital retinal telangiectasia)	• Unilateral hyperdense vitreous • Normal-sized globes	• Secondary retinal detachment • Commonly seen in children of 5–9 years of age
Norrie's disease (retinal dysplasia)	• Bilateral hyperdense vitreous chambers with blood fluid level • Retrolental mass may be seen along with retinal detachment • Microphthalmia, optic nerve atrophy, shallow anterior chamber, and small lens are the other associated features	It is invariably seen in males due to X-linked recessive inheritance
Warburg's syndrome	• It is characterized by bilateral retinal detachment with subretinal hemorrhage often with blood fluid levels and vitreous hemorrhage • Microphthalmia may be associated	It is associated with hydrocephalus, agyria, and with or without encephalocele
Persistent hyperplastic primary vitreous	• It is characterized by hyperdense vitreous in a small, deformed globe without calcification • There is an enhancing cone-shaped central retrolental hyperdensity extending from lens through vitreous to back of orbit just lateral to optic nerve, optic nerve is small • Retinal detachment may be seen and it may be associated with fluid levels	• It is a rare condition with persistent and subsequent hyperplasia of hyaloid vascular system • The condition is usually unilateral

Contd...

Contd...

Diseases	Differentiating features	Comments
Retrolental fibroplasia	• Bilateral microphthalmia with hyperdense vitreous • Calcification in the lens and choroid can be seen as a late feature	It is seen in premature infants with respiratory distress on oxygen therapy
Coloboma	• Posterior defect usually at the site of optic nerve attachment • Cystic outpouching of vitreous humor is seen at the site of defect • The condition is associated with microphthalmia	It is a congenital condition
Scleritis	Unilateral or bilateral thickened sclera with intense and persistent contrast enhancement	• Idiopathic or associated with connective tissue, disease is seen more often in women • Posterior scleritis may mimic uveal melanoma
Endophthalmitis	• Unilateral uveal-scleral thickening is the most common finding • Vitreous is usually hyperdense due to exudates	
Sclerosing endophthalmitis	• Formation of intravitreal mass • Focal uveal-scleral thickening with contrast enhancement and hyperdense vitreous • Calcification is uncommon	Usually bilateral; unilateral involvement may simulate a noncalcified retinoblastoma

Contd...

Contd...

Diseases	Differentiating features	Comments
Posterior hyaloid detachment	Fluid or blood accumulating in the most dependent part of the globe often with fluid-level fluid	Common in adults over 50 years of age
Retinal detachment	It is seen as homogeneous, hyperdensity, either crescent-shaped at the periphery of the globe (partial) or in "V"-shaped configuration with the apex toward optic disc (complete)	
Choroidal detachment	• It is seen as a smooth elevation of choroid by serous fluid with a density similar to vitreous, or a focal elevation by underlying hematoma • In contrast to retinal detachment the choroidal leaves do not converge toward the optic disc	Occurs after intraocular surgery, penetrating ocular trauma or inflammatory disease of uvea or sclera (Figs. 12A and B)
Retinoblastoma	• It is characterized by solid, smoothly marginated, lobulated retrolental hyperdense mass in endophytic type • Rarely in the exophytic type, tumor grows subretinally causing retinal detachment • Calcification is nodular • Vitreous is commonly hyperdense • Extraocular extension with optic nerve enlargement, abnormal soft tissue in orbit, intracranial extension • Contrast enhancement is common	• Most common intraocular malignancy in childhood • It is bilateral in 40% cases • Trilateral retinoblastoma is association of bilateral retinoblastoma with pinealoblastoma • Quadrilateral RB-associated suprasellar mass lesion

Contd...

Orbital Lesions

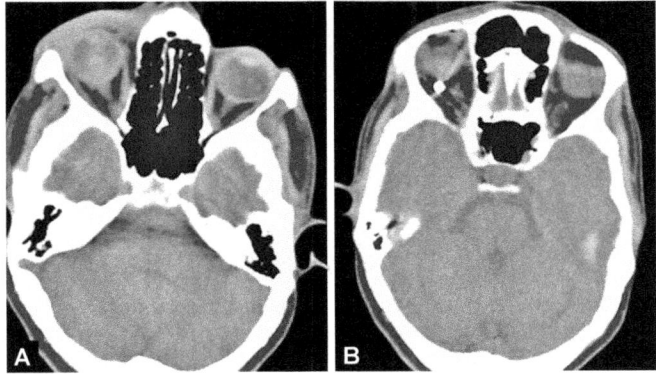

Figs. 12A and B: Transaxial contrast-enhanced computed tomography image shows hemorrhage in the posterior chamber of right eyeball following firearm injury to right orbit.

Contd...

Diseases	Differentiating features	Comments
Uveal melanoma (Figs. 13A and B)	It is seen as ill-defined thickening of the wall of the globe/bulging toward the vitreous or a well-defined hyperdense, solid, enhancing mushroom-shaped mass, protruding into the vitreous	<ul><li>Most common primary intraocular malignancy of adults (50–70 years)</li><li>Usually unilateral and most commonly arises from choroid</li></ul>
Ocular metastasis	It is usually bilateral and multiple with focal areas of wall thickening and is often associated with subretinal fluid	<ul><li>It is commonly seen in posterior temporal portion of the uvea near the macula</li></ul>

Contd...

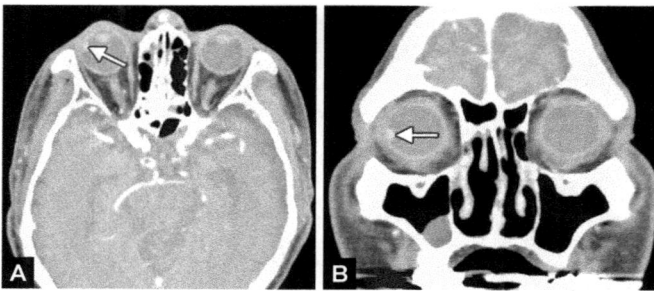

Figs. 13A and B: Axial and coronal contrast-enhanced computed tomography images show a small enhancing mass lesion in temporal wall of right globe bulging toward vitreous—uveal melanoma.

Contd...

Diseases	Differentiating features	Comments
		• Most common primary metastases are from breast and lung. In children, neuroblastoma is most common
Choroidal hemangioma	• It is seen as a sessile, intensely enhancing with focal area of thickening • Retinal detachment is frequent	• Majority are found at posterior pole temporal to optic disc • Commonly seen at 10–20 years • May be associated with Sturge-Weber syndrome

Contd...

Contd...

Diseases	Differentiating features	Comments
Retinal angioma	• CT findings are similar to choroidal hemangioma • It is bilateral in about half of the cases	• Commonly associated with von Hippel-Lindau disease • Usually associated with tuberous sclerosis or neurofibromatosis where they may be bilateral
Astrocytic hamartoma (retinal astrocytoma)	• It is usually seen as single or multiple, often calcified, hyperdense retinal nodules with cystic degeneration • Mild-to-moderate enhancement may be seen	
Medulloepi-thelioma	It is seen as a hyperdense, soft tissue mass arising from ciliary body	It is usually seen in children
Choroidal osteoma	It is characterized by sessile, intraocular mass with curvilinear calcification	It is a rare tumor occurring in young women
Choroidal cyst	• It is seen as a cystic lesion in the choroid • It may be associated with retinal detachment	It is a very rare lesion
Choroidal nevus	• It is most often missed on CT; but when detected, mimic small uveal melanoma • Most common location is posterior third of choroid	• It is a benign entity • Most often seen under 10 years of age
Macular degeneration	• It is seen as a focal, wall thickening or mass in the macular region with moderate to intense contrast enhancement	It is the most common cause of blindness in elderly

Contd...

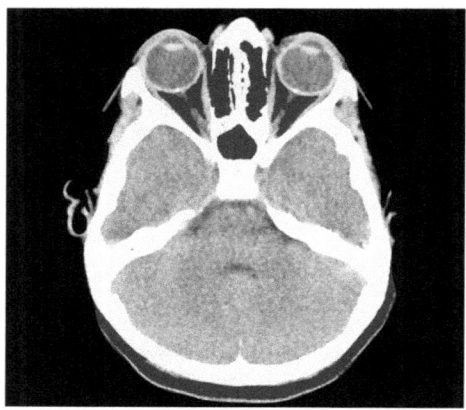

Fig. 14: Axial noncontrast-enhanced computed tomography image shows focal nodular calcifications in region of bilateral optic discs—optic disc drusen.

Contd...

Diseases	Differentiating features	Comments
	• Complication by hemorrhage, retinal, or posterior hyaloid detachment is common	
Drusen (Fig. 14)	• It is characterized by discrete, sessile, round calcification of the optic nerve disc • It is bilateral in three-fourths of the cases	It represents the accretion of hyaline-like material on surface of optic disc
Ocular hemorrhage of optic disc	The CT appearance depends upon the stage of the hemorrhage as hematoma evolves with time	It may be spontaneous or post-traumatic

(CECT: contrast-enhanced computed tomography; CSF: cerebrospinal fluid; RB: retinoblastoma)

Chapter 5

Nasal or Paranasal Sinus Lesions

Common causes of nasal or paranasal sinus lesions are described in Tables 1 to 6.

TABLE 1: Common causes of nasal or paranasal sinus lesions.

Cystic/fluid lesions	Soft tissue lesions	Bony lesions

• Without bone destruction
• *Air fluid level*:
  – Acute sinusitis
  – Sinus lavage
  – Sinus bleed
  – Baro-trauma
• Mucus retention cyst
• With sinus expansion
• Without bone destruction
• Maxillary dentigerous cyst
• Mucocele
	• Without bone destruction
	• *Mucosal thickening*:
	  – Chronic sinusitis
	  – Allergic sinusitis
	• *Soft tissue mass*:
	  – Antrochoanal polyp
	  – Sinonasal polyposis
	  – Fungiform papilloma
	  – Neurogenic tumors
	• With bone destruction
	• *Granulomatous diseases*:
	  – Fungal sinusitis
	  – Wegener's granulomatosis (Figs. 2A and B)
	  – Stewart's granuloma
	• Tumors
	• *Benign*:
	  – Inverted papilloma (Fig. 3)
	  – Chondromesenchymal hamartoma of the nose
		• Without bone destruction
		• *Benign (sclerotic)*:
		  – Fibrous dysplasia
		  – Ossifying fibroma
		  – Osteoma (Fig. 1)
		  – Paget's disease
		  – Odontoma
		• With osteolysis
		• Benign
		• Eosinophilic granuloma
		• Aneurysmal bone cyst
		• Chondroma
		• Plasmacytoma
		• Brown tumor
		• Giant cell tumor

Contd...

Contd...

Cystic/fluid lesions	Soft tissue lesions	Bony lesions

	• *Malignant*:
	  – Carcinoma paranasal sinus
	  – Esthesioneuroblastoma (Fig. 4)
	  – Lymphoma
	  – Rhabdomyosarcoma
	  – Extramedullary plasmacytoma
		• *Malignant*:
		  – Ameloblastoma
		  – Osteosarcoma
		  – Chondrosarcoma
		  – Ewing's sarcoma
		  – Neurogenic
		  – Metastases

HYPERDENSITIES ON NONCONTRAST-ENHANCED COMPUTED TOMOGRAPHY IN SINONASAL REGION

- Rhinolith
- Radiopaque radiodense foreign body
- Hematoma
- Displaced fracture fragments
- Inspissated secretions in chronic sinusitis
- Fungal sinusitis
- Chondromesenchymal hamartoma of the nose
- Carcinoma nose and paranasal sinuses.

TABLE 2: Common causes of opacification and mass lesions of sinonasal cavity without bone destruction and their relevant CT findings.

Diseases	NECT/CECT findings	Comments
Acute sinusitis	• Mucosal thickening • Air fluid level is characteristic • Blocked sinus ostia by thickened mucosa • Uniform enhancement of mucosa is seen if bacterial in nature • Frontal lobe abscess, orbital cellulitis, abscess and osteomyelitis may occur as complications	• Most common cause of sinus opacification • Usually viral

Contd...

Nasal or Paranasal Sinus Lesions

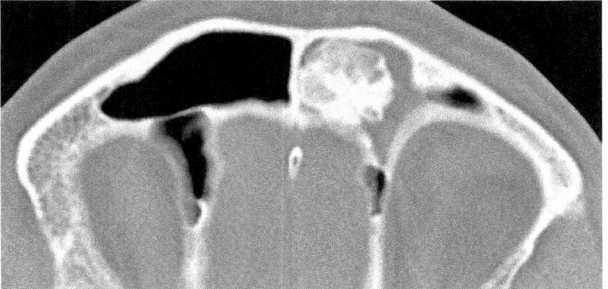

Fig. 1: A frond-like exostotic lesion arising from inner table of frontal sinus on left side with osseous appearing matrix, and collection in frontal sinus—frontal osteoma.

Contd...

Diseases	NECT/CECT findings	Comments
Chronic sinusitis (Figs. 5 and 6)	<ul><li>Mucosal thickening >5 mm</li><li>Bone remodeling and sclerosis</li><li>Multiple polyps may be present</li><li>Hyperdense lesions on NECT due to inspissated secretions</li><li>Usually no contrast enhancement</li><li>Underlying bone destruction may suggest development of osteomyelitis (Fig. 7)</li></ul>	Mild mucosal thickening is incidental on CT
Allergic sinusitis	<ul><li>Involves multiple sinuses</li><li>Bilaterally symmetrical</li><li>Sinonasal polyposis is common with inferior turbinate hypertrophy</li><li>Roomy nasal cavities in atrophic variety</li><li>Uniform enhancement of mucosa on CECT</li></ul>	It is seen in 10% of population

Contd...

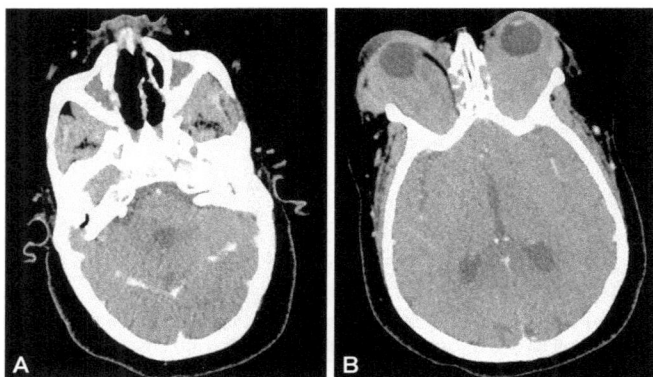

Figs. 2A and B: Axial CT images of a patient with Wegener's graulomatosis showing destruction of the nasal septum, granulomatous masses in bilateral maxillary antrum, and retrobulbar soft tissues.

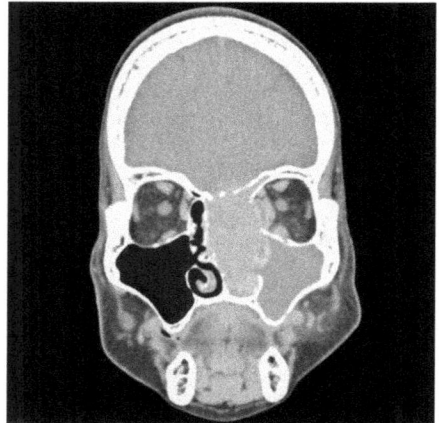

Fig. 3: Coronal CT image of inverted papilloma showing a large soft tissue mass lesion filling the left nasal cavity, displacing the nasal septum toward right and causing bony remodeling of the lateral wall of nasal cavity. The lesion is obstructing the left osteomeatal complex with resultant left maxillary secretions.

Nasal or Paranasal Sinus Lesions

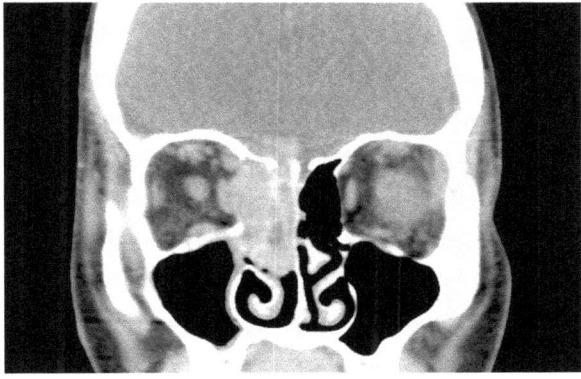

Fig. 4: Coronal CT image of esthesioneuroblastoma showing enhancing lobulated soft tissue mass lesion in right nasal cavity causing destruction of the ethmoidal bony septae and cribriform plate with resultant intracranial extension.

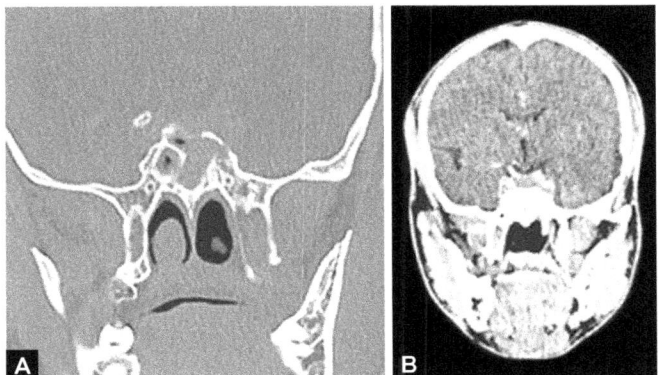

Figs. 5A and B: Osteomyelitis of sphenoid bone with hypophysitis.

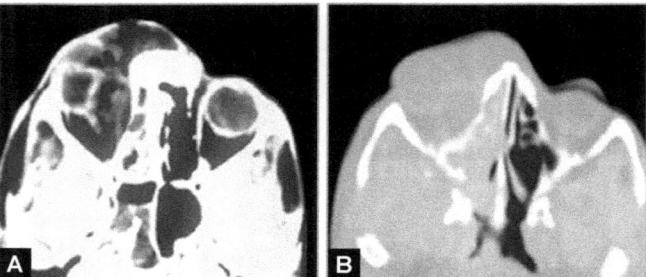

Figs. 6A and B: Axial CT images showing ethmoid sinusitis on right side with extension of the process into the right orbit with abscess formation.

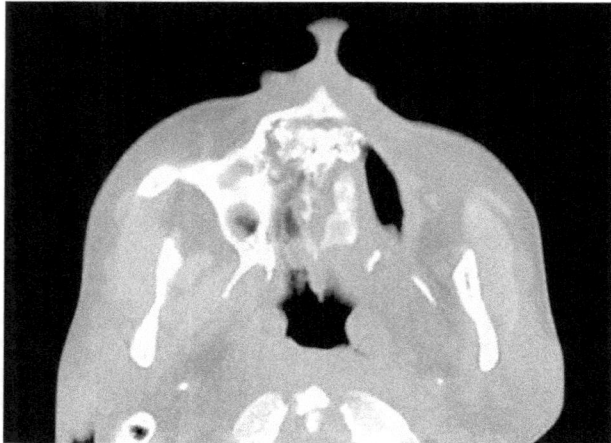

Fig. 7: Transaxial CT image shows actinomycotic osteomyelitis of maxilla and hard palate.

Nasal or Paranasal Sinus Lesions

Contd...

Diseases	NECT/CECT findings	Comments
Maxillary dentigerous cyst	• Cystic expansile lesion in relation to the crown of an unerupted tooth • It encroaches on the maxillary sinus cavity to the extent of complete obliteration	Most common site is the third molar of the maxillary teeth

Mucocele (Figs. 8A and B)	• Most common in frontal sinus followed by ethmoid (Figs. 9A and B) and maxillary, rarely in sphenoid
	• Soft tissue density mass with expansion of sinus cavity
	• Bone demineralization, remodeling, and thinning with Rim calcifications in few cases:
	  – Uniform enhancement of thin rim if inflamed
	  – Unilateral proptosis is common with hypertelorism
		Most common lesion to cause expansion of sinus obstructed as a sequelae to chronic sinusitis

Mucus retention cyst	• Most commonly seen in the floor of maxillary sinus • Smoothly marginated soft tissue density mass with no contrast enhancement	Due to obstruction of seromucinous glands
Antrochoanal polyp	• Soft tissue density mass with sinus expansion • Smooth mass enlarging the sinus ostium and extending into the nasal cavity and may reach the choanae and nasopharynx	Benign polyp seen in teenagers and young adults

Contd...

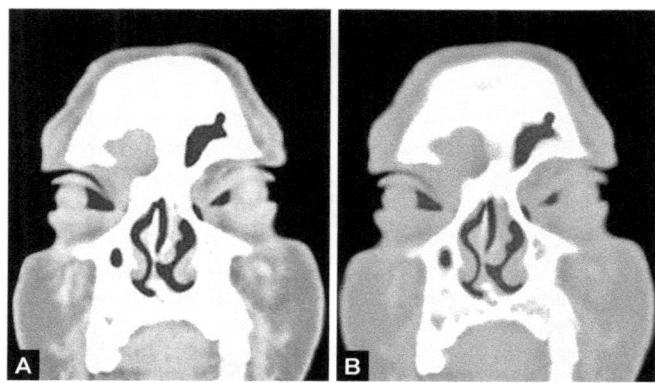

Figs. 8A and B: Mucocele of the frontal sinus with bony remodeling.

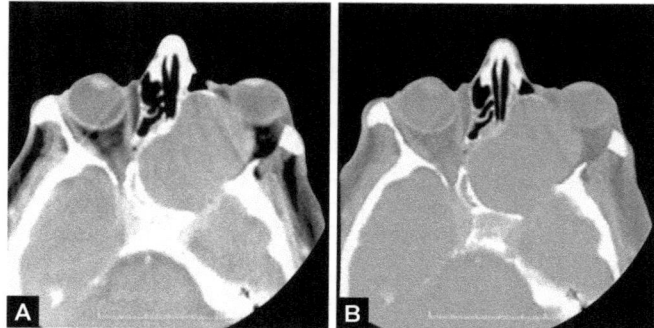

Figs. 9A and B: Axial CT images in soft tissue and bony window, showing cystic distension of left ethmoid sinus with associated bony remodeling—ethmoid mucocele. Note the left-sided proptosis due to mass effect.

Nasal or Paranasal Sinus Lesions

Contd...

Diseases	NECT/CECT findings	Comments
	• Thinning and pressure atrophy of bony turbinates and with or without DNS to the contralateral side • Minimal to mild contrast enhancement seen	
Sinonasal polyposis (Figs. 10 and 11)	• Rounded or lobulated soft tissue attenuation masses in the nasal cavity and multiple sinuses • Enlarging sinus ostium • Expansion of sinus seen • Thinning of bony trabeculae • Usually peripheral, occasionally uniform enhancement seen on CECT	• Benign lesions seen in cases of allergic sinusitis • Hypertelorism is seen with ethmoid involvement
Fungiform papilloma	• Nearly always arise from the nasal septum • Usually solitary and unilateral • Usually show minimal to mild contrast enhancement • Have irregular mucosal surface • Needs to be differentiated from inverted papilloma	• It is due to obstruction to the outflow of mucus-secreting Bowman's glands • Most common form of papilloma seen in nasal cavity • Have no premalignant potential

Contd...

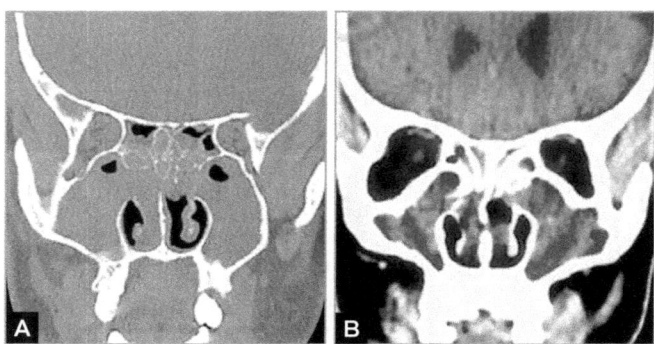

Figs. 10A and B: Coronal CT images showing sinonasal polyposis. Note the hyperdensities within likely doe to superadded fungal infection or inspissated chronic secretions.

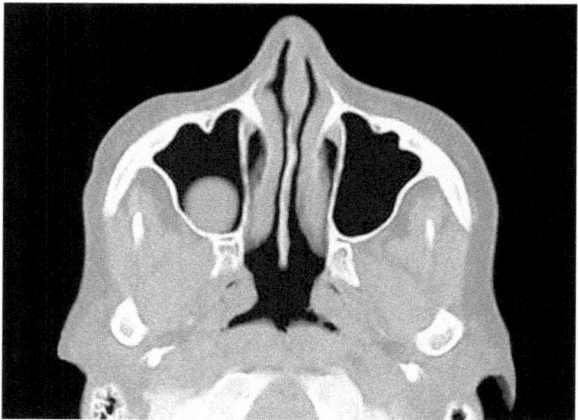

Fig. 11: Transaxial CT image shows benign antral polyp on right side.

Contd...

Diseases	NECT/CECT findings	Comments
Neurogenic tumors	• Benign encapsulated slow-growing tumor • Fusiform or rounded low attenuation soft tissue mass with mild to moderate contrast enhancement • May cause anterior bowing and remodeling of posterior wall of the maxillary sinus • It needs to be differentiated from angiofibroma that usually involves pterygopalatine fissure	Rare in sinonasal cavity
Sinus hemorrhage	• There is collection of hyperdense blood in the sinus cavity • An air-blood level may be seen • There is diffuse mucosal thickening	Secondary to barotrauma or in patients on anticoagulation

(CECT: contrast-enhanced computed tomography; NECT: noncontrast-enhanced computed tomography)

TABLE 3: Common causes and CT findings in primary bone lesions.

Diseases	NECT/CECT findings	Comments
Fibrous dysplasia (Fig. 12)	• There is facial asymmetry • Characteristically, there is unilateral overgrowth of facial bones with encroachment on sinus cavity leading to ostial blockage and secondary infections • Lytic lesions with ground-glass appearance and sclerosis • Cherubism (Figs. 13A and B) is a special variant occurring as an autosomal dominant disorder presenting in childhood more severely in males with symmetric involvement of mandible and maxilla, there is spontaneous regression in adolescence	• Sphenoid, frontal, maxillary, ethmoid bones are more commonly involved in decreasing order of frequency; the occipital and temporal bones are less commonly involved • Craniofacial form is also known as leontiasis ossea and is more common in polyostotic form 50% and less common in monostotic form 10–25%
Ossifying fibroma (Figs. 14A and B)	• Areas of increased and decreased attenuations are seen • It is a slow-growing expansile lytic lesion with central calcification • Usually unilateral and monostotic	• Mixture of osseous and fibrous tissue, impossible to differentiate from fibrous dysplasia • Maxillary, frontal, ethmoid, and mandible are involved in decreasing order of frequency, rarely seen elsewhere

Contd...

Nasal or Paranasal Sinus Lesions

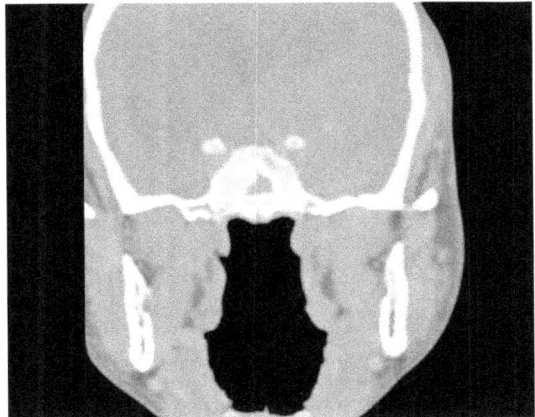

Fig. 12: Fibrous dysplasia of the sphenoid bone.

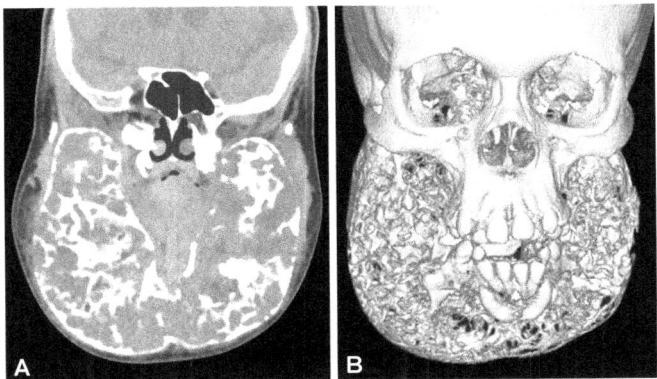

Figs. 13A and B: Coronal NECT and volume reformatted images of grossly expanded mandible with abnormal bony texture—cherubism.

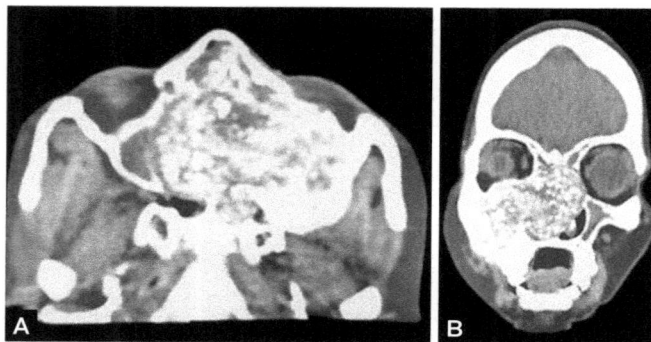

Figs. 14A and B: Axial and coronal MPR CT images of PNS showing soft tissue lesion involving left maxillary sinus and left side nasal cavity with foci of calcifications in a case of ossifying fibroma.

Contd...

Diseases	NECT/CECT findings	Comments
Osteoma (Fig. 15)	• Hyperdense (ivory) polypoidal compact bony mass • Sometimes partially calcified cancellous mass may be seen • May lead to ostial obstruction and mucocele formation, erode cribriform plate, and lead to CSF rhinorrhea • Multiple osteomas may be seen in Gardner's syndrome	Most common in frontal sinuses followed by ethmoid sinuses
Paget's disease	• Bilateral and asymmetrical • The facial bones become thickened and sclerotic with cotton-wool appearance (mixed lytic and blastic lesion) and encroachment on the sinuses	More common in patients aged 55 years and above

Contd...

Nasal or Paranasal Sinus Lesions

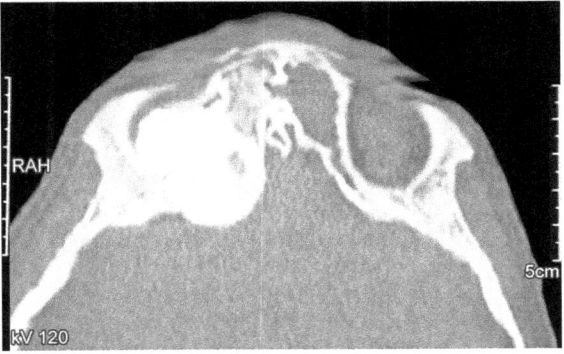

Fig. 15: Axial CT image of PNS showing hyperdense lobulated lesion arising from right frontal sinus suggestive of osteoma.

Contd...

Diseases	NECT/CECT findings	Comments
Odontoma	• It encroaches on the maxillary sinuses • Well-defined hyperdense mass lesion containing undifferentiated dental elements	
Eosinophilic granuloma	• Round to oval punched out lesion with serrated beveled edges which is sharply marginated without a sclerotic rim except in healing phase • Button sequestrum is central bone density within the lytic lesion; sometimes, a floating tooth may be seen inside • Soft tissue masses may be seen overlying the bony lytic lesion	Most benign variety of histiocytosis X localized to bone seen in 5–10 years of age (range 2–30 years)

Contd...

Contd...

Diseases	NECT/CECT findings	Comments
Ameloblastoma	• Unilateral or more commonly multiloculated lesion with coarse trabecular pattern, may be associated with impacted tooth • Leads to cortical expansion and sometimes breach with soft tissue extensions	Locally aggressive lesion, most common in mandible followed by maxilla
Brown tumor/ Giant cell tumor	Lytic expansile destructive lesion of the bone	Giant cell granuloma/reparative granuloma occurs frequently in the mandible
Plasmacytoma	• It presents as a lytic expansile lesion of the bone • Extramedullary variety presents as a predominant well-defined, moderately to intensely enhancing soft tissue mass in the sinonasal cavity with slight expansion and bone remodeling with occasional erosion	Extramedullary variety is commoner in the sinonasal region
Chondroma	It is seen as a sharply demarcated, lytic bone lesion with stippled calcification	• It usually arises in the nasal cavity of the young adults • It can mimic a meningioma when it occurs adjacent to the roof of the nasal cavity and sphenoid bone

Contd...

Contd...

Diseases	NECT/CECT findings	Comments
Osteosarcoma	Extensive bone destruction, new bone formation with aggressive periosteal reaction and large soft tissue mass	Most often arise from alveolar ridge
Chondrosarcoma	• Presents as multilobulated sharply demarcated lytic lesion with a large soft tissue component • Characteristic chondroid matrix calcification is seen	Most often arise from alveolar ridge of the maxilla
Ewing's sarcoma	There is permeative bone destruction, aggressive periosteal reaction, and a large soft tissue component	
Aneurysmal bone cyst	Multiloculated lytic expansile bone lesions sometimes seen with air-blood levels	

TABLE 4: Common causes of lesions of sinonasal cavity with bone destruction and their relevant CT findings.

Diseases	NECT/CECT findings	Comments
Fungal sinusitis (Figs. 16 and 17)	• Nodular or polypoidal thickening of mucosa, lesion/fungal ball • Hyperdense branching hyphae seen • Punctate calcifications may be seen • Spotty bone destruction with periosteitis and sclerosis • Extension into cranial cavity, orbits, and vascular structures as cavernous sinuses may be seen	Most commonly seen in diabetic and immunocompromised

Contd...

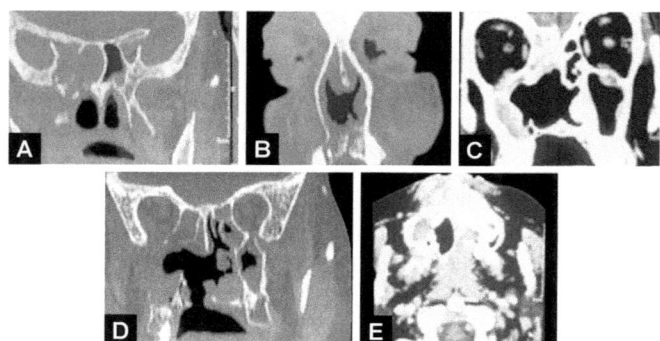

Figs. 16A to E: CT images showing fungal sinusitis and its complications.

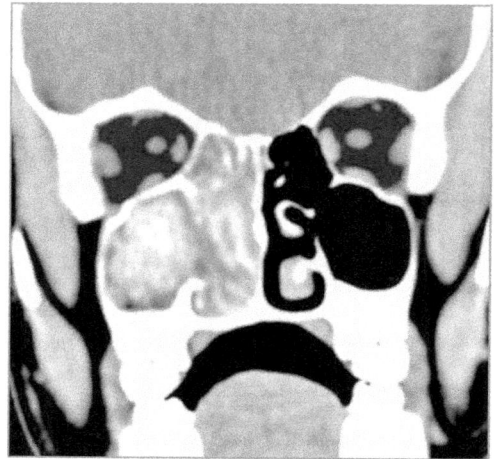

Fig. 17: Coronal CT image shows antronasal fungal polyposis.

Contd...

Diseases	NECT/CECT findings	Comments
Wegener's granulomatosis	<ul><li>Nodular ulcerated mucosa especially of maxillary sinus</li><li>Necrosis and perforation of nasal septum</li><li>Extensive bone destruction</li><li>Large soft tissue masses may be seen</li></ul>	<ul><li>Autoimmune systemic disease characterized by necrotizing granulomatous angiitis</li><li>Associated pulmonary lesions favor the diagnosis</li></ul>
Stewart's granuloma (lymphoma-like lesion)	<ul><li>Extensive and severe midfacial mutilation is seen with severe bone destruction and relatively small soft tissue mass</li><li>Extension into orbits may cause proptosis</li></ul>	Also midline granuloma or polymorphic reticulosis confined to the midfacial region and sinuses only
Inverted papilloma	<ul><li>Uniquely unilateral, most often arising from lateral nasal wall with extension into the maxillary or ethmoid sinuses; rarely, it may be present at nasal septum</li><li>There is widening of infundibulum and outflow tract of antrum with destruction of the medial antral wall/lamina papyracea of orbit, anterior cranial fossa in up to 30% of cases</li><li>Septum may be bowed to opposite side (no invasion)</li><li>Homogeneous enhancement seen</li></ul>	Commonly occurs after nasal surgery

Contd...

Contd...

Diseases	NECT/CECT findings	Comments
Esthesioneuroblastoma/ esthesioneurocytoma/ esthesioneuroepithelioma	• Polypoidal slow-growing tumor • Moderately to intensely enhancing mass seen in the nasal vault occasionally with punctate calcifications and sclerosis and remodeling of adjacent bone • May spread into the ethmoid and sphenoid sinuses and the anterior cranial fossa destroying intervening bones	Malignant tumor arising from olfactory mucosa seen in adolescents
Carcinoma paranasal sinus (Fig. 18)	• Poorly marginated soft tissue-enhancing mass with areas of necrosis • Extensive destruction of underlying and neighboring bone • Nodal metastasis is seen in regional nodes (retropharyngeal, submandibular, jugular) • May invade pterygopalatine fossa, orbits, middle cranial fossa, maxillary alveolar ridge, hard palate, buccal space, and nose	Most common in maxillary sinus
Lymphoma	• Bulky infiltrating homogeneous soft-tissue masses are seen that may show some contrast enhancement • Remodeling of adjacent bone with occasional erosion may be seen	• Most common sarcomas involving the sinonasal tract, vast majority are non-Hodgkin's type • The nasal cavity and the maxillary sinus are the most common sites

Contd...

Nasal or Paranasal Sinus Lesions

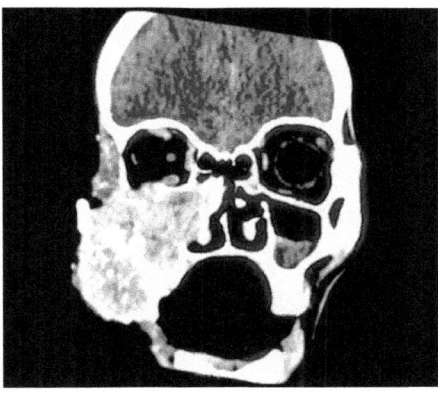

Fig. 18: Coronal CT image showing carcinoma of maxilla with soft tissue extension.

Contd...

Diseases	NECT/CECT findings	Comments
Chondro-mesenchymal hamartoma of the nose (Figs. 19A and B)	<ul><li>Polypoidal mass of heterogeneous attenuation</li><li>May contain chondroid and osseous elements</li><li>May reveal erosion of the adjacent bone with occasional extension into the skull base and orbital region or adjacent sinuses, especially the ethmoid sinus</li><li>Intensely enhancing tumor on CECT</li></ul>	Very rare tumor seen in young children
Metastases	It is seen as expansion along the margins of the sinus rather than as mucosal thickening	Most common primary metastasis is renal cell carcinoma that markedly enhances on CECT with expansion and remodeling of bone

Contd...

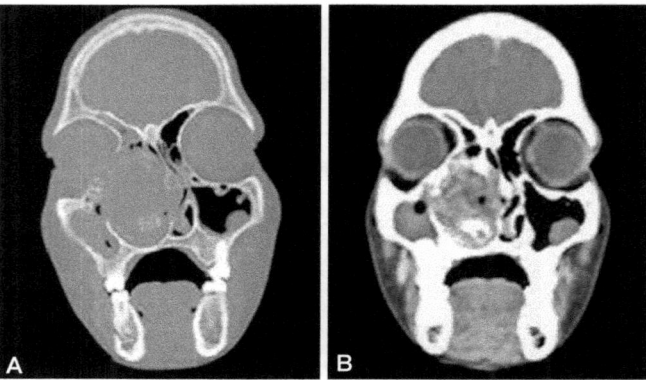

Figs. 19A and B: Coronal CT images showing features of chondromesenchymal hamartoma of the nose.

Contd...

Diseases	NECT/CECT findings	Comments
Rhabdomyosarcoma	These are seen as aggressive soft tissue, enhancing masses with bone destruction and remodeling	These are the most common soft tissue sarcomas in infants and children

TABLE 5: Common causes of nasopharyngeal lesions.

Cystic	Soft tissue/solid
Benign: • Thornwaldt's cyst • Mucus retention cyst • Meningocele • Encephalomeningocele • Chronic abscess/hematoma (Fig. 20)	*Benign:* • Adenoids • Polyp • Hematoma (secondary to trauma) • Rhinocerebral mucormycosis • Hemangioma • Angiofibroma • Encephalocele • Pleomorphic adenoma *Malignant:* • Carcinoma • Lymphoma • Chordoma • Rhabdomyosarcoma

Nasal or Paranasal Sinus Lesions

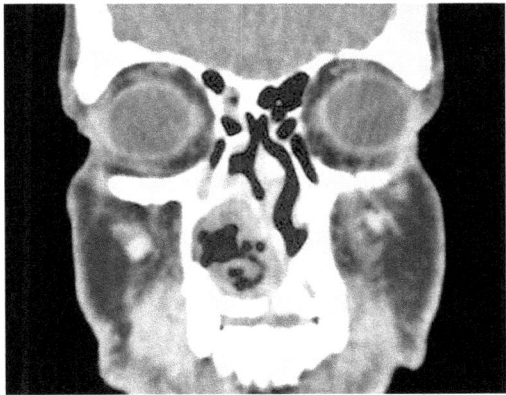

Fig. 20: Coronal CT image of PNS showing soft tissue lesion with areas of air density in left side of nasal cavity suggestive of an abscess.

TABLE 6: Differentiating features of common nasopharyngeal lesions.		
Diseases	*Differentiating features*	*Comments*
Nasopharyngeal carcinoma	• Polypoidal or papillary, mild to moderately enhancing mass • Bone destruction and invasion of the adjacent structures such as Eustachian tube through sinus of Morgagni, into foramen lacerum, encasement of ICA, extension into cavernous sinus, posterior nasal cavity, pterygopalatine fossa, along lateral pharyngeal walls, tonsillar pillars and masticator space is common • Metastases to the supraclavicular space is frequent	• Usual age at presentation is 40–50 years • The epicenter of the mass is around the tubal openings or the area adjacent to the posterior part of the turbinates

Contd...

Contd...

Diseases	Differentiating features	Comments
Juvenile angiofibroma (Figs. 21A to C)	• Intensely enhancing soft-tissue mass • Widening of pterygo-maxillary fissure or widening of the sphenopalatine foramen are pathognomonic sign • Anterior bowing of posterior antral wall is characteristic due to spread of the tumor to the pterygopalatine fossa • Invasion of sphenoid sinus through erosion of its floor and widening of inferior and superior orbital fissure may occur due to spread into orbit and middle cranial fossa	• Mean age 15 years • Almost exclusively seen in males
Hematoma	• They reveal attenuation values according to the stage • The evolution with time is characteristic • Fractured bone fragments may be seen	Fracture of the base of skull and upper cervical vertebrae are the usual associated injuries
Adenoids	Soft tissue attenuating mass along the posterior nasopharyngeal wall with mild to moderate postcontrast enhancement	Usually seen in childhood

Contd...

Nasal or Paranasal Sinus Lesions

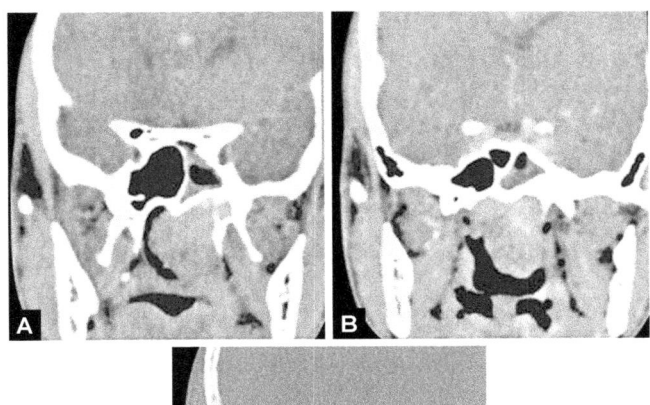
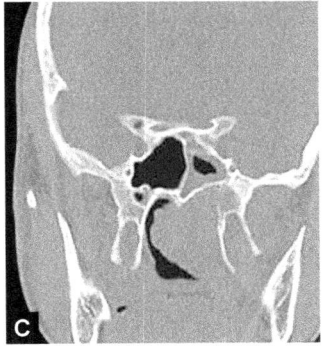

Figs. 21A to C: Coronal CT images showing features of nasopharyngeal angiofibroma.

Contd...

Diseases	Differentiating features	Comments
Lymphoma	• Usually seen as bulky masses isodense to hypodense with mild to moderate contrast enhancement • Late involvement of parapharyngeal spaces may be seen	Presence of adenopathy elsewhere in the body is highly suggestive

Contd...

Contd...

Diseases	NECT/CECT findings	Comments
Polyp	• Usually seen as rounded mass projecting into the lumen • Thinning of adjacent bones but with no aggressive bone destruction • Usually peripheral but sometimes heterogeneous enhancement	Usually in younger population
Rhabdomyosarcoma	• Bulky mass isodense with brain on noncontrast images with uniform intense enhancement • Extension into cranial vault through fissures and foramina and usually involves cavernous sinus • Bone destruction can be marked	Usually seen in less than 15 years of age but peak age of presentation is 2–5 years
Rhinocerebral mucormycosis	• It is characterized by nodular thickened mucosa • Hyperdense branching lesions may be seen on noncontrast images with moderate enhancement on CECT • Marked bone destruction • It spreads along vessels and may lead to venous cerebral infarcts, cavernous sinus and ophthalmic vein thrombosis, and invasion of orbits and sinuses	• Old debilitated or immunosuppressed or patients with diabetes mellitus (DM) are the most common susceptibles • Nasal septum and turbinates are usually destroyed
Meningocele and encephalocele (Figs. 22A and B)	Defect in skull base is usual in these cases	Usually present in infancy or young childhood

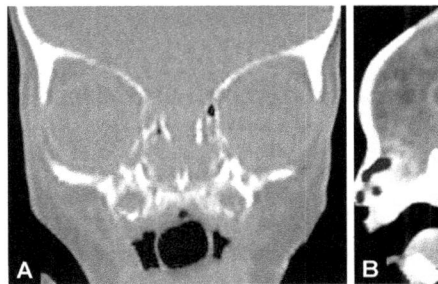
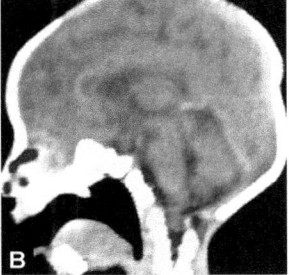

Figs. 22A and B: Coronal and sagittal CT images showing frontoethmoidal encephalocele.

Contd...

Diseases	NECT/CECT findings	Comments
Chordoma	• Midline, hypodense soft tissue mass • Destruction of basisphenoid with specks of calcifications • Variable degree of enhancement • Usually an intracranial extension is evident	It is seen in older age group of 30–70 years with peak age of presentation being 60 years

NORMAL DEVELOPMENT OF PARANASAL SINUSES (TABLE 7)

TABLE 7: Development of paranasal sinuses.

Sinuses	Status at birth	First radiological evidence	Reaches adult size by
Maxillary sinus	Present at birth	4–5 months after birth	15 years
Ethmoid sinus	Present at birth	1 year	12 years
Sphenoid sinus	Not present	4 years	15 years to adult age
Frontal sinus	Not present	6 years	Size increases until teens

ANATOMICAL VARIANTS OF PARANASAL SINUSES (TABLE 8)

TABLE 8: Anatomical variants of paranasal sinuses.

- Septal deviation
- Septal spurs
- Paradoxical middle turbinate (Fig. 23)
- Concha bullosa (Fig. 24)
- Lamellar concha (Fig. 25)
- Attachment of uncinate process: lamina papyracea/middle turbinate/base of skull (Fig. 26)
- Ethmoid bulla (Fig. 27)
- Agger nasi cell (Fig. 28)
- Haller cell (Fig. 29)
- Onodi cell (Fig. 30)
- Frontal sinus extension
- Accessory maxillary ostium
- Intersinus sphenoid septation
- *Optic nerve variations*: Delano types I–IV
- *Olfactory fossa depth*: Keros types I–III

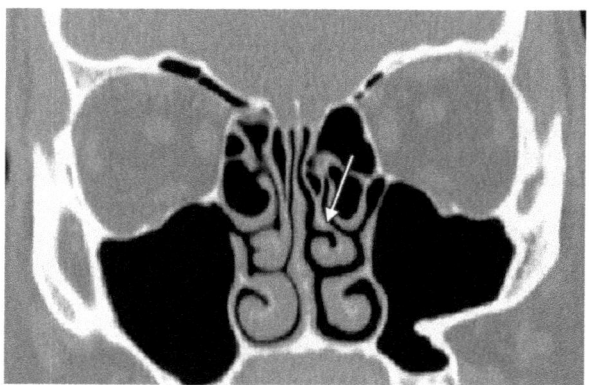

Fig. 23: Coronal CT image showing paradoxical curvature of left middle turbinate (arrow).

Nasal or Paranasal Sinus Lesions

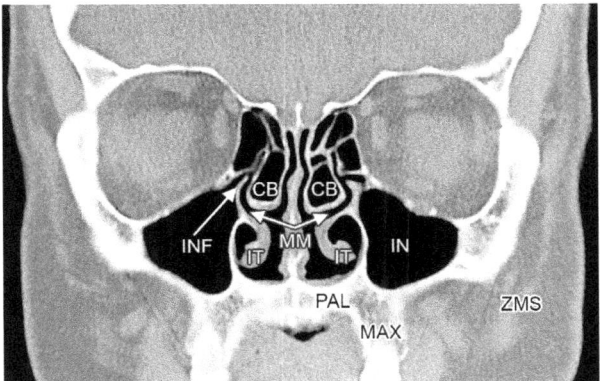

Fig. 24: Coronal CT image showing pneumatized bilateral middle turbinates—concha bullosa (CB).
[IN: infraorbital nerve and canal; INF: infundibulum; MAX: maxillary dentoalveolus (tooth-bearing area); MM: middle meatus (text label overlies the nasal septum); PAL: palate (hard); IT: inferior turbinate; ZMS: zygomaticomaxillary suture]

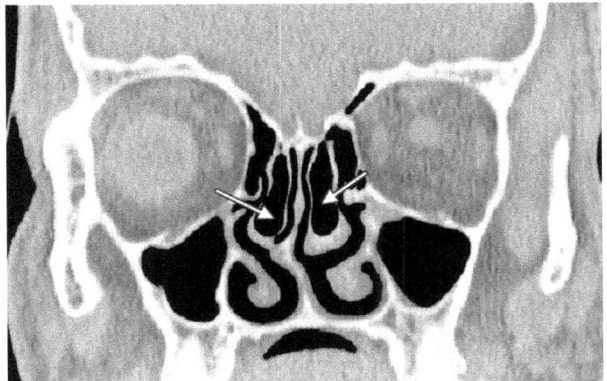

Fig. 25: Coronal CT image showing pneumatization of attachment part of bilateral middle turbinates—lamellar concha.

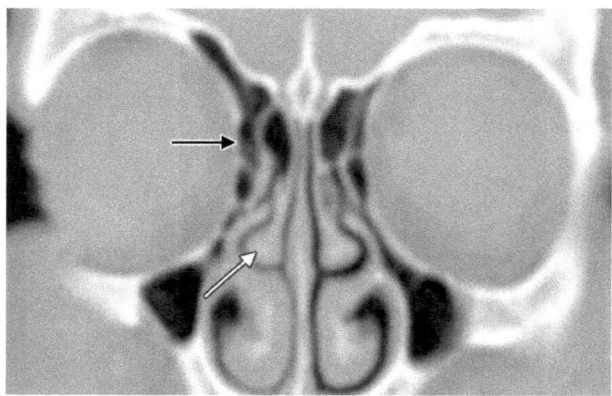

Fig. 26: Coronal CT image showing nasal structures. Middle turbinate (white arrow) and lamina papyracea (black arrow).

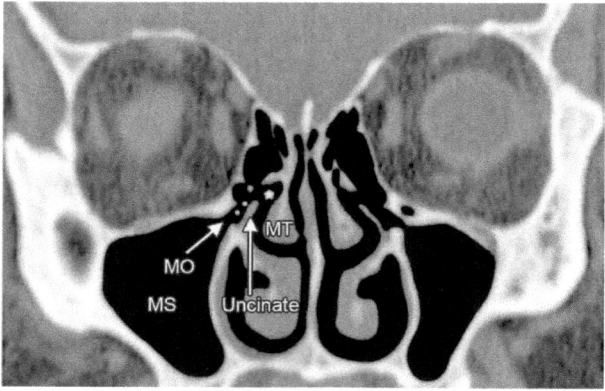

Fig. 27: Coronal CT image showing the osteomeatal complex fronto-ethmoid recess, ethmoid bulla, uncinate process, maxillary ostium and infundibulum, hiatus semilunaris, and the ethmoid infundibulum.
(MO: maxillary ostium; MS: maxillary sinus; MT: middle turbinate)

Nasal or Paranasal Sinus Lesions

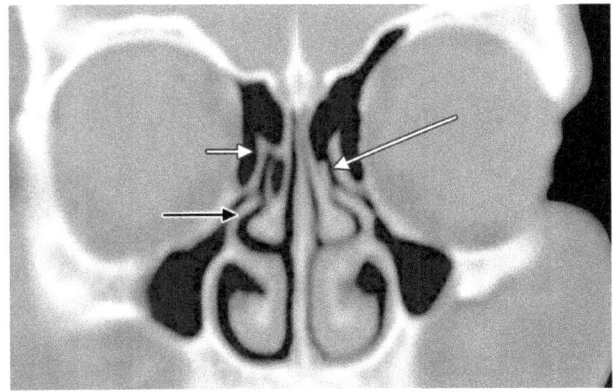

Fig. 28: Coronal CT image showing uncinate process (black arrow), Agger nasi cell (small white arrow), and frontal recess (long white arrow).

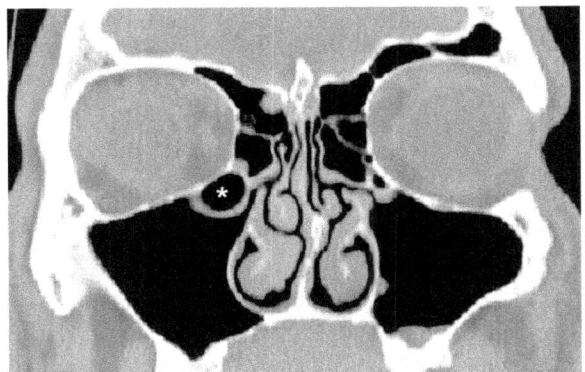

Fig. 29: Coronal CT image showing a Haller cell on right side along the floor of right orbit.

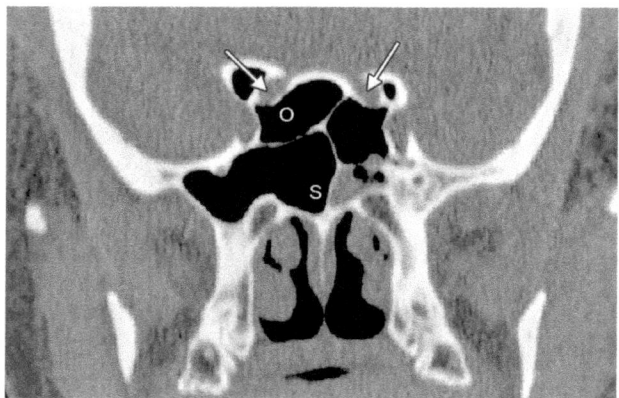

Fig. 30: Coronal CT image showing right-sided Onodi cell (O) near the right optic nerve. Note the secretion in the sphenoid sinus (S) toward left.

Chapter 6

Neck

PHARYNGEAL AND PARAPHARYNGEAL LESIONS

Pharyngeal Mucosal Space (Table 1)

It includes the mucosal surfaces and immediate submucosa of the nasopharynx, oropharynx, oral cavity, and hypopharynx. Also included in this space are lymphoid structures, minor salivary glands, constrictor muscles, and salpingopharyngeus muscle.

TABLE 1: Causes of pharyngeal and parapharyngeal lesions.		
Cystic	Solid/Complex	Calcified

• Retention cyst of the salivary gland
• Thornwaldt's cyst
• Lymphangioma
• Abscesses
• Lymph nodes
	• *Malignant:*
	  – Mucosal and submucosal malignancies
	  – Non-Hodgkin's lymphoma
	  – Salivary gland malignancies
	  – Rhabdomyosarcoma
	• *Benign:*
	  – Adenoid hypertrophy
	  – Enlarged lymph nodes
	  – Tonsillar and peritonsillar abscesses
	  – Angiofibromas
		• Postinflammatory nodal and abscess calcification
		• Postirradiation nodal calcification

Thornwaldt's Cyst

- Incidental, usually asymptomatic, midline, cystic mass located in the posterior part of the roof of nasopharynx
- No associated osseous involvement
- To be differentiated from the Rathke's pouch seen in the body of sphenoid bone, in a relatively anterosuperior location.

Angiofibroma

Markedly enhancing, ill-defined, soft-tissue mass seen almost exclusively in adolescent males arising from the fossa of Rosenmüller or sphenopalatine foramen and causing extensive bony destruction to extend into the surrounding spaces.

Squamous Cell Carcinoma (Fig. 1)

- Most common malignant tumor arising from the mucosal surfaces

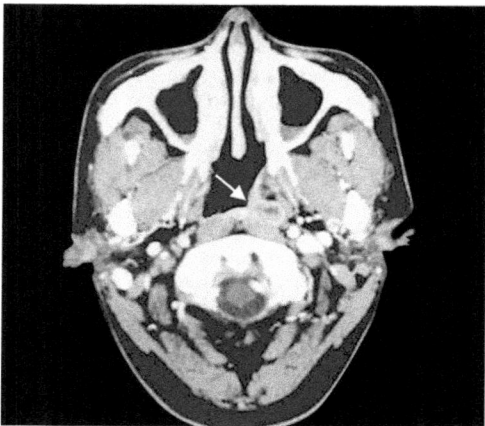

Fig. 1: Transaxial contrast-enhanced computed tomography (CECT) image shows nasopharyngeal mass on left side of midline (arrow).

- Mass has variable appearance with invasion of the parapharyngeal or retropharyngeal fat and extension into the skull base
- Lymphadenopathy in the drainage area of the lesion.

Lymphoma

- It arises from the lymphatic tissue of the Waldeyer's ring resulting in enlargement of the tonsils and adenoids
- Nodal spread is seen with involvement of multiple chains that do not fit in the lymphatic drainage
- Distant manifestations include hepatosplenomegaly and bony lesions.

Parapharyngeal Space (Tables 2 and 3)

It is triangular in axial scans with apex toward the nasopharynx. It is bounded anterolaterally by the medial pterygoid fascia and medially by the pharyngobasilar fascia. At the level of nasopharynx, the fascia of tensor vela palatini divides this space into the *pre- and poststyloid compartments*. At the level of the oropharynx, the oropharyngeal constrictors separate the compartments. Lesions of parapharyngeal space displace the carotid artery and jugular veins posteriorly.

TABLE 2: Causes of lesions in the prestyloid compartment.

Cystic	Solid/Complex	Calcified
<ul><li>Retention cyst of the salivary gland</li><li>Atypical second branchial cleft cyst</li></ul>	<ul><li>*Malignant*: – Salivary gland malignancies – Metastases</li><li>*Benign*: – Lipoma – Salivary gland tumors as pleomorphic and monomorphic adenoma</li></ul>	Calcification in granulomatous diseases of salivary glands

TABLE 3: Causes of lesions of poststyloid compartment.

Cystic	Solid/Complex	Vascular	Calcified

Neurofibroma (rarely)	• *Malignant*:
	  – Abscesses
	  – Metastases
	• *Benign*:
	  – Abscesses
	  – Enlarged lymph nodes
	  – Lipoma
	  – Paragangliomas
	  – Nerve sheath tumors as schwannomas and neurofibromas
		• Ectatic carotid artery
		• Pseudo aneurysm, dissections and thrombosis of the carotid artery
		• Ectasia of the internal jugular vein
		• Jugular vein thrombosis
			• Calcification in lymph nodes
			• Calcified plaques and thrombus

Atypical Second Branchial Cleft Cyst

Seen in a child or young adult along the posterolateral wall of the pharynx in the region of the palatine tonsil growing toward the skull base.

Salivary Gland Adenoma

Round to oval, well-circumscribed, moderately enhancing mass surrounded by fat.

Lipoma (Fig. 2)

- Well-circumscribed fatty lesion with relatively less mass effect
- Should be differentiated from dermoid that may contain calcification, fat-fluid level, and are usually seen in midline.

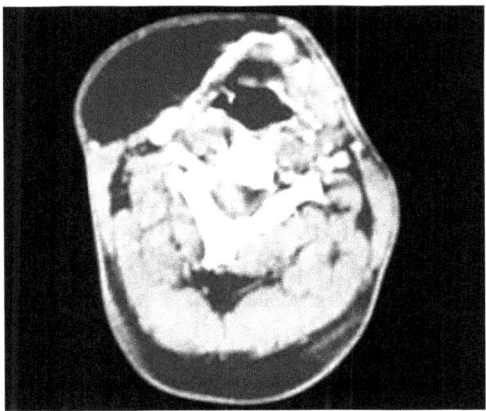

Fig. 2: Axial CECT image of neck showing well-marginated hypodense lesion of fat density on right side of neck suggesting lipoma.

Poststyloid compartment is also known as *carotid space* that extends from the base of the skull to the level of the aortic arch.

Nerve Sheath Tumors (Figs. 3A to C)

- These displace the carotid artery anteriorly and medially.
- Schwannomas are well-defined, fusiform, soft-tissue masses with varying degree and inhomogeneous contrast enhancement and cystic degeneration. May cause smooth scalloping of the jugular foramen and may be multiple in patients with neurofibromatosis.
- Neurofibromas are relatively hypodense soft-tissue masses with homogeneous enhancement. They may be multiple in patients with neurofibromatosis.
- Schwannoma needs differentiation from meningioma extending inferiorly from the jugular foramen. The latter is hyperdense and sometimes calcified. It shows greater enhancement and may demonstrate dural attachment.

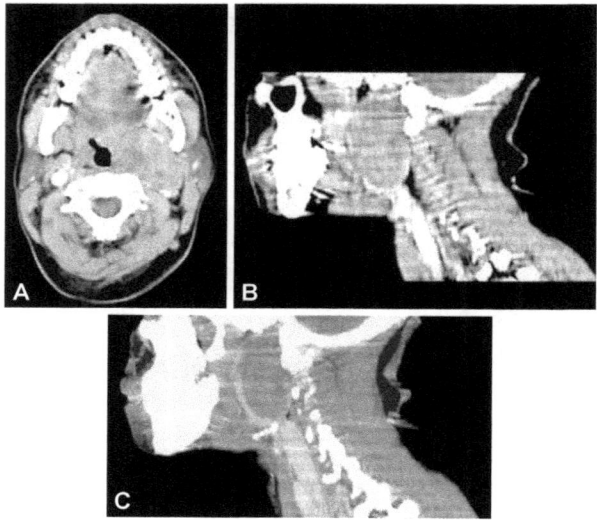

Figs. 3A to C: Axial and sagittal CT images showing a carotid sheath mass.

Paragangliomas (Glomus Tumors)

- These are slowly growing, intensely enhancing, soft-tissue mass with irregular and permeative destruction of the adjacent bone.
- They are multiple in 5% of cases and 20–30% have a family history.

Ectatic Carotid Artery

It is seen as dilated, tortuous artery that is folded on itself and is commonly seen in elderly.

NECK SPACE LESIONS

Sublingual Space (Table 4)

These are paired spaces located in the floor of the mouth and are defined by the mandible anteriorly and laterally, hyoid bone posteriorly, oral mucosa superiorly, and mylohyoid muscle inferiorly. The paired genioglossus and geniohyoid muscles lying in the sagittal plane separates the spaces. A median fat plane or septum and a lateral fat plane (lateral to the genioglossus) are normally visualized.

TABLE 4: Causes of lesions in sublingual space.

Cystic	Solid/Complex	Calcified
<ul><li>Ranulas</li><li>Retention cyst of sublingual glands (Fig. 5)</li><li>Thyroglossal cyst</li><li>Cellulitis and abscess</li><li>Lymphangioma</li><li>Enlarged lymph nodes</li><li>Dilated submandibular duct (>3 mm in diameter)</li></ul>	<ul><li>*Malignant:*<ul><li>Carcinoma extending from the floor of mouth and tongue (Figs. 4A and B)</li><li>Sublingual gland malignancies</li></ul></li><li>*Benign:*<ul><li>Dermoid and epidermoid</li><li>Hemangioma</li><li>Lingual thyroid gland</li><li>Abscesses</li><li>Enlarged lymph nodes</li><li>Pleomorphic adenoma</li></ul></li></ul>	<ul><li>Submandibular duct calculi</li><li>Calcification in nodes and abscesses</li><li>Phleboliths in hemangiomas</li></ul>

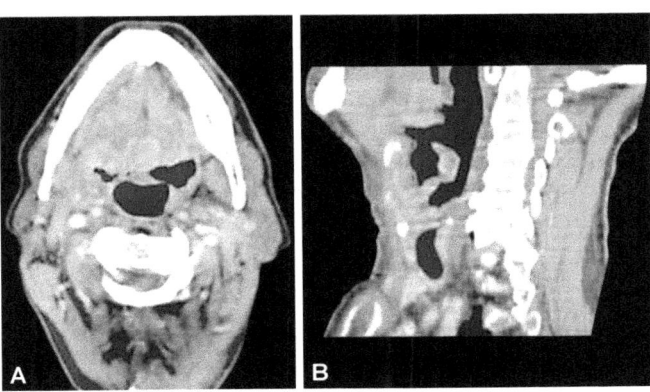

Figs. 4A and B: Axial and sagittal CT images showing a mass at the base of tongue.

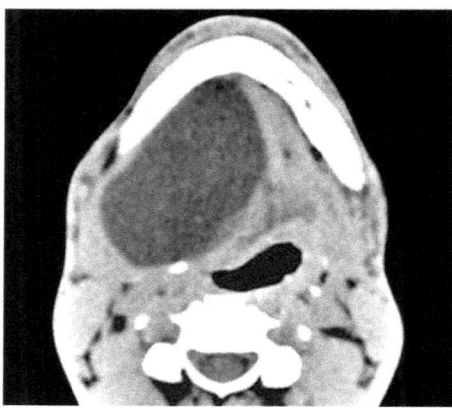

Fig. 5: Transaxial CT image shows mucocele of right sublingual gland.

Ranula

- A simple type is a unilocular, well-defined, cystic mass that in fact represents a postinflammatory retention cyst of the salivary glands.
- A diving type is characterized by a large cystic mass extending from the posterior sublingual space into the submandibular and parapharyngeal space. The bulk of the cyst is seen in the latter spaces with a characteristic thin extension into the sublingual space referred to as the "*tail sign.*" This sign differentiates it from an epidermoid or lymphangioma.
- Retention cyst of the submandibular gland can be differentiated from the ranula by the involvement of the submandibular gland in the former.

Ludwig's Angina

- It is characterized by involvement of the sublingual and submandibular space.
- Features include thickening of the overlying skin, increased attenuation of the subcutaneous fat, visualization of the

small-engorged veins, inflammation of the adjacent muscles, and obliteration of the adjacent fat and fascial planes. This may progress to frank ring enhancing lesions or abscesses.
- Mandibular osteomyelitis and submandibular calculi may be associated.

Submandibular Space (Table 5)

It lies posterolateral to the sublingual space.

TABLE 5: Causes of lesions of submandibular space.

Cystic	Solid/Complex	Calcified
<ul><li>Cystic hygroma</li><li>Second branchial cleft cyst</li><li>Thyroglossal duct cyst</li><li>Retention cyst of the salivary gland</li><li>Abscesses</li></ul>	<ul><li>*Malignant:*<ul><li>Submandibular gland malignancies as muco-epidermoid carcinoma, adenocystic carcinoma</li><li>Lymphoma</li></ul></li><li>*Benign:*<ul><li>Dermoid and epidermoid</li><li>Abscesses (Fig. 7)</li><li>Enlarged lymph nodes</li><li>Pleomorphic adenoma</li></ul></li></ul>	<ul><li>Submandibular gland calculi (Fig. 6)</li><li>Calcification in nodes and abscesses</li></ul>

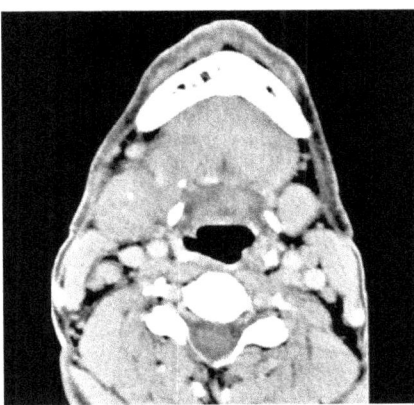

Fig. 6: Transaxial CECT image shows sialadenitis of submandibular gland.

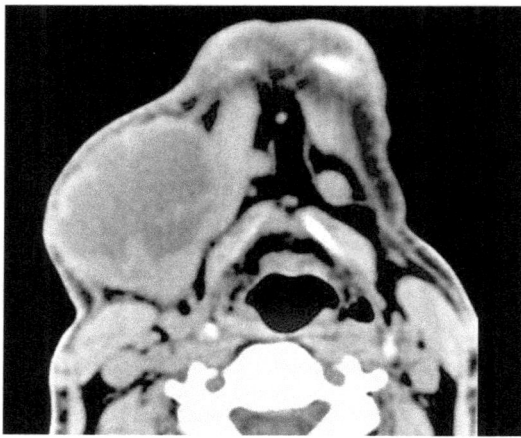

Fig. 7: Transaxial CT image shows loculated abscess in right submandibular space.

Second Branchial Cleft Cyst

- It is seen as a unilocular mass in the posterior submandibular space displacing the submandibular gland anteromedially, the sternomastoid posterolaterally, and carotid artery and internal jugular vein posteromedially.
- A beak pointing medially between the internal and external carotid arteries is pathognomonic, when visualized.
- The cyst may enlarge following infection or trauma.

Thyroglossal Cyst

Seen as a midline mass usually in infrahyoid location, followed by suprahyoid and hyoid location in the order of frequency.

Dermoid and Epidermoid

- These are seen as unilocular, hypodense lesions.
- Dermoids are seen in the midline.

Buccal Space

It is a small space and lies anterior to the masseter and lateral to the buccinator muscle. Lesions involving this space include:
- Infections and deeply invading tumors of the adjacent skin
- Infections and neoplasms from adjacent spaces such as parotid and masticator space.

Masticator Space (Table 6)

It is formed by the superficial layer of the cervical fascia.

TABLE 6: Causes of lesions of masticator space.

Cystic	Solid/Complex	Calcified
<ul><li>Dental and bony cysts</li><li>Lymphangioma (Figs. 8A to C)</li><li>Radionecrosis</li><li>Abscesses</li></ul>	<ul><li>*Malignant:*<ul><li>Soft-tissue sarcoma</li><li>Rhabdomyosarcoma</li><li>Extracranial extension of the meningioma from the middle cranial fossa</li><li>Malignant schwannoma</li><li>Metastases</li></ul></li><li>*Benign:*<ul><li>Abscesses</li><li>Accessory parotid gland</li><li>Hemangioma</li><li>Lipoma</li><li>Nerve sheath tumors as schwannomas and neurofibromas</li></ul></li></ul>	<ul><li>Osteomyelitis</li><li>Dental tumors</li><li>Osteosarcoma and other bony malignancies arising from the mandible</li><li>Phleboliths in hemangioma</li></ul>

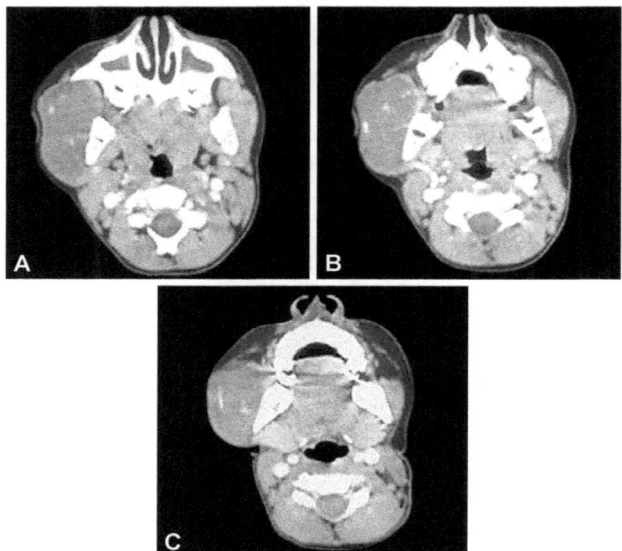

Figs. 8A to C: Axial CT images showing a large cystic lymphangioma in the right masseter.

Accessory Parotid Gland

- Seen along the lateral surface of the masseter muscle in approximately 20% of the population.
- Usually bilateral and symmetric.

Hemangioma

- Capillary type is poorly marginated while cavernous type is well marginated and both show considerable contrast enhancement.
- Capillary type is seen in infants and children and tends to be transspatial that is involving multiple contiguous spaces.
- Cavernous type is usually seen in second to fourth decades of life and often shows progressive enlargement.

Malignant Schwannoma

- It arises from the mandibular branch of the trigeminal nerve.
- It appears as a tubular mass with mandibular destruction and foramen widening.

Retropharyngeal Space (Table 7)

It lies between the middle and posterior layers of deep cervical fascia, posterior to the visceral space and extends from the base of the skull to the mediastinum. It is further subdivided into the suprahyoid and infrahyoid compartments.

Lymphadenopathy

- Multiple enlarged nodes exceeding 1 cm in diameter suggest a high possibility of metastases.

TABLE 7: Causes of lesions of retropharyngeal space.

Cystic	Solid/Complex	Air-containing lesion	Calcified

• Abscesses
• Lymph nodes
• Fluid collection secondary to lymphatic or venous obstruction
• Chronic hematomas
	• *Malignant:*
	  – Extension from mucosal carcinomas as nasopharyngeal carcinoma
	  – Metastases
	• *Benign:*
	  – Enlarged lymph nodes
	  – Hematomas
	  – Hemangiomas
	  – Lipomas
		• Emphysema secondary to trauma, foreign body aspiration or assisted ventilation
		• Abscesses
			Postinflammatory nodal and abscess calcification

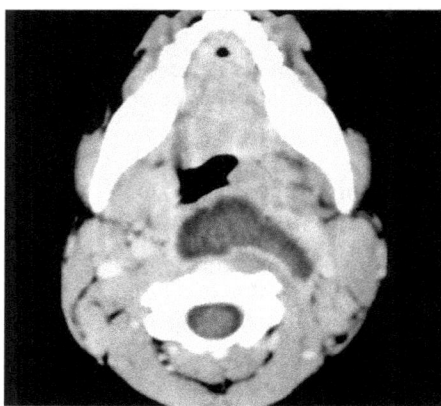

Fig. 9: Axial CECT image of neck showing enhancing soft-tissue lesion in right retropharyngeal space in case of retropharyngeal abscess.

- Reactive nodal hyperplasia is usually seen in children and young adults and the nodal diameter rarely exceeds 1 cm.

Abscesses (Fig. 9)

- Retropharyngeal abscess has a bow-tie configuration.
- It is indistinguishable from the hematoma.

Posterior Cervical Space (Table 8)

It is bounded by the carotid space posterolaterally, sternocleidomastoid muscle anterolaterally, and paraspinal muscles posteromedially.

Atypical Second Branchial Cleft Cyst

It is seen as a cystic mass along the anterior border of the common carotid artery.

TABLE 8: Causes of lesions in posterior cervical space.

Cystic	Solid/Complex	Calcified

• Abscesses
• Lymph nodes
• Cystic hygroma
• Atypical branchial cleft cyst
	• *Malignant:*
	  – Lymphoma
	  – Metastases
	  – Liposarcoma
	• *Benign:*
	  – Enlarged lymph nodes
	  – Lipomas
	  – Hypertrophic levator scapulae muscle
	  – Nerve sheath tumors as schwannomas, neurofibromas
		Postinflammatory nodal and abscess calcification

Prevertebral/Perivertebral Space

It is formed by the deep cervical fascia and is divided into anterior and posterior compartments by the fascia attaching to the transverse processes of the vertebra. The former contains the vertebral bodies, spinal cord, vertebral arteries, phrenic nerves, and prevertebral and scalene muscles. The latter contains the neural arches of the vertebrae and paraspinous muscles.

Lesions related to the structures in this space are discussed elsewhere.

PAROTID LESIONS

Parotid Space (Table 9)

It is located posterior to the masseter muscle and is formed by the superficial cervical fascia. Retromandibular vein forms a landmark between the superficial and deep parotid.

Criteria for intraparotid lesion:
- Parotid surrounds 50% or greater circumference of the lesion
- The epicenter of the lesion is seen lateral to the parapharyngeal space (Fig. 10)

TABLE 9: Causes of lesions in parotid space.

Cystic	Solid/Complex	Calcified

• Lymphoepithelial cyst
• First branchial cleft cyst
• Retention cyst of the salivary gland
• Lymphangioma
• Abscesses
• Enlarged lymph nodes
	• *Malignant:*
	  – Parotid gland malignancies as Warthin's tumor and adenocystic carcinoma
	• *Benign:*
	  – Infectious and inflammatory diseases of the parotid including granulomatous diseases, AIDS, Sjögren syndrome
	  – Enlarged lymph nodes
	• *Abscesses:*
	  – Hemangioma
	  – Lipoma
	  – Pleomorphic and monomorphic adenoma
		• Parotid calculi
		• Calcification in nodes, abscesses and granulomatous diseases
		• Phleboliths in hemangiomas

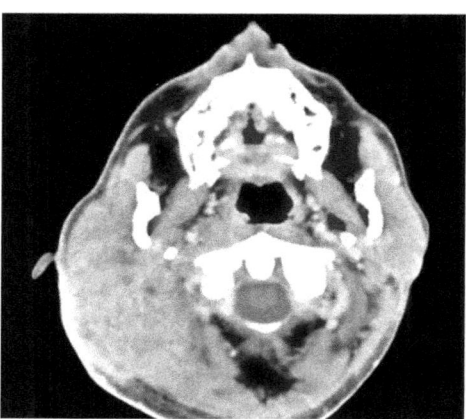

Fig. 10: Transaxial CECT image shows malignant pleomorphic adenoma of parotid gland with local invasion.

- The parapharyngeal fat is displaced medially
- The stylomandibular tunnel is widened.

Criteria for extraparotid lesion: Fat plane between the lesion and the parotid.

Lymphoepithelial Cysts

- It occurs in HIV positive patients, when it may be the earliest presentation.
- These are usually multiple with thin walls and associated cervical adenopathy.
- These are secondary to the obstruction of the intraparenchymal ducts by the lymphocytic infiltrate or may arise from the intraparotid lymph nodes.

First Branchial Cleft Cyst

- Occurs in the middle-aged women with history of multiple parotid abscesses unresponsive to treatment.
- May rupture into the external acoustic meatus resulting in otorrhea.

Hemangioma

- It is the most common parotid lesion in the infancy.
- May spontaneously regress.

Lymphangioma

- It is usually a multicystic, thin-walled lesion without contrast enhancement that does not involute spontaneously.
- Sudden increase in size may be due to hemorrhage or infection. The latter is responsible for contrast enhancement.
- Associated enlarged vessels aid differentiation between hemangioma and lymphangioma.

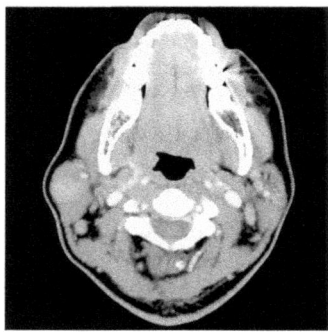

Fig. 11: Axial CECT image of neck showing enhancing lesion arising from right parotid gland in case of Warthin's tumor.

Warthin's Tumor (Papillary Cystadenoma Lymphomatosum) (Fig. 11)

- Second most common benign tumor of the parotid occurring between fourth and seventh decade of life, predominantly in males.
- May be multifocal within the parotid substance and may be bilateral as well.

LESIONS OF THE ORAL CAVITY (TABLE 10)

TABLE 10: Causes of lesions of the oral cavity.

Cystic	Solid	Complex	Calcified	Fatty
• Thyroglossal duct cyst • Ranula • Muscus retention cyst • Dermoid/epidermoid cyst • Lymphangioma	• Lingual thyroid • Hemangioma • Salivary gland tumors • Tumors of the tongue (Figs. 12A and B) • Carcinoma of the tonsil • Lymphadenopathy	• Abscess • Necrotizing fasciitis • Necrotic tumors	• Tonsillolith • Calculi in parotid and submandibular ducts	Dermoid

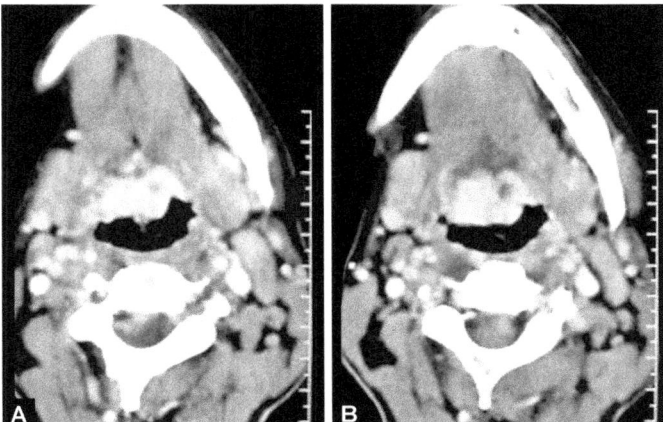

Figs. 12A and B: Transaxial CECT images showing hemangioma at base of tongue.

Lingual Thyroid

- It is seen as an intensely enhancing, soft-tissue mass in the midline of the dorsal part of the tongue.
- The attenuation values may coincide with that of the thyroid gland on both noncontrast and postcontrast images.

LARYNGEAL OR VISCERAL SPACE (TABLE 11)

It lies in the midline and is formed by the middle layer of the deep cervical fascia, and extends from the hyoid bone to the mediastinum. It contains the larynx and hypopharynx, thyroid and parathyroid, trachea and esophagus, paratracheal lymph nodes, and recurrent laryngeal nerves. Lesions of the larynx and hypopharynx are as follows.

TABLE 11: Causes of lesions in laryngeal space.

Cystic	Solid/Complex	Air-containing lesion	Calcified

• Congenital cyst
• Retention cyst of the minor salivary gland
• Laryngeal mucocele/pyocele
• Abscesses
• Lymph nodes
	• *Malignant:*
	  – Carcinomas (Figs. 13 and 14)
	  – Non-Hodgkin's lymphoma
	  – Salivary gland malignancies
	  – Fibro and liposarcoma
	  – Metastases
	• *Benign:*
	  – Enlarged lymph nodes
	  – Epiglottitis
	  – Polyps
	  – Papillomas
	  – Hemangiomas
	  – Nerve sheath tumors as schwannomas
	  – Salivary gland tumor as pleomorphic adenoma
	  – Paragangliomas
	  – Atypical carcinoid tumors
	  – Amyloidosis
		• Laryngocele
		• Abscesses
		• Enlarged pyriform sinuses
		• Prominent laryngeal ventricle
			• Tumors arising from the laryngeal cartilage as chondromas, chondrometaplasia and chondrosarcoma
			• Metastases to the laryngeal cartilage
			• Inflammatory lesions of the laryngeal cartilage as polychondritis, rheumatoid arthritis, etc.
			• Granulomatous mucosal diseases as tuberculosis
			• Postinflammatory nodal and abscess calcification
			• Postirradiation nodal calcification

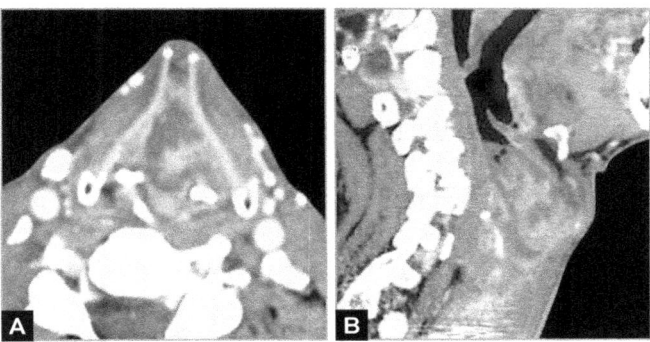

Figs. 13A and B: Axial and sagittal CT images showing carcinoma larynx completely occluding the air passage.

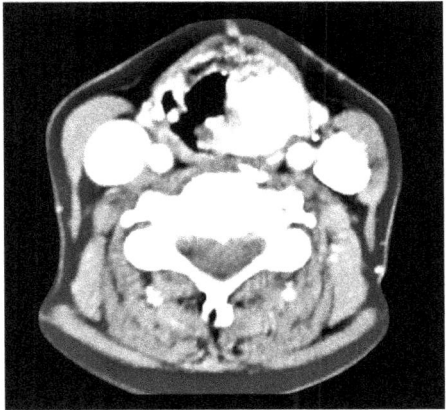

Fig. 14: Axial CECT image showing intensely enhancing mass in the left pyriform fossa.

Congenital Cyst

- It is seen as a thin-walled cyst arising in the region of the aryepiglottic fold.
- It usually develops in infancy.

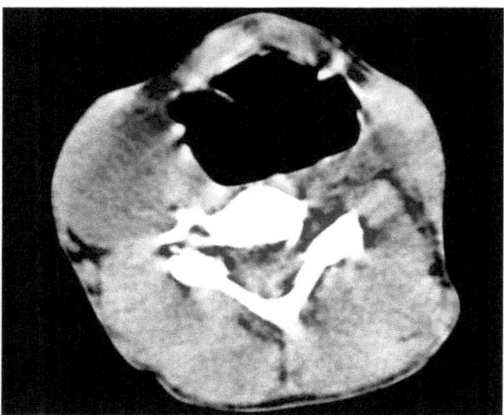

Fig. 15: Axial CT image of neck showing fluid density lesion in right paralaryngeal space, which increased in size on valsalva (not shown) suggesting external laryngocele.

- Cysts of larger sizes may bulge into the laryngeal vestibule, preepiglottic space, or the lateral part of neck.

Laryngocele (Fig. 15)

- It is an abnormal elongation and enlargement of the ventricular appendix that is filled with air.
- It is said to be *external* when it extends laterally through the thyrohyoid membrane; *internal* when it is confined by the thyrohyoid membrane; and *mixed* when both the components are present.
- Blockage at the opening of the vestibule gives rise to the fluid collection giving rise to *laryngeal mucocele* and when infected it gives rise to laryngeal pyocele.
- The differentiation is, however, to be made in cases of vocal cord paralysis that causes dilatation of the ipsilateral laryngeal ventricle.

Amyloidosis

It is characterized by submucosal thickening with nodules on the epiglottis and vocal cords.

Rheumatoid Arthritis

- It is characterized by cricoarytenoid subluxation, thickening of true vocal cords, and nodule formation.
- These findings are usually with advanced disease.

Polyp

- These are fibrous or fibroangiomatous in nature.
- They are usually seen in persons with vocal abuse.
- It is characterized by nodular lesion on the free margin of the true vocal cords at the junction of the anterior and middle third. The lesions are frequently bilateral.

Papilloma/Papillomatosis

- It is characterized by nodular lesions in the anterior half of the larynx at the level of the true vocal cords.
- These are multiple in children under 10 years of age and solitary in adults.
- The lesions may extend into the subglottic region up to the trachea and bronchi.

Chondroma

- These are seen as soft-tissue mass with scattered calcification that is arising from the laryngeal cartilages most commonly from the posterolateral surface of the cricoid cartilage.
- Rarely, chondrosarcoma may be in the same location.

Hemangioma

- It is seen as an enhancing soft-tissue mass with calcified foci (phleboliths).
- Subglottic region is the most common site in the neonates while the true vocal cords are the most common site in adults.

Other Lesions

Cervical Thymic Cyst

Usually unilateral, unilocular, or multilocular cystic lesion located anywhere between the mandibular angle and anterior mid-neck along the migratory tract of thymic tissue into the mediastinum.

Zenker's Diverticulum

It is seen as an air-distended pouch with or without fluid level originating from the pharyngoesophageal junction in relation to the posterolateral wall of the esophagus.

THYROID AND PARATHYROID GLAND LESIONS (TABLES 12 AND 13)

The average thyroid lobe measures 3 cm in greatest anteroposterior diameter and 2 cm in width.

The normal thyroid gland has a density of approximately 80–100 HU on CT due to high iodine content.

TABLE 12: Causes of thyroid and parathyroid gland lesions.	
Cystic	Solid
Colloid cyst	• Granuloma • Thyroiditis • Adenomatous hyperplasia • Adenoma • Carcinoma • Lymphoma • Metastases

Neck

TABLE 13: Differentiating features of various thyroid and parathyroid lesions.

Diseases	Differentiating features	Comments
Colloid cyst	It is seen as solitary, cystic mass with a smooth regular wall within thyroid gland	It results from colloid accumulation in macrofollicles
Thyroiditis	• *Graves' disease* is seen as diffuse enlargement of gland without nodular lesions • Prominent pyramidal lobe may be seen • NECT density is actually decreased due to decrease iodine content with marked postcontrast enhancement • *Hashimoto's thyroiditis*; marked thyroid enlargement and show inhomogeneous contrast enhancement • *De Quervain's thyroiditis*: On NECT mild thyroid enlargement is seen and has lower than normal attenuation • *Suppurative thyroiditis*: Focal or diffuse enlargement with or without abscess formation (low-density center with rim enhancement)	• Autoimmune thyroiditis • Third to fourth decade with female preponderance • Presents as hyperthyroidism • Autoimmune thyroiditis • Fourth to fifth decades may also be present in children • Present as hypothyroidism • Self-limited inflammatory process • Occurs following a viral URTI • Second to fifth decades • Uncommon and typically occurs due to bacterial infection
Thyroid granuloma	Single or multiple well-circumscribed nodules which may be calcified	Rare

Contd...

Contd...

Diseases	Differentiating Features	Comments
Adenomatous hyperplasia	Cystic (colloid degeneration or hemorrhage) or solid (degenerative) lesion in an asymmetric enlarged thyroid	Most common cold nodule in scintigraphy
Thyroid adenoma	Inhomogeneous well-circumscribed mass measuring 1–4 cm in diameter within the thyroid gland. May contain coarse calcification with irregular distribution or along periphery of lesion	• Toxic and non-functioning adenomas also found in goiters • Sudden enlargement may be seen due to spontaneous hemorrhage

Thyroid carcinoma (Figs. 16A and B)	Heterogeneous hypodense unilateral intrathyroidal mass with infiltrating margins obscuring adjacent soft-tissue planes or mass with well-defined margins simulating benign lesion. Areas of hemorrhage and necrosis may be seen. Punctate or linear calcification at the periphery are seen in approximately. 50% of cases (psammomatous bodies—most commonly in papillary carcinomas). Lymphatic spread to regional lymph nodes occurs early. Hematogenous spread more often to lung and bone	• The majority of histological classification of thyroid carcinoma includes; Papillary carcinoma; 80–90%
		  – Low-grade malignancy
		  – Cervical lymph node spread seen in 50% cases
		  – "cold" nodule in 50% cases
		• Follicular carcinoma
		  – 5% well-differentiated low-grade malignancy
		• Anaplastic carcinoma
		  – Elderly women

Contd...

Contd...

Diseases	Differentiating features	Comments
		– Highly aggressive – Associated necrotic lymph nodes seen in majority of patients
Thyroid lymphoma and metastasis	Infiltrating or well-marginated hypodense mass within the thyroid. Thyroid lymphoma more commonly present as solitary mass	• Metastasis–Rare – Lung breast and kidney are the most common site of thyroid metastasis • Lymphoma; uncommon – Increased incidence is seen with Hashimoto's thyroiditis

(URTI: upper respiratory tract infection)

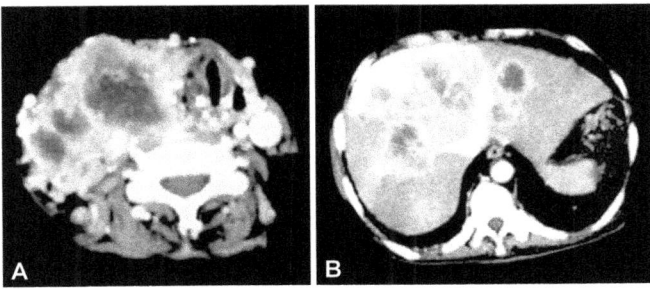

Figs. 16A and B: Axial CT images showing a large carcinoma of thyroid with hypervascular metastases in the liver.

Parathyroid Lesions

Parathyroid Cyst

- Usually located in relation to the inferior pole of the thyroid posteriorly
- Usually seen in fourth to fifth decades of life.

Parathyroid Mass

- Seen as well-circumscribed mass embedded in the thyroid bed or located at ectopic location that may be in the cervicothoracic junction or the upper mediastinum.
- Adenomas cannot be differentiated from carcinomas. The latter has a much lower occurrence than the former.

LYMPH NODES IN THE NECK

Nodes in the neck are embedded in the fat that surround the vessels and form planes separating major cervical muscles. There are ten major groups of nodes in the neck, which are broadly divided into superficial and deep group.

Superficial

- *Submental*—inferior to the anterior mandible and mylohyoid and between the digastric muscles
- *Submandibular*—in submandibular space
- *Parotid*—within the parotid gland and usually not seen, unless enlarged
- *Occipital*—in the occipital region
- *Mastoid*—near the mastoid bone
- *Facial*—along the facial vessels.

Deep

- *Retropharyngeal*—in the suprahyoid retropharyngeal space, along the lateral border of the longus capitis muscle

- *Sublingual*—deep in the floor of the mouth in the sublingual space and consists of a median group lying between the genioglossus muscles and a lateral group along the course of the lingual artery
- *Anterior*—in the anterior triangle
- *Lateral*—its superficial group is along the external jugular vein and its deep group is further subdivided into:
    - *Spinal accessory*—found in the fat of the posterior triangle and posterior cervical space lateral and posterior to the spinal accessory nerve between the trapezius and sternocleidomastoid
    - *Transverse cervical*—in the supraclavicular region
    - *Internal jugular*—along the course of internal jugular vein and further subdivided into:
        - *High*—from base of skull to carotid bifurcation/hyoid bone and includes the jugulodigastric node
        - *Middle*—from carotid bifurcation/hyoid bone to omohyoid/cricoid cartilage
        - *Low*—from omohyoid/cricoid cartilage to the clavicles and includes the nodes of Virchow.

As per the American Joint Committee on Cancer, the cervical lymph nodes are divided into seven levels based on the prognostic importance. These are:
- *Level I*—submental and submandibular nodes
- *Level II*—high internal jugular nodes
- *Level III*—middle internal jugular nodes
- *Level IV*—low internal jugular nodes
- *Level V*—spinal accessory and transverse cervical nodes
- *Level VI*—pretracheal, paratracheal and prelaryngeal nodes
- *Level VII*—nodes in the tracheoesophageal groove and upper mediastinum.

Size Criteria for Lymphadenopathy

- At levels I and II, the maximum transaxial diameter is >1.5 cm and the minimum transaxial diameter is >1.1 cm.

- At levels III to VII, the maximum and minimum transaxial diameters is >1 cm.
- Clusters are seen as three or more contiguous, ill-defined nodes at the same level ranging from 8 mm to 15 mm in diameter.
- The ratio of the maximum longitudinal to maximal transaxial diameter (L/T) of the enlarged nodes is also significant. Ratio of <2 suggests a high possibility of malignancy while a ratio of >2 suggests a high possibility of benign process.

Shape Criteria

- Round nodes tend to be neoplastic.
- Elliptical or bean-shaped nodes are normal or hyperplastic.

Central Hypodensity in Nodes

- Suppuration
- Metastatic (Fig. 17)
- Fatty change seen in hilum of normal nodes, but may also be seen secondary to infection or irradiation.

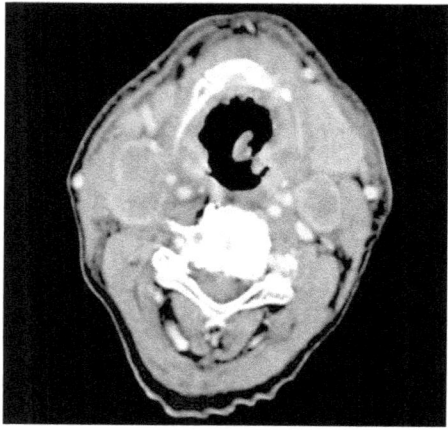

Fig. 17: Axial CT image showing bilateral metastatic lymphadenopathy.

Calcification in Nodes

- Granulomatous diseases as tuberculosis
- Previously irradiated neoplastic nodes
- Metastatic tumors as thyroid carcinoma.

DIFFERENTIAL DIAGNOSIS OF THYROID DISEASES (TABLE 14)

TABLE 14: Differential diagnosis of thyroid lesions.

Diseases	Differentiating features	Comments
Thyroglossal duct cyst	<ul><li>Isodense to water</li><li>Hyperdense when there is high protein content</li></ul>	<ul><li>Infrahyoid—65%</li><li>At hyoid—15%</li><li>Suprahyoid—20%</li></ul>
Graves' disease	<ul><li>Enlarged thyroid demonstrates avid enhancement</li><li>Noncontrast CT density is actually decreased, reflecting a decrease in iodine concentration even though there is an overall increase in the iodine content of the gland</li></ul>	<ul><li>*Peak incidence*: Third to fourth decades with female predominance</li><li>There is marked enlargement of thyroid without focal nodules (diffuse toxic goiter). Also there may be prominent enlargement of pyramidal lobe</li><li>Vascularity is increased</li></ul>
Hashimoto's thyroiditis (chronic lymphocytic thyroiditis)	<ul><li>There is an inhomogeneous distribution of iodine</li><li>Following contrast administration, it shows enhancement</li></ul>	<ul><li>Painless diffuse enlargement of gland in young or middle-aged women</li><li>Antibodies develops against thyroglobulin, thyroperoxidase, and TSH receptors</li></ul>

Contd...

Contd...

Diseases	Differentiating features	Comments
De Quervain's thyroiditis (subacute granulomatous thyroiditis)	Shows lower than normal attenuation	• Self-limited inflammatory process occurs following viral URTI by coxsackievirus and mumps • Present with fever, goiter, and pain on palpation
Acute suppurative thyroiditis	Affected portion will be enlarged and heterogeneous in CT density	• Caused by bacterial infection • Infection usually begins in perithyroidal tissue
Riedel's thyroiditis (struma)	On CT thyroid may be hypodense	• Rare form of chronic thyroiditis characterized by a fibrosing reaction similar to that seen in retroperitoneal fibrosis, which destroys thyroid and extends into adjacent soft tissue • Confused with malignancy (anaplastic variety)
Thyroid goiter	• Asymmetric gland with multiple low density areas reflecting regions of hemorrhage, cyst formation, or necrosis • Focal region of hyperdensity are common reflecting calcification, hemorrhage, or colloid	• Goiter—any clinical enlargement of thyroid gland • Simple goiter • Multinodular goiter—characterized by nodularity, focal hemorrhage, focal calcifications, cyst formation, and scarring

Contd...

Contd...

Diseases	Differentiating features	Comments
Colloid cyst	Solitary cystic mass with a smooth regular wall within the thyroid gland	- Colloid accumulation in macrofollicle - These simple cysts are extremely uncommon
Adenomatous hyperplasia	Cystic (colloid degeneration or hemorrhage) or solid (degenerative) lesions in an asymmetrically enlarged thyroid	Most common "cold" nodule in scintigraphy
Thyroid adenoma	- Inhomogeneous well-circumscribed mass measuring 1–4 cm in diameter within thyroid gland - May contain coarse calcifications with irregular distribution	- Most result in no thyroid dysfunction - <10% develops autonomy and may cause thyrotoxicosis. - Most adenomas are solitary, but may also develops as a part of a multinodular process
Papillary carcinoma	- Imaging appearance may include a dominant nodule, multiple nodules, diffuse infiltration of gland that manifest as heterogeneous hypodensity, or normal appearing gland on CT - Metastatic lymph node may be calcified, cystic, hemorrhagic, or may contain colloid	Accounts for 60–70% of all thyroid malignancies commonly spreads along the rich lymphatic system within and adjacent to the thyroid gland accounting for the multifocal nature of the tumor within the thyroid gland and its spread to regional lymph nodes

Contd...

Contd...

Diseases	Differentiating features	Comments
Follicular carcinoma	Cannot be differentiated from follicular adenoma on imaging	• Capsular and vascular invasion on histopathology is required for diagnosis • Hematogeneous seeding is more common than lymphatic spread
Medullary carcinoma	• Associated coarse calcification • At presentation, 50% of cases have nodal metastases and 15–25% have distant metastases to liver, lungs, and bone	Medullary carcinoma is believed to arise from parafollicular C-cells that secrete thyrocalcitonin may be associated with MEN syndrome
Anaplastic carcinoma	Punctate calcifications and necrosis are frequently present nodal or distant metastases in 80% of patients; the involved lymph nodes show evidence of necrosis	• Anaplastic carcinoma is one of the most aggressive head and neck cancers and has a grave prognosis • Patients frequently present with signs and symptoms of airway compression
Thyroid lymphoma and metastases	Infiltrating or well-marginated mass within the thyroid similar to thyroid carcinoma	Rare

(TSH: thyroid-stimulating hormone; URTI: upper respiratory tract infection; MEN: multiple endocrine neoplasia)

DIFFERENTIAL DIAGNOSIS OF PAROTID LESIONS (TABLE 15)

TABLE 15: Differential diagnosis of parotid lesions.

Diseases	Differentiating features	Comments
Acute parotitis	Enlarged gland, abnormal attenuation or intensity, and avid enhancement	Main predisposition factor are dehydration and poor dental hygiene
• Viral (mumps and cytomegalovirus) • Bacterial (*Staphylococcus* and *Streptococcus*)	• Central ducts are dilated and wall of duct shows enhancement • There is usually inflammatory stranding into the overlying subcutaneous tissue and thickening of the investing deep cervical fascia	Infection may progress to an abscess
Granulomatous sialadenitis (tuberculosis, candida, catscratch fever)	Unilateral or less commonly bilateral diffuse enlargement of the parotid gland, multiple small nodular densities distributed throughout the gland, or a solitary mass	• Presents usually as progressive, localized, or diffuse painless glandular enlargement • Associated with sarcoidosis, tuberculosis, etc.
Chronic recurrent sialadenitis	Unilateral, diffusely enlarged, often slightly denser than normal parotid gland. Dilated Stensen duct with or without calculi may be evident	• Recurrent painful swelling • Usually associated with incomplete obstruction of the Stensen duct

Contd...

Contd...

Diseases	Differentiating features	Comments
Sialosis	• Slightly enlarged parotid gland which may appear dense or fatty depending upon the dominant pathologic change • CT sialogram is normal except for intraglandular splaying of the ducts by the increased volume	• Sialosis is a noninflammatory, nonneoplastic, recurrent, painless salivary gland swelling, usually bilateral • Sialosis has been described in connection with endocrine diseases, malnutrition, hepatic cirrhosis, chronic alcoholism, or different deficiency diseases (e.g. avitaminoses)
Sjögren syndrome	• Appearance ranges from normal findings to glandular enlargement with increased attenuation at CT • Advanced Sjögren disease typically has a "salt and pepper" or "honeycomb" appearance • CT sialogram reveals a normal central duct system and numerous punctate collections of contrast material uniformly scattered throughout the gland	• Sjögren syndrome is a chronic autoimmune disease predominantly affecting women over 40 years of age • It is characterized by intense lymphocytic and plasma cell infiltration and destruction of salivary and lacrimal glands • Frequently associated with both reactive and neoplastic lymphoproliferative disease

Contd...

Contd...

Diseases	Differentiating features	Comments
First branchial cleft cyst	• Cystic mass with varying wall thickness depending on the degree of inflammation • Lesion is located either within parotid gland or at its periphery	Occurs most often in middle-aged women presenting with a history of "multiple parotid abscesses unresponsive to treatment"
Hemangioma	• Capillary hemangiomas—CECT demonstrates a well-defined mass with uniform, intense enhancement • Cavernous hemangiomas—NCCT • Phleboliths are occasionally seen • After contrast material administration, there is a variable pattern of enhancement	• Congenital capillary hemangiomas represent 90% of parotid gland tumors during the first year of life, whereas cavernous hemangiomas rarely involve the parotid gland • Capillary hemangiomas manifest as a soft mass noted shortly after birth
Lymphangioma	• Heterogeneous with septations and cystic areas • Often contains fluid-fluid levels, and solid portions of the lesion may enhance	Lymphangiomas are classified on the basis of the size of the cystic spaces as lymphangioma simplex, cavernous lymphangioma, or venolymphatic malformations

Contd...

Contd...

Diseases	Differentiating features	Comments
Pleomorphic adenomas	Small tumors are more homogeneous and well-defined with higher attenuation with strong enhancement after contrast medium administration whereas larger tumors tend to have pedunculated outgrowth from the main lesion (lobulated contour and are more heterogeneous including necrotic and hemorrhagic areas	• Most common benign salivary gland tumor in adults fourth to fifth decades. F>M usually solitary and unilateral grow slowly and may be asymptomatic. Pleomorphic adenomas may contain small calcifications • Nontreated cases may undergo malignant transformation after decades
Warthin's tumor	• Present as well-circumscribed, small, ovoid, smoothly marginated masses, partly cystic, partly solid lesions often located in the tail of the parotid gland • Enhancement after contrast medium administration is often relatively poor	• Adenolymphoma or papillary cystadenoma lymphomatosum • It is the second most common benign parotid gland neoplasm in adults and children fifth to sixth decades M>F • Warthin's tumor is usually solitary, unilateral, and slow growing

Contd...

Contd...

Diseases	Differentiating features	Comments
		• In about 10–60% of cases, tumors may occur bilaterally or multifocally (most common salivary gland tumor to present with multifocal or bilateral involvement)
Mucoepider-moid carcinoma	Low-grade lesions are well circumscribed, whereas high grade lesions tend to have poor margins and infiltrate surrounding tissues	The most common malignant tumors in children and adults third to fifth decades
Adenoid cystic carcinoma	On CECT widened nerve may be seen in a widened bony neural canal and obliterating the normal fat present at the extracranial opening of these canals	It usually presents as an infiltrating mass with a high propensity for perineural spread Perineural disease can also present with "skip" lesions distally in a nerve that seems to be normal
Other carcinomas of parotid	Low-grade lesions are benign in appearance with well-delineated smooth borders	Includes acinic cell carcinoma, salivary duct carcinoma, adenocarcinoma, etc.

Contd...

Contd...

Diseases	Differentiating features	Comments
Lymphoma	• CT demonstrate focal masses confined to an intraparotid lymph node or diffuse parotid infiltration • CT usually demonstrates slight homogeneous enhancement following contrast material administration	• Primary lymphoma of the salivary glands most often involves the parotid gland and is classified as a MALToma, indicating its origin from mucosal lymphoid tissue • Secondary lymphoma of the salivary glands is also rare, but like primary disease most commonly involves the parotid gland
Metastases	One or multiple homogeneous focal lesions or diffuse infiltration of entire gland	• Metastases to salivary glands are mainly observed in the parotid gland due to the presence of intraglandular lymph nodes, which drain the face, external ear, and scalp • Skin malignancies (melanoma, squamous cell carcinomas) are the most common primary tumors metastasizing to the salivary glands

Chapter 7

Chest

PULMONARY NODULAR AND CAVITATING LESIONS

Solitary Pulmonary Nodule

A solitary pulmonary nodule (SPN) is defined as a single discrete pulmonary opacity smaller than 3 cm that is surrounded by normal lung tissue and is not associated with adenopathy or atelectasis.

Malignant Lesions (Table 1)

- Bronchogenic carcinoma
- Carcinoid
- Solitary metastasis.

Benign Lesions (Table 1)

- *Benign neoplasms*: Hamartoma, lipomas, and fibroma
- *Vascular lesions*: Arteriovenous malformation
- *Infectious granuloma*: Tuberculosis, atypical mycobacterial infection, histoplasmosis, coccidioidomycosis, and blastomycosis
- *Other infections*: Bacterial abscess, echinococcal cyst, aspergilloma, ascariasis, and filariasis
- *Noninfectious granuloma*: Rheumatoid arthritis, Wegener's granulomatosis, and sarcoidosis
- *Developmental lesions*: Bronchogenic cyst and pulmonary sequestration

- *Other conditions*: Hematoma, bronchiolitis obliterans, organizing pneumonia, pseudotumor, pulmonary infarction, rounded atelectasis, and mucoid impaction.

There are various features on CT scan, which can be helpful in differentiating benign and malignant nodules.

TABLE 1: Differentiating features of benign and malignant lesions on CT.

Characteristic	Benign	Malignant	Remarks
Nodule size growth (doubling time)	<2 cm 20–30 days or >400 days (stability of the lesion size over a 2-year period is a very reliable indicator)	>3 cm 30–400 days (meta-stases can have a shorter doubling time)	• Doubling time is the time required for a nodule to double in volume (26% increase in nodule diameter) • Small lung malignancies can double in volume and yet appear radiologically stable. Hence, assessment of growth rate is better by measurement of volume
Margins	Well-circumscribed smooth borders	Irregular, lobulated, or spiculated (corona radiata) borders	• Spiculated border is the most sensitive in predicting malignancy • Lobulation occurs in up to 25% of benign nodules

Contd...

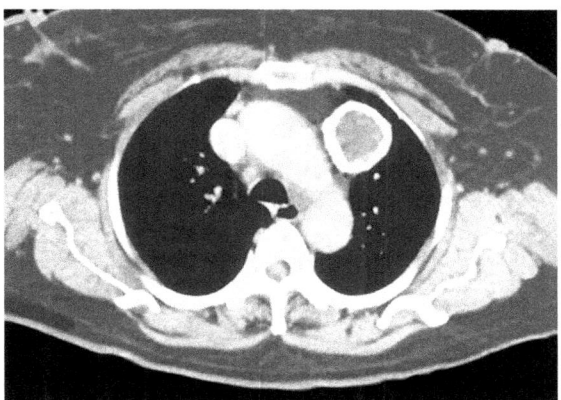

Fig. 1: Axial contrast-enhanced computed tomography (CECT) image of chest showing soft tissue lesion with concentric calcification in left upper lobe suggesting calcified granuloma.

Contd...

Characteristic	Benign	Malignant	Remarks
Calcification pattern	Five patterns of calcification are seen commonly, including diffuse, central, laminar, concentric (chondroid) (Fig. 1) and popcorn calcifications	Stippled or eccentric pattern	Calcification within a nodule is more likely to be seen in a benign nodule; however, approximately 10% of malignant nodules demonstrate calcification
Intranodular fat	Present	Absent	Fat is seen at CT in up to 50% of hamartoma and is best visualized at thinner sections CT

Contd...

Contd...

Characteristic	Benign	Malignant	Remarks
Cavitation wall thickness	Smooth, thin and regular walls <4 mm	Nodular, thick, irregular walls >16 mm	Abscesses may have slightly nodular walls but the thickness is less relative to the malignant lesions
Pseudocavitation	Absent	Present (in bronchiolo-alveolar cell carcinoma and lymphoma)	Small, focal, low-attenuation regions within or surrounding the periphery of a nodule and air bronchograms within a nodule
Feeding vessel sign	Present in septic emboli, AVM, etc.	Present in metastatic emboli	
Contrast enhancement	<15 HU	>20 HU	Assessment of enhancement involves repeated measurement of attenuation of a nodule over a 5-minute period

(AVM: arteriovenous malformation; HU: Hounsfield unit)

Solitary pulmonary nodule with calcification includes:
- Congenital—hamartoma and vascular malformation.
- Infections/infestation—granuloma (tubercular, histoplasmosis), hydatidosis, filariasis, and dracunculiasis
- Tumors—benign (teratoma, carcinoid, adenoma), malignant (bronchogenic tumor, metastases—osteosarcoma, chondrosarcoma, mucinous adenocarcinoma, germ cell tumors, thyroid carcinoma, and synovial sarcoma).

Solitary pulmonary nodule can be grouped based on the location into various categories (Table 2).

TABLE 2: Classification and differentiating features of solitary pulmonary nodule (SPN) according to zones in lungs.

Upper zone	Lower zone
Tuberculoma: <ul><li>More common on the right side</li><li>0.5–4 cm, rounded nodules that usually have surrounding associated satellite lesions</li><li>Cavitation is uncommon and when present is small and eccentric</li></ul> *Carcinoma especially with necrosis*: <ul><li>They have eccentric cavitation</li><li>More commonly seen in squamous cell carcinoma with peripheral location</li></ul> *Progressive massive fibrosis*: <ul><li>Usually multiple</li><li>Begin peripherally and move centrally; also involves the mid-zones</li><li>Background nodularity of pneumoconiosis may be present</li></ul>	*Pulmonary sequestration*: <ul><li>Two-thirds occur in the left lower lobe and one-third in the right lower lobe</li><li>Emphysematous elements may be present, and adjacent atelectasis often exists</li><li>Most lesions appear hypervascular</li><li>Mucoid impaction of a bronchus surrounded by hyperinflated lung is believed to be characteristic of intralobar type</li><li>Lesions of extralobar type (ELS) may occur above or below the diaphragm, sometimes in the retroperitoneum</li></ul> *Bronchogenic cyst*: <ul><li>Two-thirds are intrapulmonary and lie in medial one-third of lower lobes. It is usually intrapulmonary and mediastinal</li></ul>

Lower zone

Histoplasmosis:
- Venous collaterals can be seen, indicative of long-standing venous occlusion.
- Stippled or dense central calcification within the mass giving a target appearance is present in most of these patients with fibrosing mediastinitis.

Contd...

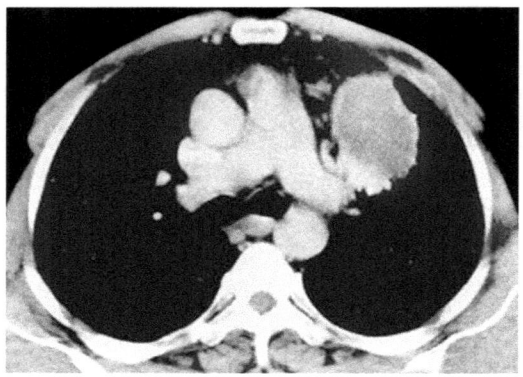

Fig. 2: Transaxial CT image shows hydatid cyst in left lung anteriorly.

Contd...

Hydatid cyst (Fig. 2):
- The *meniscus sign*, or *crescent sign*, is characterized by the presence of air between the pericyst and the laminated membrane, appears as growth continues and the cysts erode adjacent bronchioles.
- Cystic rupture may result in different radiologic signs. The *cumbo sign*, or *onion peel sign*, is defined as the presence of the meniscus sign and an air-fluid level within the endocyst. The *water lily sign* represents an endocyst floating in a partially fluid-filled cyst, whereas an endocyst floating in a completely fluid-filled cyst is said to have a "mass within the cavity" appearance.

Pulmonary infarction (Figs. 3A and B):
- Usually associated with a pleural effusion or elevation of the hemidiaphragm
- *Arteriovenous malformation (Figs. 4A and B):*
    - Well-defined, rounded, or lobulated mass of variable diameter
    - It has predilection for the inner third of the lungs
    - Demonstration of the feeding artery and veins is diagnostic.
- *Pulmonary varix:*
    - Well-defined, rounded or lobulated mass of variable diameter
    - Present in close proximity to left atrium
    - Contrast enhancement simultaneously with the left atrium is diagnostic

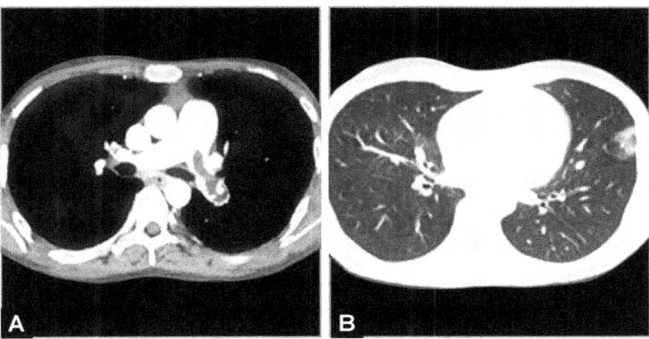

Figs. 3A and B: Axial CT images showing thrombus in the left pulmonary artery with extension into the lobar artery with resultant pulmonary infarct in the left upper lobe.

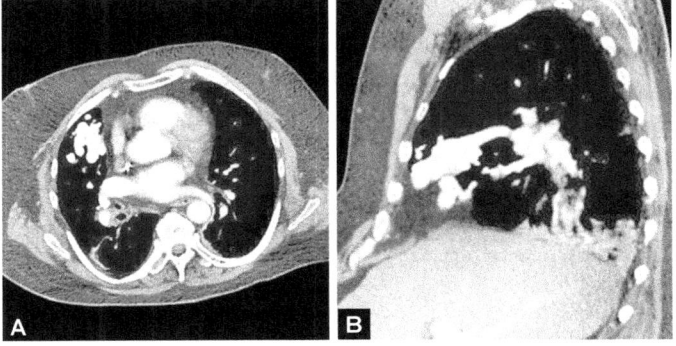

Figs. 4A and B: Axial and sagittal CECT images showing presence of arteriovenous malformation in right lung.

Solitary pulmonary nodule can be seen in peripheral or central location (Table 3).

TABLE 3: Classification and differentiating features of SPN according to location in lungs.

Central lesions	Peripheral lesions
Bronchial carcinoid: • 80% arise in the main, lobar, or segmental bronchi • Calcification is common • Lesions are highly vascular and usually demonstrate marked homogeneous enhancement • Large polypoidal lesions, which partly obstruct the bronchus, may produce a ball-valve affect, resulting in hyperinflation or expiratory air trapping *Squamous cell carcinoma:* • Most likely to cavitate. Squamous cell carcinomas grow intraluminally and are least likely to metastasize distantly *Small cell carcinoma*	*Metastasis:* • 25% of pulmonary nodules are solitary • Calcification is rare but occurs with metastatic osteosarcoma, chondrosarcoma, etc. • Hilar adenopathy and effusions are uncommon • They may be ill-defined or well-defined; ill definition suggests prostate, breast, or stomach *Adenocarcinoma (Figs. 5A and B):* • It may arise from a previous scar and rarely cavitates • An eccentric pattern of calcification may be evident • An early propensity is noted of metastases to the lymph nodes, pleura, adrenal glands, central nervous system, and bone *Large cell carcinoma:* • The lesion grows rapidly with early metastases and a poor outcome

Contd...

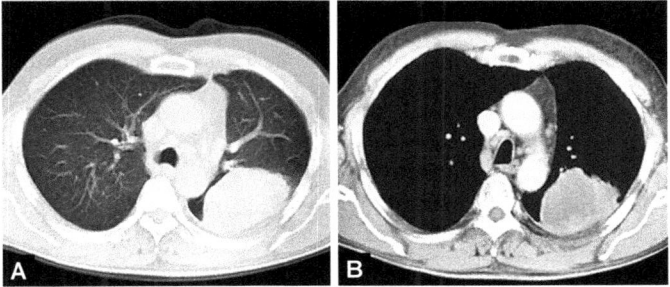

Figs. 5A and B: Axial CT images of chest show heterogeneously enhancing peripheral mass lesion abutting the pleura in a biopsy proven adenocarcinoma lung.

Contd...

Peripheral lesions

Hamartoma:
- Show varying patterns of calcification, including irregular popcorn, stippled, or curvilinear pattern, or even a combination of all three
- On high-resolution computed tomography, fat attenuation is detectable in 34% of tumors, and fat and calcium in 19%.
- The finding of both fat and calcification is a specific combination for hamartoma, particularly in tumors smaller than 2.5 cm in diameter.

Hematoma:
- Peripheral, smooth, and well-defined, 2–6 cm, slow resolution over several weeks

Adenoma:
- Well-defined, rounded lesion with postcontrast enhancement

Localized form of alveolar cell carcinoma:
- When small, it presents as a well-defined nodule with pleural tags
- Larger lesions show air bronchogram and irregular margins (sunburst pattern).

Age

Our main aim is to exclude the malignant lesion, incidence of which increases with age in the following manner:
- Risk of 3% at age 35–39 years
- Risk of 15% at age 40–49 years
- Risk of 43% at age 50–59 years
- Risk of greater than 50% in patients older than 60 years.

Lesions

Lesions, which are commonly seen in pediatric age group, include:
- *Pneumonia*:
    - Simple consolidation, especially pneumococcal. Air bronchogram will be seen.
    - Rounded pneumonia/atelectasis is commonly seen in the lower lobes in the posterior segments. It has Ill-defined margins with air bronchogram.
- Hydatid disease
- *Bronchogenic cyst*:
    - A bronchogenic cyst appears as a single, smooth, round, or elliptical mass with an imperceptible wall and uniform attenuation
    - Commonly located in perihilar region
    - It demonstrates water or soft-tissue density. Cysts do not enhance after administration of intravenous (IV) contrast
    - The attenuation value is dependent on the contents of the cyst and can vary from water attenuation to soft-tissue attenuation. The value can be >100 HU owing to a high protein level or calcium oxalate in the mucoid cyst.
    - Air within the cyst is uncommon and suggestive of secondary infection and communication with the tracheobronchial tree.
    - Calcification occurs occasionally in the wall or within the cyst contents.
- Pleuropulmonary blastoma
- Rhabdomyosarcoma
- Bronchogenic carcinoma

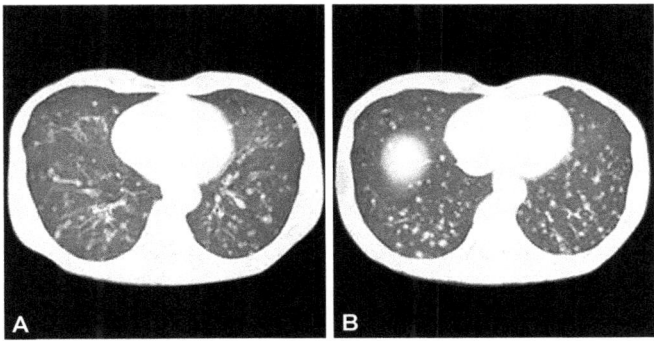

Figs. 6A and B: Axial CT images showing pulmonary metastases.

- *Metastases (Figs. 6A and B):*
  - Majority of lung nodules are benign even in child with known malignancy; one-third of new lung nodules may be benign.
  - Common primary tumor metastasizing to the lungs includes osteosarcoma, Ewing sarcoma, Wilms' tumor, etc.

Cavitatory lesions can be divided into the various categories (Table 4).

TABLE 4: Causes of various cavitatory lesions.	
Malignant	*Benign*

• Squamous cell
• Adenocarcinoma
• Lymphoma
• Metastatic carcinoma (Fig. 7)
	• *Infections:*
	  – *Staphylococcus aureus*
	  – *Streptococcus species*
	  – *Mycobacterium tuberculosis*
	  – *Fusobacterium species*
	  – *Klebsiella pneumoniae*
	  – Aspergillosis
	  – Paragonimiasis
	  – *Bacteroides* species
	  – *Cryptococcus*
	  – *Entamoeba*

Contd...

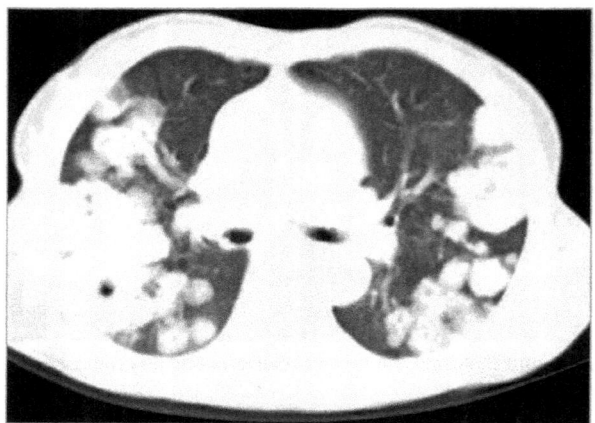

Fig. 7: Axial CT image showing multiple pulmonary metastases with necrosis noted in some of the lesions.

Contd...

Malignant	Benign

	• *Autoimmune disease*:
	  – Wegener syndrome granulomatosis
	  – Sjögren syndrome
	  – Necrobiotic nodule of rheumatoid disease
	• *Trauma*:
	  – Pulmonary laceration
	  – Pneumatocele
	  – Hematoma
	• *Congenital*:
	  – Bronchogenic cyst
	  – Sequestration of lobe
	  – Diaphragmatic hernia (Figs. 8 and 9)
	  – Cystic adenomatoid malformation (Types I and II)

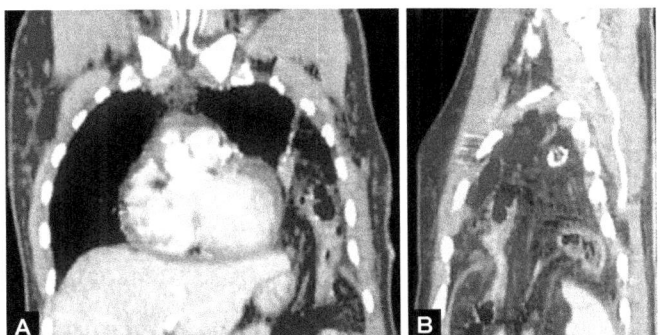

Figs. 8A and B: CT scans showing a left-sided diaphragmatic hernia with intrathoracic herniation of the stomach and splenic flexure along with mesenteric fat and vessels.

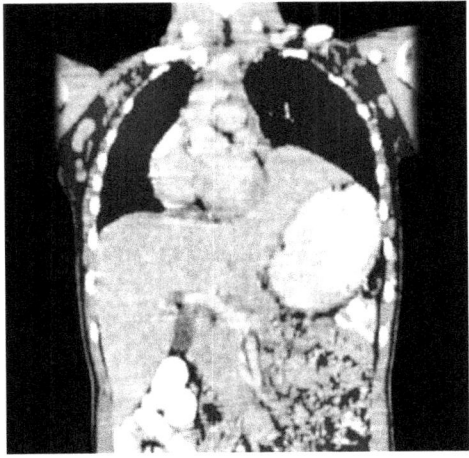

Fig. 9: Coronal CT image showing eventration of left dome with left hepatic lobe herniation that is a close differential diagnosis of diaphragmatic hernia.

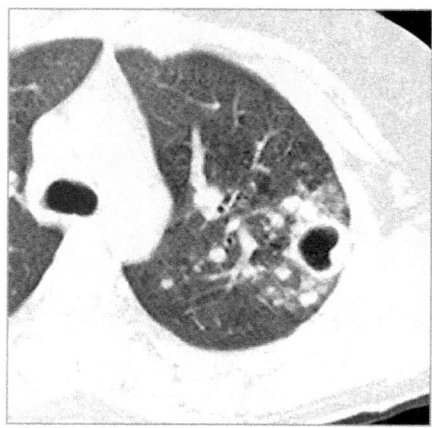

Fig. 10: A peripheral cavitating lesion with thick walls with an eccentric nodule and multiple surrounding satellite nodules highly suggestive of an abscess.

Cavitatory lesions can be divided into thin or thick walled:
- *Thick walled includes*:
    - Bacterial abscess (Fig. 10)
        - Thick-walled with a ragged inner lining
        - Associated with effusion and empyema or pyopneumothorax
        - Almost invariable in children not so common in adults
        - Pneumatoceles may also be seen during the resolution phase.
    - Blastomycosis/actinomycosis/cryptococcosis/nocardiosis
        - Usually reveal focal lung opacities in the lower lobes often nodular in character
        - Cavitation occurs less commonly in patients with blastomycosis than in patients with tuberculosis or chronic histoplasmosis.

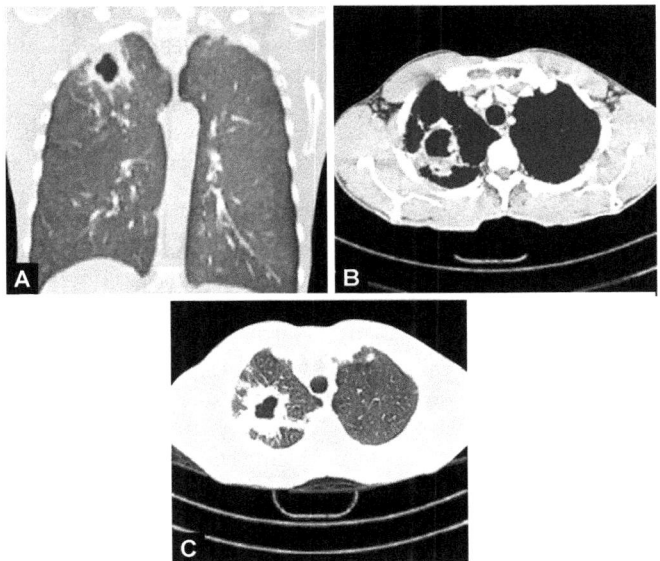

Figs. 11A to C: Coronal and axial CT images showing a thick-walled cavity (biopsy showed squamous cell carcinoma).

- Wegener granulomatosis
    - Widespread disease with cavitation in some of the nodules
    - Thick-walled becoming thinner with time.
- Necrotizing squamous cell carcinoma (Figs. 11A to C)
- Lymphoma
    - Thick or thin walled, and typically in an area of infiltration
    - Hilar and mediastinal lymphadenopathy is commonly associated.
- *Thin walled includes*:
    - Chronic tuberculous cavity
    - Bulla
        - There may be presence of air fluid level

- Coccidioidomycosis
  - The nodules frequently are well-defined, simulating metastasis, or they may be ill-defined
  - They have a parahilar and lower lobe distribution.
  - Focal area of ground-glass attenuation may be seen.
  - Nodules may show cavitation, foci of calcifications, and central lucency.
- Emboli
  - Aseptic cavitation is usually multiple and arises in large area of consolidation after about 2 weeks
  - If localized to a segment, the most common sites are apical segment of lower lobe.
  - Majority has scalloped inner margins and cross-cavity band shadows. Effusion may be seen.
- Paragonimiasis
  - Radiological findings in early stage include pneumothorax or hydropneumothorax (Fig. 12), focal air space consolidation, and linear opacities and are caused by the migration of juvenile worms.
  - Later findings include thin-walled cysts, dense mass-like consolidation, nodules, or bronchiectasis and are due to worm cysts.

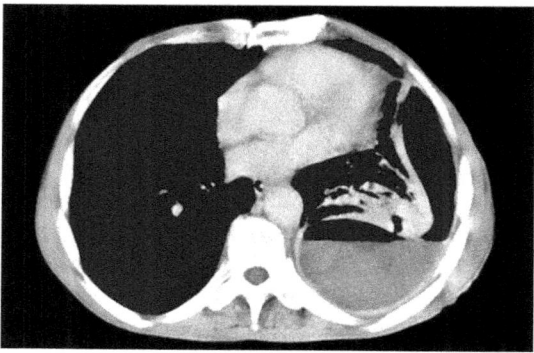

Fig. 12: Transaxial CT image shows presence of hydropneumothorax on left side.

- Hydatid/amebiasis
- Metastasis from squamous cell carcinoma
- *Pneumocystis carinii* pneumonia *(PCP)*
    - Initially, scattered foci of ground-glass opacity of air space consolidation is seen tend to decrease in size or resolve after the acute stage of the infection.
    - In treated patients with resolving of subacute infection, reticular opacities representing thickened interlobular septa and intralobular lines can be seen in association with ground-glass opacity.
    - Cysts related to PCP are usually multiple, occur most often in the upper zones of the lungs.
- Post-traumatic cysts
    - Single or multiple, may be unilocular or multilocular
    - Distinguished from cavitating hematomas as they present early, within hours of the injury.
- Pneumatoceles
- Cystic fibrosis.

MASS WITHIN A CAVITY

- Blood clot in a cavity
- Hydatid cyst (ectocyst separation from a pericyst)
- Debris within an abscess (e.g. septic emboli)
- Fungal ball in a cavity (mobile nature may be demonstrable with change in posture)
- Necrotic tissue in a cavitating pulmonary neoplasm.

Some important points about wall thickening:
- *<1 mm*: Virtually always benign
- *1–5 mm*: 96% benign
- *5–15 mm*: 50% benign/50% malignant
- *>15 mm*: 92% malignant
- More irregular and thicker the wall, greater probability of neoplastic disease.

INTERSTITIAL LUNG DISEASES

The various interstitial lung diseases can cause five main radiographic patterns (Figs. 13 and 14; Table 5).

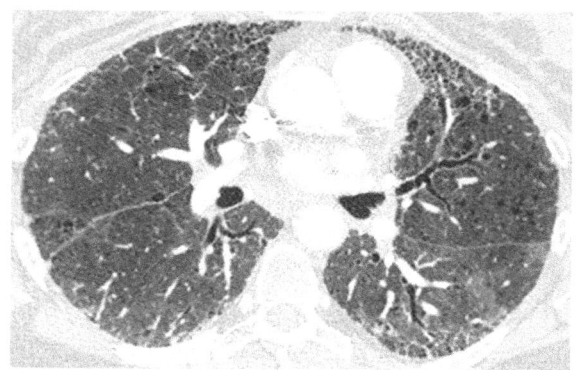

Fig. 13: Axial high-resolution CT scan showing features of interstitial disease.

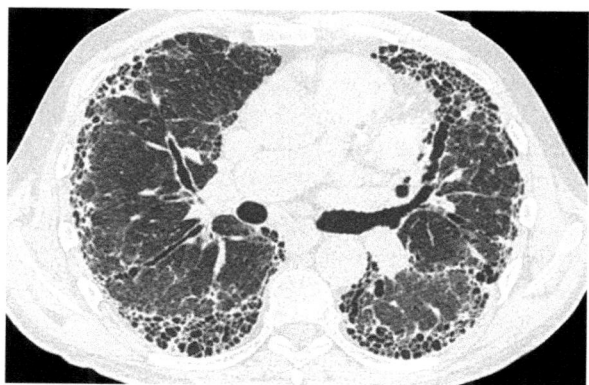

Fig. 14: Axial high-resolution CT scan of lungs showing subpleural honeycomb cysts in interstitial lung disease.

TABLE 5: Common causes of interstitial lung diseases according to radiographic patterns.

Septal pattern		Reticular pattern	Nodular pattern	Reticulonodular pattern	Ground-glass pattern
Smooth	Beaded				
• Interstitial pulmonary edema • Lymphocytic interstitial pneumonia • Leukemia	• Lymphangitis carcinomatosa • Sarcoidosis • Fibrosing alveolitis • Sarcoidosis	• Chronic extrinsic allergic alveolitis • Asbestosis • Langerhans' cell histiocytosis • Drug-induced pneumonitis (methotrexate, gold salts) • Radiation pneumonitis • Collagen vascular diseases (rheumatoid arthritis, SLE, ankylosing arthritis)	• Perilymphatic (sarcoidosis) • Centrilobular (subacute extrinsic allergic alveolitis, bronchiolitis) • Bronchovascular (leukemia, lymphoma, Kaposi's sarcoma) • Random (silicosis, coal workers' pneumoconiosis, granulomatous disease) • Cavitating (tuberculosis, fungal, septic emboli, metastases, Wegener's granulomatosis)	• Langerhans' cell histiocytosis • Sarcoidosis • Lymphangitis carcinomatosa	• Subacute extrinsic allergic alveolitis • *Pneumocystis carinii* pneumonia • Desquamative interstitial pneumonia • Nonspecific interstitial pneumonia • Idiopathic pulmonary hemorrhage and edema • Lymphocytic interstitial pneumonia

(SLE: systemic lupus erythematosus)

Pulmonary Edema

- Intrapulmonary vessels lose their normally sharp margins due to edema fluid in the surrounding lymphatic spaces. This is seen as perivascular "cuffing." Peribronchial cuffing is also seen.
- Septal edema becomes visible when edema fluid enters into the interlobular septa. Kerley B lines represent these thickened septa and are seen in the periphery of the lungs, perpendicular to the pleural surface, no longer than 2 cm in length.
- Less commonly seen are Kerley A lines, which are due to edema fluid in the central pulmonary septa. These are lines radiating from the hila, 2–6 cm long, thin, and nonbranching. They are best seen in the upper zones.
- Kerley C lines are short lines, seen centrally at the lung bases.
- Alveolar pulmonary edema is seen as a generalized hazy air space opacification. It may occur in the right lung first, and tends to be perihilar in distribution initially, before becoming bilateral and generalized.

Lymphangitis Carcinomatosa

- There is uniform often nodular thickening of the interlobular septa and irregular thickening of the bronchovascular bundles in the central portions of the lungs.
- There is often patchy air space shadowing. Nodular shadows may be seen scattered throughout the parenchyma.
- It may involve all zones or may be predominantly central or peripheral.
- Hilar lymph node enlargement is seen in only some patients.

Fibrosing Alveolitis (Idiopathic Pulmonary Fibrosis)

- It is characterized by fine reticular pattern that is symmetric and most prominent at the bases with ground-glass opacification.
- The distribution of disease is in subpleural location and at bases.

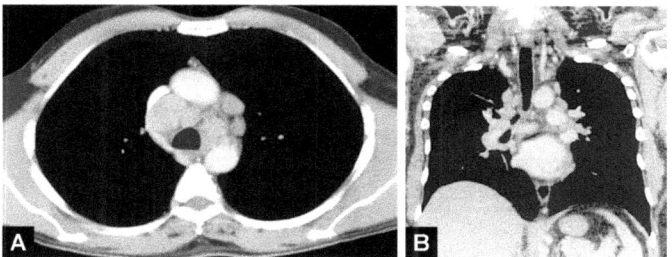

Figs. 15A and B: Axial and coronal CECT images showing mediastinal lymphadenopathy in sarcoidosis.

- As the "fibrosis" progresses, the reticular pattern becomes coarser, and there is progressive loss of lung volume.
- In the end stage, there is honeycombing and dilated pulmonary arteries due to pulmonary arterial hypertension.

Sarcoidosis (Figs. 15A and B)

- There is perilymphatic distribution of lesions in the form of thickening of bronchovascular bundle, septal thickening, and subpleural nodules.
- Presence of bilateral and symmetric hilar and mediastinal lymphadenopathy are helpful for the diagnosis of sarcoidosis.
- Patchy areas of ground-glass opacity are sometimes that is usually considered to correlate with disease activity.

Extrinsic Allergic Alveolitis (Hypersensitivity Pneumonitis)

Subacute

- The subacute phase occurs from several days to months after exposure. In this phase, diffuse ground-glass opacities and small (1–5 mm) centrilobular and poorly defined nodules often

affect all zones, though middle and upper lobe predominance is often seen.
- Associated areas of ground-glass opacification are common and often produce a mosaic pattern of attenuation. The areas of ground-glass attenuation are usually diffuse, but they may spare the periphery.

Chronic

- It commonly demonstrates intralobular interstitial thickening and centrilobular nodules predominantly involving the mid and upper lung zones.
- Usually present is relative sparing of the lung apices and the costophrenic sulci, which aids in distinguishing this disorder from idiopathic pulmonary fibrosis.
- Honeycombing is found in about 75% of patients with end-stage lung disease due to hypersensitivity pneumonitis.

Asbestosis

- Common high-resolution computed tomography (HRCT) findings in early asbestosis are intralobular small rounded or branching opacities, thickened interlobular septa, subpleural curvilinear lines, and parenchymal bands.
- With progression of disease, honeycombing is seen.
- The findings predominantly involve the subpleural regions of the lower lung zones.
- The CT study should include images with the patient in the prone position to differentiate normal dependent parenchymal opacity from mild subpleural fibrosis.

Langerhans' Cell Histiocytosis

- Early stage of the disease is characterized by the abundance of nodules and cavitating nodules, whereas cysts are few and do not tend to be confluent.

- Advanced disease is characterized by a small number of nodules, whereas cysts have increased in number and size and are confluent.
- The following sequence of abnormalities seen with CT corresponds to the evolution of the disease: nodules, cavitating nodules, thick-walled cysts, cysts, and confluent cysts, rupture, or collapse of cysts with or without pneumothorax.

Lymphangioleiomyomatosis

- Numerous thin-walled lung cysts, surrounded by relatively normal lung parenchyma, characterize it.
- The walls of the lung cysts usually range from being faintly perceptible to 4 mm in thickness.
- In the majority of patients, the cysts are distributed diffusely throughout the lungs, and no lung zone is spared. Rupture of these cysts can result in pneumothorax. Chylous pleural effusion may be seen.

Silicosis

- It consists of small, well-circumscribed nodules that are usually 2–5 mm in diameter but range from 1 mm to 10 mm, mainly involving the upper and posterior lung zones.
- The appearance of large opacities or hyperattenuating areas over 1 cm in diameter indicates the presence of complicated silicosis. These masses tend to develop in the mid-zone or periphery of the upper lung and migrate toward the hila, leaving overinflated emphysematous spaces between the conglomerate mass and the pleura. They are often bilateral, symmetric, and calcified and can demonstrate cavitation.
- Eggshell calcifications in hilar and mediastinal lymph nodes are occasionally seen.

Coal Workers' Pneumoconiosis

- It is characterized by sharply demarcated, rounded nodules or irregular, contracted nodules that are centrilobular or subpleural in distribution.
- Nodules are present diffusely and bilaterally, but upper lobe and posterior predominance of nodules is seen.

Pneumocystis Carinii Pneumonia

- The most characteristic finding at HRCT is ground-glass attenuation.
- There is often a mosaic or geographic pattern with relatively normal secondary pulmonary lobules adjacent to diseased ones.
- The distribution may be diffuse, perihilar, or upper lobe.
- Other features include a miliary pattern, small nodules, focal masses, interstitial disease with reticulation, septal thickening, and small cystic lesions.
- Hilar adenopathy and pleural effusion are distinctly unusual.

Desquamative Interstitial Pneumonia

- Areas of ground-glass opacity are predominantly seen at the periphery of lower lung zone.
- Irregular lines of attenuation, cystic changes, and traction bronchiectasis may also be seen but are usually not prominent.

Nonspecific Interstitial Pneumonia

- It predominates in the middle and lower lungs.
- Ground-glass attenuation is the salient feature of nonspecific interstitial pneumonia.
- The ground-glass attenuation is frequently associated with traction bronchiectasis, suggesting lung fibrosis.
- Honeycombing, consolidation, and less commonly nodules are also seen.

Idiopathic Pulmonary Hemorrhage

- Findings include air space consolidation or ground-glass opacities with air bronchograms, which has perihilar predominance with a tendency to spare the lung apices.
- The differential diagnosis depends on the patient's immune status. The most common causes in the immunocompetent patient are antiglomerular basement membrane disease (Goodpasture's syndrome), collagen vascular disease, and idiopathic pulmonary hemorrhage. In immunocompromised patients, diffuse pulmonary hemorrhage is almost always associated with an underlying infection or lung injury.

Collagen Vascular Disease (Fig. 16)

- These are characterized by features of fibrosis (as septal thickening, traction bronchiectasis, and honeycombing) and ground-glass opacity.

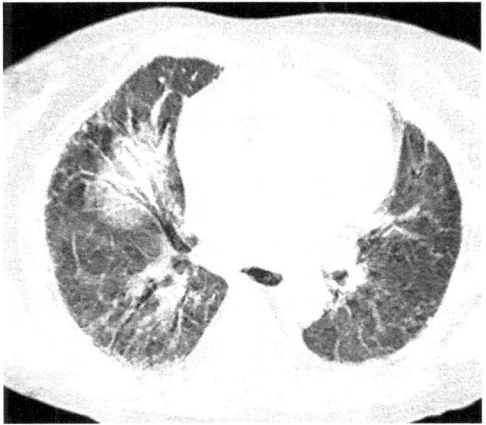

Fig. 16: Axial CT (lung window) image of the right lung shows consolidation and bilateral interlobular septal thickening and dilated esophagus in a case of systemic sclerosis.

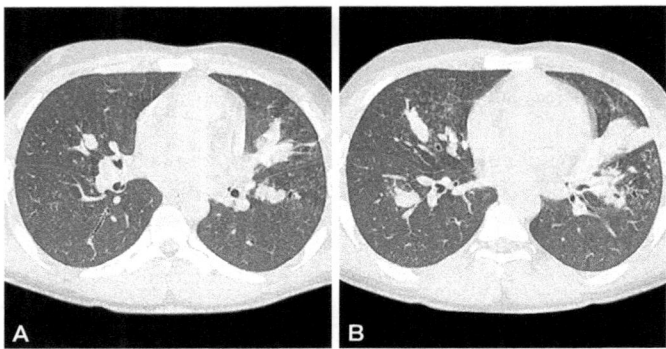

Figs. 17A and B: Transaxial CT images in pulmonary window setting show branching bronchoceles in allergic bronchopulmonary aspergillosis.

- Lesions are predominantly seen in lower peripheral zones except in ankylosing spondylitis where the upper zones are predominantly involved in the early stages and in late stages, it may mimic chronic tuberculosis.
- Other findings are pleural thickening, pleural effusion, and nodules (small—centrilobular; large—cavitating).

Tree-in-bud Appearance

- Infections with endobronchial dissemination of disease (tuberculosis)
- Noninfectious disorders include:
  - Allergic bronchopulmonary aspergillosis (Figs. 17A and B)
  - Aspiration pneumonitis
  - Bronchiolitis.

CYSTIC PULMONARY DISEASES* (TABLES 6 AND 7)

TABLE 6: Common cystic pulmonary diseases and their characteristic findings.

Diseases	Findings	Remarks
Idiopathic pulmonary fibrosis	Honeycomb cysts with basal and subpleural involvement; patchy distribution; cysts show decrease in size with forced expiration	Irregular lines (fine or coarse) of attenuation predominantly in subpleural and basal location
Histiocytosis	Thin-walled cysts with random distribution with sparing of bases; intervening parenchyma is normal with preservation of pulmonary volume	Reticulonodular (usually in the early stages; with regression in the late stage) appearance is usually associated
Tuberous sclerosis	Thin-walled cysts with random and diffuse distribution; intervening parenchyma is normal with preservation of pulmonary volume	Associated angiomyolipoma are seen in various organs
Lymphocytic interstitial pneumonitis	Thin-walled cysts with basilar distribution and subpleural involvement is unusual	Associated ground-glass attenuation is common
Lymphangioleiomyomatosis	Thin-walled, uniform-sized cysts with random and diffuse distribution with equal involvement of upper and lower lung zones; intervening parenchyma is normal with preservation of pulmonary volume	Characteristically seen in women of childbearing age; chylous effusion is associated

*These diseases have to be differentiated from the mimickers that are tabulated in the following section.

TABLE 7: Common conditions and their characteristics for drugs simulating cystic pulmonary diseases.

Diseases	Findings	Remarks
Cystic bronchiectasis (Fig. 18)	Cystic structures contiguous with the bronchial tree; disease may be diffuse or focal depending upon the etiology	Signet ring appearance with air-fluid level are characteristic
Centrilobular emphysema	Cystic lesions without discernible wall with vascular structure within it	Associated features of chronic pulmonary airway disease
Paraseptal emphysema	Subpleural cystic spaces without discernible wall with upper lobe predominance	Typically a single layer of cysts is seen in the subpleural location

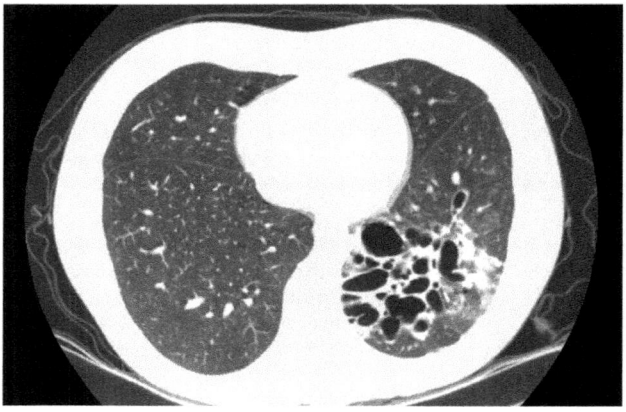

Fig. 18: Axial CT scan shows cystic bronchiectasis.

CT Angiogram Sign

Visualization of pulmonary vessels on contrast-enhanced computed tomography within an airless, fluid-filled portion of the lung. It can be seen in:
- Bronchoalveolar carcinoma
- Lymphoma
- Pulmonary edema
- *Pneumonia*:
    - Obstructive
    - Lipoid
    - Bacterial.

Differential Diagnosis of Opacity with an Air Bronchogram

They can be classified into the following categories:
- *Infective*:
    - Pneumonia
- *Inflammatory*:
    - Radiation pneumonitis
        - HRCT shows cicatrization atelectasis of right upper lobe with traction bronchiectasis giving the air bronchogram sign.
        - There is no proximal obstructing lesion.
        - There are multiple patchy nodular consolidation in right lower lobe superior segment and linear consolidation in right middle lobe medial segment.
    - Progressive massive fibrosis
        - The appearance of large opacities or hyperattenuating areas over 1 cm in diameter indicates the presence of progressive massive fibrosis on the background of silicosis or coal workers' pneumoconiosis.

- These masses tend to develop in the mid-zone or periphery of the upper lung and migrate toward the hila, leaving overinflated emphysematous spaces between the conglomerate mass and the pleura.
- *Neoplastic*:
  – Alveolar cell carcinoma
    - It typically has one of the three radiological patterns. Those are a solitary nodule (43%), consolidation (30%), and multicentric or diffuse disease (27%).
    - Other associated features are pleural effusion and hilar or mediastinal lymphadenopathy.
    - Solitary nodules are located in the periphery of the lung and show spiculated borders (star pattern, due to infiltrative tumor growth, localized lymphangitic spread, or desmoplastic reaction), pleural tags, and bubble-like lucencies or pseudocavitation. Segmental or lobar consolidation can be caused by the combination of tumor growth along the alveolar wall and secretion of mucin.
    - Production of mucin can cause swelling of the lobe, leading to bulging of interlobar fissure, and heterogeneous attenuation in small masses or uniform low attenuation with CT angiogram sign in more confluent consolidation.
    - In the third form, bronchioloalveolar cell carcinoma may have a widespread multinodular pattern.
  – Lymphoma/lymphosarcoma (Figs. 19A to D)
    - Multiple or solitary pulmonary lesions.
    - Diffuse pulmonary infiltration may be present.
    - Lesions include masses or mass-like areas of consolidation and pulmonary nodules.
    - Associated findings are air bronchograms, airway dilatation, a positive angiogram sign, and a halo of ground-glass shadowing at lesion margins.

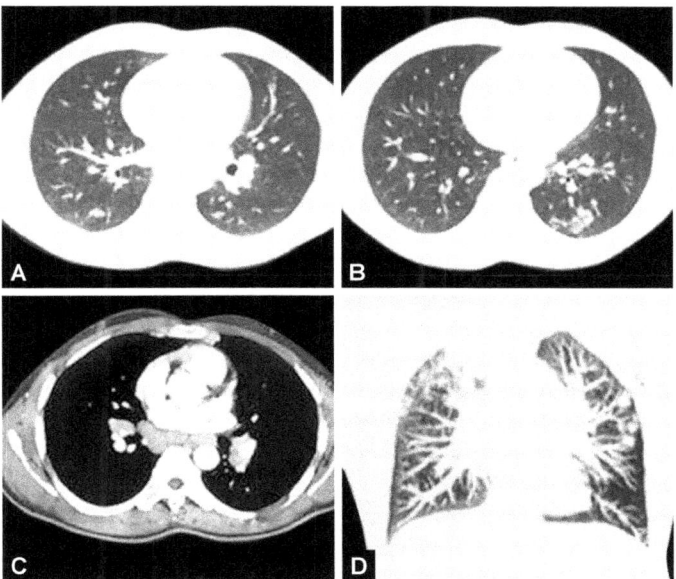

Figs. 19A to D: Axial CT scans showing posterior mediastinal and bilateral lymphadenopathy with pulmonary lesions in form of nodules and consolidation suggestive of lymphoma.

- Peribronchovascular thickening, hilar or mediastinal lymph node enlargement, and pleural effusions or thickening may also be seen.

MEDIASTINAL MASSES

They can be divided into anterior, middle, and posterior mediastinal masses.

Anterior Mediastinal Masses (Tables 8 and 9)

TABLE 8: Causes and differentiating features of anterior mediastinal masses in children.

Diseases	Differentiating features	Additional features
Congenital		
Normal thymus	In children and adolescent, the thymus is isodense to the muscle while in adults it is isodense to fat	Maximum total thickness of thymic tissue under 20 years of age should not exceed 1.8 cm; while after 20 years, it should not be more than 1.3 cm
Cystic hygroma/ lymphangiomas	• Smooth, unilocular or multilocular, thin-walled, lobulated mass, which may mold to or envelop, rather than displace, the adjacent mediastinal structure • Homogeneous low attenuation similar to that of water, but can have higher attenuation or consist of a combination of fluid, solid tissue, and fat	• Primary mediastinal lymphangioma are rare but they are usually seen as extension of the cystic hygroma of the neck • Calcification is rare • Thickened septa can be secondary to superadded infection as can be thickened enhancing walls
Morgagni hernia	Fat-containing cardiophrenic angle mass with associated omental or mesenteric vessels	It is almost invariably seen on the right side but occasionally bilateral
Neoplastic		
Lymphoma* and leukemia	*Hodgkin disease*: • Multiple, usually discrete, mild to moderately enhancing, nodal masses are	• Most common neoplastic anterior mediastinal mass • Usually the age is >10 years

Contd...

Contd...

Diseases	Differentiating features	Additional features
	seen in the anterior mediastinum and the paratracheal region • Superior mediastinum is almost invariably involved	• Disease more commonly involves the thymus rather than the lymph nodes in the anterior mediastinum
	Non-Hodgkin lymphoma: • Nodal masses are seen similar to that seen in Hodgkin disease but superior mediastinal involvement is less common • Middle mediastinum involvement is more common	• The nodal involvement is noncontiguous and is usually seen in the higher age group relative to the Hodgkin disease • Pleural and pericardial effusion is present in about one-third
Germ cell tumor		
Benign teratoma/ dermoid	It is seen as a well-defined, usually lobulated, heterogeneous mass with thick walls that may enhance and may even show curvilinear calcification. Admixture of soft-tissue, fluid, fat, and calcium attenuation is usually present	• About 76% of all teratomatous lesions contains some fat • Presence of fat-fluid level and malformed teeth are pathognomonic
Malignant teratoma/ teratocarcinoma	These most often demonstrate nodular/ irregular or poorly defined margins with invasion of mediastinal fat and adjacent structures. It can mold to and compress surrounding structures	• These demonstrate fat less often (40%) whereas benign teratomas shows fat about 90% and malignant are more likely to appear solid

Contd...

Contd...

Diseases	Differentiating features	Additional features
Thymoma		
Benign	• Homogeneous, oval, rounded or lobulated soft-tissue masses with mild uniform enhancement • Areas of decreased attenuation may be present and correspond to cystic changes or foci of hemorrhage and necrosis • It usually grows asymmetrically to one side of the anterior mediastinum	• Thymoma is commonly associated with red cell aplasia, hypogamma-globulinemia, etc. • Calcification is seen in 25% of cases that can be curvilinear, punctate or linear
Invasive	Irregular borders between the mass and the adjacent mediastinal structures and pleura suggest the diagnosis	• Pulmonary parenchymal and chest wall involvement is very rare • Pleural involvement may be nodular or sheet-like mimicking mesothelioma but associated pleural effusion is rare in thymoma
Inflammatory		
Lymphadenopathy (Fig. 20)	• These are most often seen as conglomerate masses with ill-defined borders and heterogeneous enhancement	• Inflammatory lymph node enlargement is less common than neoplastic involvement in the anterior mediastinum

Contd...

Chest

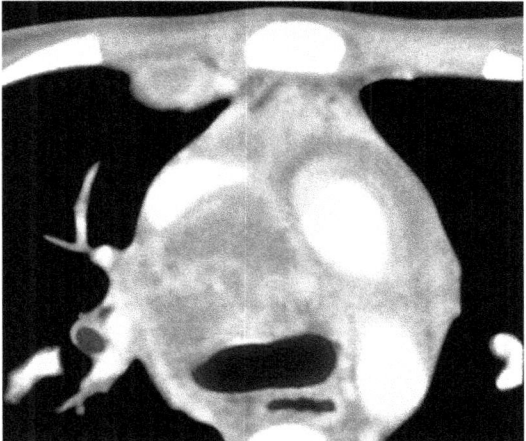

Fig. 20: Characteristic mediastinal adenopathy with rim enhancement and central necrosis suggestive of tuberculosis.

Contd...

Diseases	Differentiating features	Additional features
	• Rim enhancement with central hypodensity is due to necrosis • Calcification is seen in chronic infections	• Most common causes are tuberculosis and histoplasmosis • In tuberculosis, associated lesions in the lungs are usually seen and the lymph nodes will reveal caseous necrosis in the center

*Nodal masses elsewhere in the body (neck, abdomen) and invasion of the anterior chest wall supports the diagnosis.

TABLE 9: Causes and differentiating features of anterior mediastinal masses in adults.

Diseases	Differentiating features	Additional features
Retrosternal goiter (Figs. 21A and B)	The typical CT features of intrathoracic goiter can be summarized as follows: • Continuity with the cervical thyroid gland, well-defined borders • Punctate, coarse, or ring-like calcifications • Nonhomogeneity often with minimal or nonenhancing, well-defined, low-density areas • Precontrast attenuation values often at least 15 HU greater than adjacent musculature with at least 25 HU enhancement after intravenous contrast	Patterns of extension of the goiter into the mediastinum with cradling of the goiter by the right and left brachiocephalic vessels high in the mediastinum and extension behind the great vessels to the paratracheal or retrotracheal region
Thymoma (Fig. 22)	As above	It is commonly associated with autoimmune diseases especially myasthenia gravis
Teratoma	As above	
Inflammatory lymph nodes	As above	
Vascular tortuous innominate artery	Contiguous scans reveal the true nature of the lesion	A common finding in elderly

Contd...

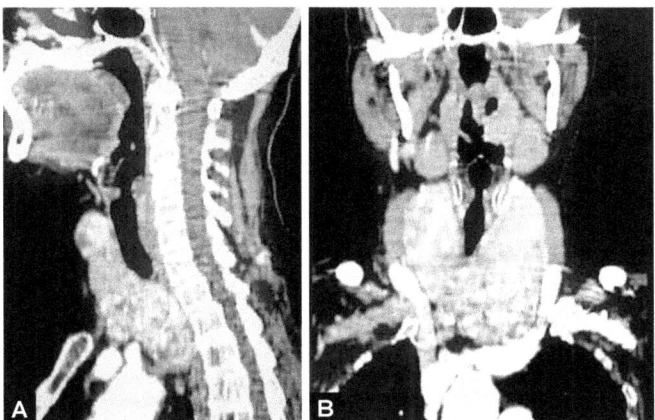

Figs. 21A and B: Contrast-enhanced computed tomography sagittal and coronal MPR images of neck showing multinodular goiter extending into mediastinum retrosternaly.

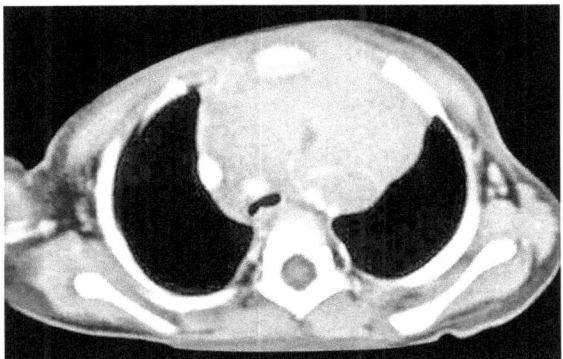

Fig. 22: Axial CT scan showing a large thymic mass suggestive of thymoma.

Contd...

Diseases	Differentiating features	Additional features
Aneurysm of the ascending aorta	It is seen as dilatation of the aorta with a diameter greater than 4 cm. Craniocaudal extent of aneurysm, presence of intraluminal thrombus are accurately depicted by CT	It is the least common site of aortic aneurysm
Germ cell tumors (choriocarcinoma, seminoma, embryonal cell carcinoma, endodermal sinus tumor)	• Irregular soft tissue mass with central necrosis/degeneration • Invasion of the adjacent structures is common • Intratumoral calcification may be seen	• Seen in young adults in third to fourth decades more commonly in males • Transpleural spread suggests a high probability of lymphoma/invasive thymoma rather than germ cell tumor
Anterior cardiophrenic angle masses		
Pericardial fat pad	It demonstrates the fat density	• Seen especially in obese people • Rare in adults
Morgagni hernia	As above	The majority of these arise in the anterior cardiophrenic angle, more frequently on the right side, but they can be seen as high in the pericardial recesses at the level of the proximal aorta and pulmonary arteries
Pleuropericardial cyst/Springwater cyst	• The cyst appears as a single, smooth, round or elliptical mass with enhancing wall and uniform fluid attenuation • These cysts may demonstrate different shapes when studied at different times	Occasionally, cysts are pedunculated

Middle Mediastinal Masses (Table 10)

TABLE 10: Causes and differentiating features of middle mediastinal masses.

Diseases	Differentiating features	Additional features
Children		
Congenital		
Bronchogenic cyst	• It appears as a single, smooth, round, or elliptical mass with an imperceptible/thin wall and uniform attenuation • The attenuation value is dependent on the contents of the cyst and can vary from water attenuation to soft-tissue attenuation	• They may occur in any part of the mediastinum, but most are near the carina or posterior mediastinum • The HU value of the internal contents can be >100 HU owing to a high protein level or calcium oxalate in the mucoid cyst • Air within the cyst is uncommon and suggestive of secondary infection and communication with the tracheo-bronchial tree
Esophageal duplication cyst	• Their appearance at CT imaging is identical to that of bronchogenic cysts except that the wall of the lesion may be thicker and in more intimate contact with the esophagus • It can be tubular in shape	The majority are detected in infants or children, usually adjacent to or within the esophageal wall
Cystic hygroma	As above	

Contd...

Contd...

Diseases	Differentiating features	Additional features
Inflammatory		
Lymphadenopathy	As above	It is common in tuberculosis, histoplasmosis, and sarcoidosis
Neoplastic	• Most middle mediastinal tumors are extension of those, which arise, primarily in the anterior mediastinum • Findings therefore correspond to the primary tumor	
Adults		
Hiatus hernia (Fig. 23)	• It appears as a retrocardiac mass with or without an air-fluid level • The mass usually can be traced into the esophageal hiatus on sequential scans	Herniation of omentum through the esophageal hiatus may result in an increase in the fat surrounding the lower esophagus
Achalasia	Moderate-to-marked esophageal dilatation with normal wall thickness	CT may be invaluable in confirming the diagnosis or in detecting atypical features that may indicate the presence of other diseases or superimposed benign or malignant

Contd...

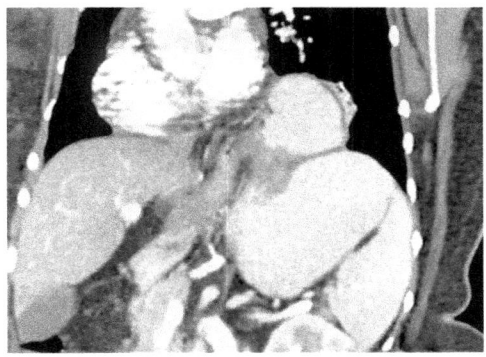

Fig. 23: Oblique coronal multiplanar reconstruction CT image showing sliding hiatus hernia.

Contd...

Diseases	Differentiating features	Additional features
Epiphrenic esophageal diverticulum	A thin-walled, air or air-fluid filled structure communicating with the esophagus	However, those not associated with a distal esophageal obstruction (stricture, achalasia) may remain contracted in resting state and thus may not be visible
Lymphadenopathy	As above	
Carcinoma of the bronchus (Figs. 24A and B)	Ill-defined, hetero-geneously enhancing mass in and around the bronchi with features of malignancy as described above	<ul><li>Associated paren-chymal changes in the form of distal obstructive consolidation, atelectasis or emphysema may be seen</li><li>Associated bony and adrenal masses may be highly suggestive</li></ul>

Contd...

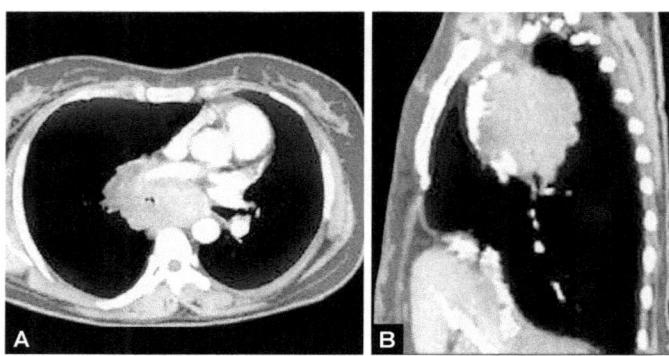

Figs. 24A and B: Carcinoma bronchus with invasion of the right pulmonary artery, pericardium, and esophagus.

Contd...

Diseases	Differentiating features	Additional features
Aneurysm of the aorta (Figs. 25A and B)	As above	
Bronchogenic cyst	As above	
Esophageal masses (leiomyoma and leiomyosarcoma) (Figs. 26A and B)	• Leiomyoma is seen as well-defined enhancing mass inseparable from the wall • Leiomyosarcoma is seen as large, heterogeneously enhancing mass with a large exophytic component with central necrosis or ulceration	

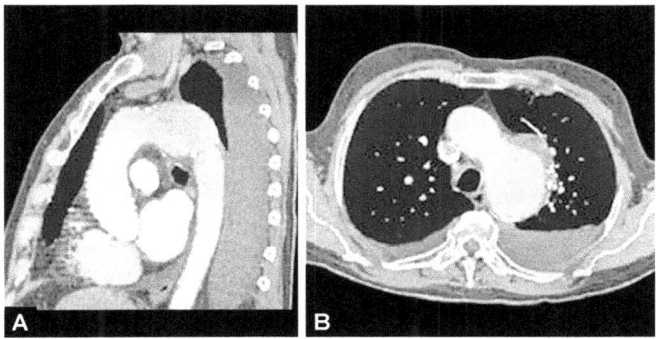

Figs. 25A and B: Sagittal and axial CT images showing aortic arch aneurysm.

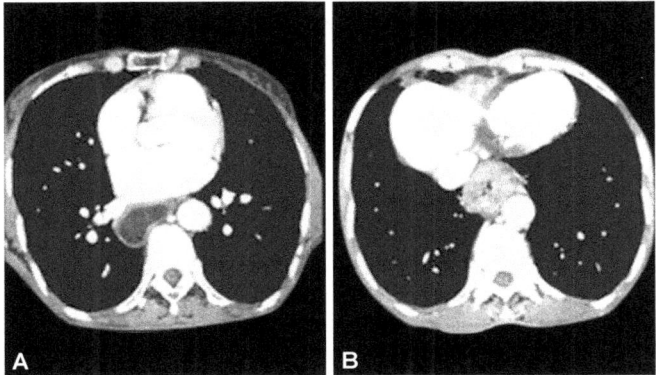

Figs. 26A and B: Axial CT images showing proximal esophageal dilatation due to distal carcinoma of the esophagus.

Posterior Mediastinal Masses (Table 11)

TABLE 11: Causes and differentiating features of posterior mediastinal masses.

Diseases	Differentiating features	Additional features
Children		
Neurogenic masses (Tumors) [These originate from autonomic ganglia and include ganglioneuroma (benign), ganglioneuroblastoma, and neuroblastoma (malignant)]	• A well-defined, oval- or crescent-shaped mass with low or intermediate attenuation • Discrete punctate calcification (20%) • Little (80%) or no enhancement (20%) • Thinning of posterior ribs, separation of ribs, and enlargement of intervertebral foramina are characteristics	If suspected ganglioneuromas have components that show atypical findings, malignant or aggressive elements due to neuroblastoma, ganglioneuroblastoma or pheochromocytoma should be considered

Bochdalek's hernia (congenital diaphragmatic hernia—CDH)	• *The classic appearance is:*
	  – The left hemithorax filled with cyst-like structures (loops of bowel)
	  – The mediastinum shifted to the right
	  – The abdomen is relatively devoid of gas
	  – The stomach remains visible within the abdomen but may be in an abnormal location, often more central
		• Bochdalek's hernias occur on the left side 75% of the time
		• The abnormal positioning of the stomach may be helpful in differentiating CDH from those few cases of congenital cystic adenomatoid malformation in which the cysts are large enough to mimic the air-filled intestinal loops

Contd...

Contd...

Diseases	Differentiating features	Additional features
Neuroenteric cyst	• It is seen as a thin-walled, well-defined cystic mass in the paravertebral with communication with the spinal canal • The internal contents are water dense in the absence of infection or hemorrhage	• Usually right-sided • May also be located in the middle mediastinum • It is associated with • vertebral body anomalies (hemi-vertebra, butterfly vertebra, and secondary scoliosis) and are usually superior to the cyst
Extramedullary hematopoiesis	• Typically bilateral, well-circumscribed, lobulated, paravertebral mass lesions usually located caudal to the D6 vertebrae • Widening of the ribs especially at the vertebral end • The vertebral body is devoid of bony erosion, has a lacy appearance with fat attenuation. Transverse process are also expanded	• May be seen as single or multiple, sometimes unilateral paravertebral mass lesions • The absence of calcification and the presence of adipose tissue are characteristic

Adults

Neurogenic tumors

Schwannoma and neurofibroma	• Homogeneous density mass with mild-to-moderate enhancement growing along the course of the parent nerve	• Calcification is rare • Plexiform neurofibroma appear as low density, infiltrating mass

Contd...

Contd...

Diseases	Differentiating features	Additional features
	• Schwannoma may demonstrate central hypodensity due to high lipid content or cystic degeneration • Widened intervertebral foramina and posterior rib pressure erosion are common	• Ill-defined, necrosis, hemorrhage within the mass and adjacent osseous destruction and sudden increase in size suggests malignant transformation
Paragangliomas (chemodectoma and pheochromocytoma)	They are rounded masses with intense, homogeneous contrast enhancement	• Chemodectoma are commonly located in the region of the aortic arch (aortic body tumor) • Pheochromocytoma can also be seen adjacent to the heart and pericardium
Lateral thoracic meningocele	• They appear as well-defined, homogeneous, hypoattenuating paravertebral masses • Other findings include enlargement of intervertebral foramina and associated vertebral and rib anomalies and scoliosis • CT myelography shows filling of the meningocele	
Abscess	• Ring enhancing, complex mass with thick nodular/irregular walls	Usually associated with inflammation of disk and vertebral body destruction

Contd...

Contd...

Diseases	Differentiating features	Additional features
	• Fat stranding in the adjacent mediastinal fat • Air and sometimes air-fluid level may be seen in cases of active infection	
Hiatus hernia	As above	
Aortic aneurysm	• It is seen as fusiform or saccular dilatation of the aorta with diameter exceeding 4 cm • Most demonstrate lining thrombus and curvilinear calcification • Adjacent vertebral and rib erosion may be seen	• It is seen in the descending part, arch and ascending part in the order of decreasing frequency • More than 6 cm suggests significant and more than 10 cm diameter suggests a 50% risk of rupture

Mediastinal Masses Containing Fat

- Teratoma and teratocarcinoma
- *Lipoma*:
    - They occur predominantly in the anterior mediastinum.
    - They have homogeneous fat attenuation of approximately –100 HU and well-defined margins with minimal or no mass effect.
    - Presence of enhancing soft-tissue masses within suggests a sarcomatous change.
- *Lipomatosis*:
    - It is seen as excessive unencapsulated infiltrative fat deposition.
    - It is commonly associated with obesity and exogenous steroid administration.

- *Thymolipoma*:
    - These are rare, benign, slow-growing tumors in the anterior part of the superior mediastinum that contain an admixture of thymic parenchyma and mature adipose tissue, with the former accounting for 10–33%.
    - They appear as primarily fatty tissue mixed with soft-tissue attenuation that represents thymic.
    - The sharp borders of the lesion delineate a well-defined capsule, with no invasion of surrounding structures.
- *Lipoblastoma*:
    - These are rare soft-tissue mesenchymal tumors of embryonic white fat that occur during infancy and early childhood.
    - These tumors are divided into two categories. The more common superficial well-defined mass is known simply as a lipoblastoma. The second form is a deep, unencapsulated infiltrative lesion known as lipoblastomatosis.
    - Myxoid liposarcomas may have a similar CT appearance but are relatively uncommon in children.
    - These fat-containing lesions are characterized by predominant intratumoral stranding.
    - This tumor can often be differentiated from other mediastinal fat-containing tumors on the basis of the patient's age and clinical history.
- Diaphragmatic hernia
- Schwannoma.

Mediastinal Cysts

- Congenital—bronchogenic cyst (Figs. 27A and B), neuroenteric cyst, enteric cyst, thymic cyst
- Pericardial cyst
- *Thymic cyst*:
    - Simple congenital thymic cysts are very rare and usually appear as well-defined, unilocular, water-attenuation masses with imperceptible walls.

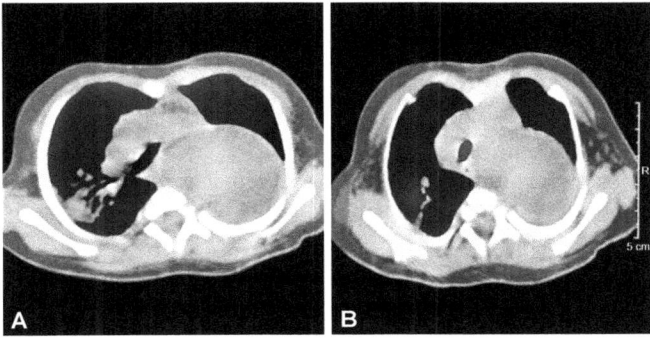

Figs. 27A and B: Axial CECT images of chest showing fluid density cystic structure involving the middle mediastinum in a child suggesting bronchogenic cyst.

- Multilocular thymic cysts may appear as well-defined, heterogeneous cystic masses with a clearly seen wall.
- Acquired thymic cysts are usually multilocular occur after radiation therapy for Hodgkin's disease, in association with thymic tumors, and after thoracotomy.
- Some thymic cysts may have increased attenuation secondary to hemorrhage or infection and may be misdiagnosed as solid masses. They can also have fat attenuation due to high cholesterol content.
- Curvilinear calcification of the cyst wall occurs in a minority.

- *Cystic tumors*:
  - Lymphangioma
  - Mature cystic teratoma
  - Mediastinal pancreatic pseudocyst
    - A cystic posterior mediastinal mass that develops over a short time in a patient with evidence of pancreatitis is likely to be a pseudocyst.
    - CT shows a thin, cystic, low-attenuation mass in the posterior mediastinum or adjacent thoracic cavity associated with compression or displacement of the esophagus or splaying of the diaphragmatic crura.

- Cyst contents can be isoattenuating or hyperattenuating relative to water, depending on the presence of hemorrhage or infection.
- An abdominal component is common but is not invariably present.

- *Cystic Schwannoma*:
  - Schwannoma appears as a well-marginated, smooth, rounded or elliptical mass in the paravertebral region or along the courses of intercostal nerves.
  - Schwannomas have heterogeneous attenuation, including low-attenuation areas caused by the coalescence of interstitial fluid, xanthomatous change, or cystic degeneration secondary to infarction.
  - Enlargement of neural foramina with or without extension into the spinal canal may be associated with paravertebral tumors.
- *Meningocele*:
  - They appear as well-defined, homogeneous, low-attenuation paravertebral masses with communication with the spinal canal more readily demonstrable on CT myelography.
- *Mediastinal abscess*:
  - They are uncommon and are usually related to surgery, esophageal perforation, or spread of infection from an adjacent region.
  - The abscesses may appear as a low-attenuation mass owing to fluid content.
  - Air bubbles, contiguity or communication with an empyema or subphrenic abscess, and clinical features usually permit differentiation from true cysts or neoplasms.
  - However, percutaneous needle aspiration may be required to distinguish an abscess from an uninfected postoperative seroma or hematoma.

CLASSIFICATION OF REGIONAL INTRATHORACIC LYMPH NODES (TABLE 12)

Nodal enlargement is commonly defined as >1 cm in short-axis diameter.

Chest

TABLE 12: Classification of regional intrathoracic lymph nodes.

Stations	Groups	Remarks
1	Highest mediastinal nodes	These lie cranial to the superior aspect of the left innominate or brachiocephalic vein where the vein crosses the trachea
2	Upper paratracheal nodes	These nodes are located below the inferior boundary of station-1 nodes and cranial to the superior aspect of the aortic arch
3	Prevascular and retrotracheal nodes	• Prevascular nodes are anterior to the great vessel branches and cranial to the superior aspect of the aortic arch • Retrotracheal nodes are posterior to the trachea, inferior to the thoracic inlet, and cranial to the inferior aspect of the azygos vein
4	Lower paratracheal nodes	The lower right paratracheal nodes lie to the right of the tracheal midline. They are caudal to the superior aspect of the aortic arch and cranial to the superior aspect of the right upper lobe bronchus. The lower left paratracheal nodes lie to the left of the tracheal midline. They are caudal to the superior aspect of the aortic arch and cranial to the superior aspect of the left upper lobe bronchus. The lower paratracheal nodes are further divided into superior and inferior subsets. Station-4 superior nodes are cranial to the superior aspect of the azygos arch, whereas station-4 inferior nodes are caudal to the superior aspect of the azygos arch.
5	Subaortic or aortopulmonary window nodes	These nodes lie lateral to the ligamentum arteriosum and are medial to the origin of the first branch of the left pulmonary artery

Contd...

Contd...

Stations	Groups	Remarks
6	Para-aortic (ascending aortic or phrenic) nodes	These nodes are anterior and lateral to the aortic arch at levels caudal to the superior aspect of the aortic arch
7	Subcarinal nodes	These nodes are caudal to the tracheal carina between the main bronchi
8	Paraesophageal nodes	These nodes are adjacent to the wall of the esophagus and to the right or left of the tracheal midline
9	Pulmonary ligament nodes	These nodes are within the pulmonary ligament
10	Hilar nodes	These nodes are the proximal lobar nodes. Right hilar nodes are caudal to the superior aspect of the right upper lobe bronchus and lie adjacent to the right main bronchus and the proximal bronchus intermedius. Similarly, the left hilar nodes are caudal to the superior aspect of the left upper lobe bronchus adjacent to the left main bronchus
11	Interlobar nodes	These nodes are between lobar bronchi and are adjacent to the proximal lobar bronchi
12	Lobar nodes	These nodes are located adjacent to distal portions of the lobar bronchi
13	Segmental nodes	These nodes are adjacent to the segmental bronchi
14	Subsegmental nodes	These nodes are adjacent to the subsegmental bronchi in the lung parenchyma

MEDIASTINAL LYMPHADENOPATHY (TABLE 13)

TABLE 13: Differentiating features of various causes of mediastinal lymphadenopathy according to characteristic patterns.

Characteristic patterns	Conditions	Features
Calcified lymph nodes	• Granulomatous disease	• Healed granulomatous disease are usually responsible for calcified hilar or mediastinal lymph nodes
	• Pneumocystis carinii infection	• Disseminated *Pneumocystis carinii* infection in AIDS patients, especially in those who have received prophylaxis with aerosolized pentamidine • *Pneumocystis carinii* organisms are found in the calcified lymph nodes
	• Metastases	• Metastases from osteosarcoma, mucinous ovarian or colonic carcinoma, papillary carcinoma of the thyroid or bronchogenic carcinoma may contain calcification
Eggshell calcification (shell-like calcification up to 2 mm thick in the periphery of at least two lymph nodes; calcification may be solid or broken)	• Silicosis	• Seen in approximately 5% of silicotics. Predominantly hilar nodes but may also be observed in the anterior and posterior mediastinal lymph nodes, cervical, and intraperitoneal lymph nodes. Lungs show multiple small nodular shadows or areas of massive fibrosis.

Contd...

Contd...

Characteristic patterns	Conditions	Features
	• Coal miner's pneumoconiosis	• Occurs in only 1% of cases • Associated pulmonary changes include miliary shadowing or massive shadows
	• Sarcoidosis	• Calcification of lymph nodes occurs in 5% of patients • Calcification appears about 6 years after the onset of the disease • It is almost invariably associated with advanced pulmonary disease and in some cases with steroid therapy
	• Lymphoma after radiotherapy	• Usually appears at 1–9 years post-RT
	• Amyloidosis	• Egg-shell calcification is rarely seen • The characteristic CT findings are circumferential wall thickening with calcification of the trachea and central bronchial tree with substantial narrowing of the main, lobar, and segmental bronchi
Hypodense lymph nodes	• Metastases	• Most mediastinal and hilar lymph node metastases arise from a primary thoracic neoplasm, most commonly bronchogenic carcinoma • Generally, the lymphadenopathy is unilateral

Contd...

Contd...

Characteristic patterns	Conditions	Features
		• Usually, the CT reveals a lung nodule or mass in lungs • In patients with extra-thoracic neoplasm, intrapulmonary metastases are at least 10 times more common than nodal metastasis • The most common tumors associated with intrathoracic metastasis are renal, testicular, head and neck, breast, and melanoma
	• Lymphoma	• These may be seen either at the time of initial diagnosis or following treatment • Necrosis is seen most commonly in the nodular sclerosing and mixed cellularity cell types of lymphoma
	• Tuberculosis (TB)	• Unilateral hilar and/or mediastinal lymphnode enlargement in TB is characteristically seen in childhood primary TB • In adults, similar findings may be seen as a manifestation of either primary or reactivation disease • In TB right paratracheal and tracheobronchial lymph nodes are involved most frequently

Contd...

Contd...

Characteristic patterns	Conditions	Features
	• Fungal infections	• In infections like histoplasmosis a low attenuation mass is seen, usually in the right paratracheal and subcarinal region
Enhancing lymph nodes	• Vascular metastasis	• Metastases in this category include primaries of renal cell carcinoma, melanoma, and papillary thyroid carcinoma • The hila and right paratracheal nodal groups are most commonly involved • Lymph node involvement is usually asymmetric, but bilateral hilar, with or without mediastinal lymphadenopathy may be seen • Isolated lymphadenopathy, without associated parenchymal involvement, is seen in approximately 60% of cases
	• Castleman's disease	• It is also known as angiofollicular hyperplasia or giant lymph node hyperplasia • It is a rare disorder of lymphoid tissue with unclear etiology and pathogenesis • CECT shows a dense uniform enhancement

Contd...

Contd...

Characteristic patterns	Conditions	Features
		• CT shows one of three morphologic patterns in the decreasing order of frequency: a solitary mass, a dominant infiltrative mass with associated lymphadenopathy or diffuse lymphadenopathy confined to a single mediastinal compartment • Dynamic CT demonstrates early rapid enhancement and washout in the delayed phase, phase, which is considered typical and differentiates this disease from other mediastinal tumors such as lymphoma • Tumors greater than 5 cm in diameter generally demonstrate heterogeneous enhancement
	• Angioimmunoblastic lymphadenopathy	• It is a type of peripheral T-cell lymphoma with high pyrexia and generalized adenopathy • Features include bilateral mediastinal and hilar lymphadenopathy, pleural effusion, and atelectasis • Diffuse CT contrast enhancement of lymph nodes can aid in diagnosing angioimmunoblastic lymphadenopathy

LESIONS OF TRACHEOBRONCHIAL TREE

Congenital Lesions (Table 14)

TABLE 14: Common causes and differentiating features of various congenital lesions of tracheobronchial tree.

Diseases	Differentiating features	Remarks
Tracheomalacia	<ul><li>The caliber according to the phase of respiration</li><li>There is expiratory collapse resulting in a functional obstruction and hence the lung fields appear hypoattenuating</li></ul>	Cine CT provides dynamic assessment in these cases
Tracheal stenosis	<ul><li>Long segment stenosis is associated with bilateral pulmonary hypoplasia</li><li>Short segment stenosis consists of narrowing in the lower third with normal distal end of trachea and bronchi</li></ul>	It may be associated with other anomalies especially pulmonary artery sling complex

Contd...

Contd...

Diseases	Differentiating features	Remarks
Tracheal bronchus	This anomalous bronchus usually exits the right lateral wall of the trachea >2 cm above the major carina and can supply the entire upper lobe or its apical segment	The anomalous bronchus may end blindly and is called tracheal diverticulum
Bronchial atresia	The bronchus distal to the site of atresia is seen as a water-density mass that correspond to the bronchocele with an area of focal air trapping	Expiratory CT clearly depicts the pathology
Tracheoeso-phageal fistula	3D CT and virtual bronchoscopy allow accurate location of the site of fistula and can show the length of gap between the proximal and distal esophageal pouches	It is commonly associated with vertebral, tracheoesophageal, complex, and renal anomalies complex

Acquired Lesions (Table 15)

TABLE 15: Common causes and differentiating features of various acquired lesions of tracheobronchial tree.

Diseases	Differentiating features	Remarks
Tracheal stenosis	CT demonstrates the site and severity of the narrowing	• Tuberculosis may cause fibrosis and chronic tracheal stenosis • Fibrosing mediastinitis, which is due to tuberculosis or histoplasmosis, can cause both tracheal and bronchial stenosis (Fig. 28) • Saber-sheath trachea occurs in older men and is almost invariably associated with COPD. It affects the intrathoracic part of the trachea • Tracheal stenosis may be the result of previous injury like prolonged tracheal intubation or tracheostomy

Contd...

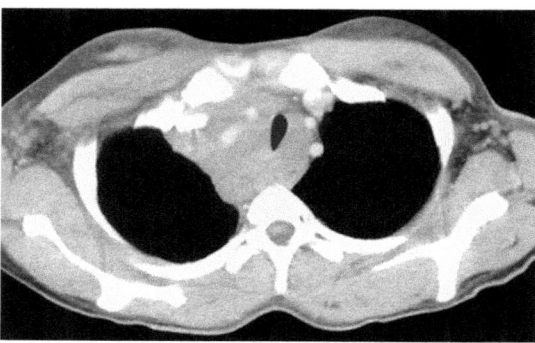

Fig. 28: Transaxial CT image shows fibrosing mediastinitis with tracheal and vascular stenosis.

Contd...

Diseases	Differentiating features	Remarks
Bronchiectasis	• The internal bronchial diameter > diameter the adjacent artery • Lack of bronchial tapering (same diameter as the parent branch for >2 cm) • Bronchi seen within 1 cm of costal pleura or abutting mediastinal pleura • Bronchial wall thickening may be seen	• In cylindrical bronchiectasis, bronchi coursing horizontally are seen as parallel lines, and vertically oriented bronchi are seen as circular lucencies larger than the adjacent pulmonary artery (*signet ring appearance*) • Varicose bronchiectasis may be seen as nonuniform bronchial dilatation • A cystic cluster of thin-walled cystic spaces may be present, often with air-fluid level in cystic variety
Emphysema	Centrilobular emphysema is seen as small, round areas of low attenuation, several mm in diameter, grouped near the centers of secondary pulmonary lobules, and lacking visible walls	Centrilobular emphysema is most severe in upper lung zones

Contd...

Contd...

Diseases	Differentiating features	Remarks
	In panlobular emphysema the characteristic is decreased lung attenuation, with few visible pulmonary vessels in the abnormal regions; bullae or cysts are characteristically absent	Panlobular emphysema is almost always most severe in the lower lobes
	Paraseptal emphysema is characterized by involvement of the distal part of the secondary lobule. The bullae or air cysts are commonly seen in these patients with thin walls	Most striking in a subpleural location
Constrictive bronchiolitis (obliterative bronchiolitis, bronchiolitis obliterans)	It demonstrates mosaic areas of decreased attenuation and vascularity with evidence of air-trapping and peripheral cylindrical bronchiectasis	

Contd...

Contd...

Diseases	Differentiating features	Remarks
Acute bronchiolitis	It demonstrates small, ill-defined centrilobular nodules representing bronchioles impacted with inflammatory material and peribronchiolar inflammation, branching linear opacities corresponding to inflamed airway walls, and focal areas of consolidation due to bronchopneumonia	
Cryptogenic organizing pneumonia (idiopathic BOOP)	• It has patchy, unilateral or bilateral, areas of air-space consolidation or ground-glass attenuation with nodules being less common • Subpleural or peribronchial distribution is demonstrated in up to 50% of cases • Linear or reticular opacities may be seen in some subjects	A small number of patients with cryptogenic organizing pneumonia will progress to honeycombing

Contd...

Contd...

Diseases	Differentiating features	Remarks
Primary tumors	• Benign tumors present as small well-defined intraluminal nodules • Malignant tumors of the trachea tend to occur close to the carina and are seen as ill-defined masses with destruction of the walls	• Benign tumors are mostly papilloma, fibroma, chondroma, or hemangioma • Malignant tumors are mostly squamous, adenoid cystic or adenocarcinoma
Foreign body	It is seen as a nonenhancing lesion occupying the lumen of bronchus	Most common lesion in the pediatric age group

(BOOP: Bronchiolitis obliterans organizing pneumonia; COPD: Chronic obstructive pulmonary disease)

PLEURAL LESIONS

Pleural Calcification (Table 16)

TABLE 16: Causes and differentiating features of pleural calcification.	
Disease entities	*Features*
Old empyema and old hemothorax (Fig. 29)	• Amorphous bizarre, plaques, often with a vacuolated appearance near the inner surface of greatly thickened pleura • Usually unilateral

Contd...

Chest

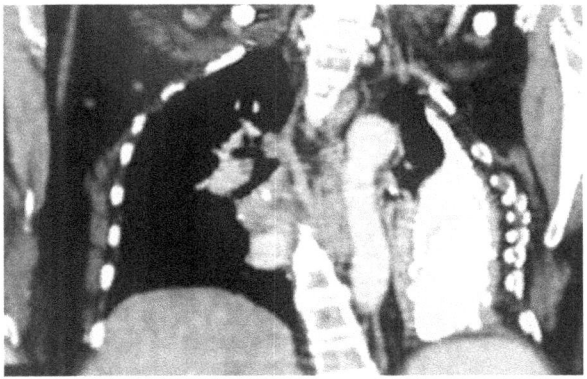

Fig. 29: Coronal CT image of chest showing calcified empyema left side in an old case of tuberculosis.

Contd...

Disease entities	Features
Asbestosis	• *Pleural plaques* appear as discrete well-defined areas of localized pleural thickening (Fig. 30). They are usually multiple, bilateral, and located adjacent to rigid structures, such as the ribs, midportion of the chest, aponeurotic portion of the diaphragm, mediastinum, and paravertebral regions. Lung apices and costophrenic angles typically are spared • *Diffuse pleural thickening* is defined as an uninterrupted sheet at least 5 cm wide, 8–10 cm long craniocaudally, and at least 3 mm thick. It may be bilateral and tends to involve the posterolateral surfaces of the lower thorax

Contd...

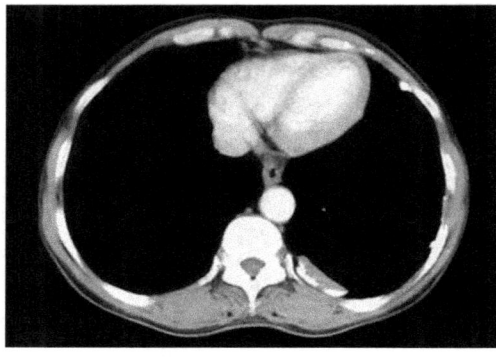

Fig. 30: Transaxial CT image shows calcified pleural plaque on left side posteriorly.

Contd...

Disease entities	Features
	- *Benign asbestos-related pleural effusion* may be unilateral or bilateral and are usually small
- The earliest abnormal HRCT finding is subpleural micronodularity, which represents early mild peribronchial and centrilobular fibrosis
- As the disease progresses, intralobular and interlobular septal thickening are seen, eventually resulting in architectural distortion, traction bronchiectasis, and honeycombing
- Mild mediastinal lymphadenopathy is found frequently with uncomplicated asbestosis
- Malignant mesothelioma is seen as irregular nodular pleural thickening, which may involve the interlobar fissures (86%), pleural effusion, loss of volume, pleural calcification, and chest wall invasion

Contd...

Contd...

Disease entities	Features
Silicosis	• Features with simple silicosis or CWP consists of small, well-circumscribed nodules that are usually 2–5 mm in diameter but range from 1 mm to 10 mm, mainly involving the upper and posterior lung zones • Pleural plaques such as asbestos exposure may be seen
Talc exposure	Appearances are usually similar to asbestos inhalation

(CWP: coal workers' pneumoconiosis; HRCT: high-resolution computed tomography)

Local Pleural Masses (Table 17)

TABLE 17: Causes and differentiating features of local pleural masses.

Nature	Diseases	Features
Benign	Loculated pleural effusion (Fig. 31)	It is seen as a fluid attenuating collection
	• Localized fibrous tumor of the pleura	• It is a rare tumor of mesodermal origin representing <5% of all neoplasia involving the pleura • Approximately 70–80% of these tumors arise from visceral pleura, with the remainder arising from the parietal pleura • These are seen as well-delineated, often lobulated soft-tissue attenuation mass in close relation to the pleural surface or fissure, and absence of chest wall invasion. The margin at the junction of the mass with the pleura usually tapers smoothly

Contd...

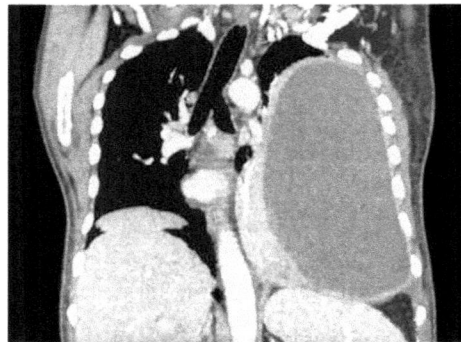

Fig. 31: Coronal CT image showing loculated pleural effusion on left side.

Contd...

Nature	Diseases	Features
		• They may demonstrate acute angles with the pleura with smooth tapering margins resulting in *beak* or *thong* sign
		• Calcifications are noted in large tumors and related to the areas of necrosis
		• The tumors have rich vascularization and shows intense and homogeneous enhancement
		• Identification of pedicle is a clue to the diagnosis. Indirect evidence of the presence of the pedicle can be seen as a change in the position of the lesion with change in posture

Contd...

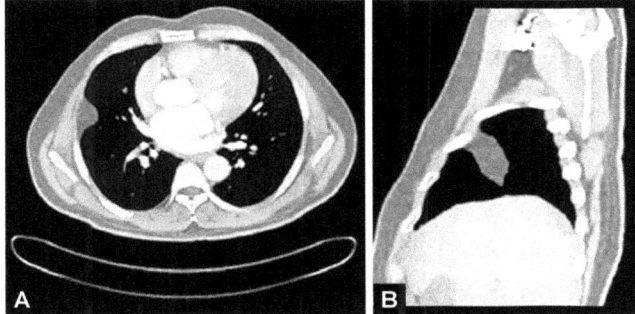

Figs. 32A and B: Axial and sagittal CT images showing pleural lipoma on right side.

Contd...

Nature	Diseases	Features
	Fibrin balls	• Develop in a serofibrinous pleural effusion and become visible following the absorption of the fluid • They are small and tend to be situated near the lung base • They may disappear spontaneously or remain unchanged for many years
	Pleural lipoma (Figs. 32A and B)	It is seen as a well-defined, homogeneous, and completely fat-attenuating mass with sometimes thin fibrous strands
Malignant	Metastases	• They can originate from intrathoracic or extrathoracic primary • Among the intrathoracic are included the bronchogenic (most common) carcinoma, thymoma, lymphoma, etc. Contact of >3 cm with the pleural surface suggests pleural invasion

Contd...

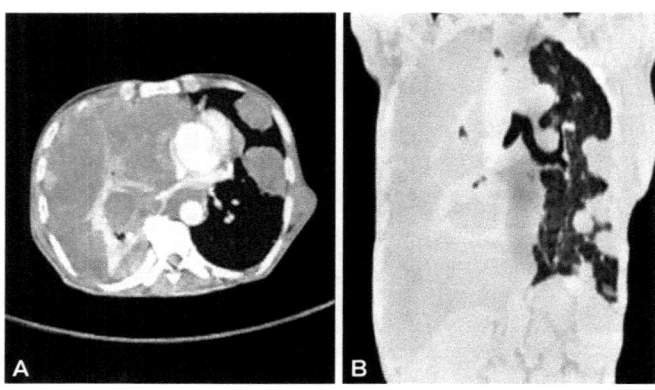

Figs. 33A and B: Axial and coronal CT images showing a mesothelioma of pleura with contralateral pulmonary metastases.

Contd...

Nature	Diseases	Features
		• Among the extrathoracic are included adenocarcinoma of breast, pancreas, ovary, gastrointestinal tract, and majority are multifocal
	Mesothelioma (Figs. 33A and B)	• A history of occupational exposure of asbestos is found in only 40–80% of patients with malignant pleural mesothelioma • Diffuse, unilateral pleural thickening occurs in up to two-thirds of patients. Sheet-like or lobulated pleural thickening may encase the lung, grow into the fissures, and create a pleural rind • Mesothelioma may also present as discrete pleural masses

Contd...

Contd...

Nature	Diseases	Features
		• Discrete pulmonary masses and hilar mass can also occur • Invasion of the chest wall occurs in far-advanced disease • Pleural effusion occurs in 30–80% of the patients with malignant mesothelioma
	Pleural lymphoma	• Involvement of the pleura by lymphoma may occur in both Hodgkin's and non-Hodgkin's disease • On CT, pleural lymphoma appears either as a solitary nodule or as multiple, broad-based pleural plaques usually associated with pleural effusion. Mass may be very large sometimes occupying the entire hemithorax • Pleural nodules represent the confluence of lymphoid tissue • Pleural effusion in lymphoma due to impaired lymphatic drainage appears to be the primary mechanism in Hodgkin's disease and direct pleural infiltration is the predominant cause in non-Hodgkin's lymphoma
	Malignant fibrous tumor of the pleura	• Usually the fibrous tumors have rich vascularization and shows intense and homogeneous enhancement • Nonenhancing areas correspond to necrosis, myxoid degeneration, or hemorrhage within the tumor • CT findings that suggest a malignant fibrous tumor include a diameter larger than 10 cm, central necrosis, and ipsilateral pleural effusion and chest wall invasion

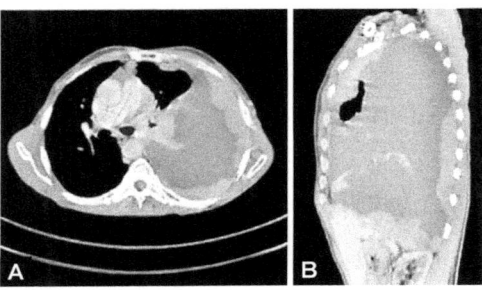

Figs. 34A and B: Axial and sagittal CT images showing nodular pleura.

Pleural Thickening (Figs. 34A and B)

Diffuse pleural thickening of the pleura is less specific to asbestos exposure than for pleural plaque development.

Diffuse pleural thickening has been defined on CT scanning as a continuous sheet more than 5 cm wide, more than 8 cm in craniocaudal extent, and more than 3 mm thick. Diffuse pleural thickening may be difficult to differentiate from multiple pleural plaques, but the following points may assist in diagnosis:
- Plaques usually spare the costophrenic angles and lung apices.
- Diffuse pleural thickening due to asbestos exposure rarely calcifies.
- Diffuse pleural thickening is ill defined and irregular from all angles, whereas plaques are well-defined.
- Plaques rarely extend over more than four rib interspaces unless multiple and confluent.

Causes

Various causes of pleural thickening include:
- *Asbestos exposure*: Diffuse pleural thickening may result from exudative pleural effusion secondary to asbestos exposure
- Hemothorax
- Tuberculosis
- Chest surgery
- Drugs such as methysergide can rarely cause diffuse pleural thickening
- Parapneumonic effusion.

Chapter 8

Abdomen

ABDOMINAL WALL LESIONS (TABLES 1 AND 2)

TABLE 1: Common causes of abdominal lesions.

Solid	Cystic	Fatty	Calcified	Air
<ul><li>Hematoma</li><li>Hemangioma</li><li>Desmoid</li><li>Pyogenic granuloma</li><li>Neurofibroma</li><li>Soft tissue sarcoma</li><li>Lymphoma</li><li>Metastases (Fig. 1)</li></ul>	<ul><li>Sebaceous cyst</li><li>Abscess</li><li>Chronic hematoma</li><li>Urachal cyst</li><li>Vitellointestinal cyst</li><li>Endometrioma</li><li>Localized collection</li></ul>	<ul><li>Lipoma</li><li>Liposarcoma</li></ul>	Tumoral calcification	<ul><li>Abscess</li><li>Necrotizing fasciitis</li><li>Bowel containing hernia</li></ul>

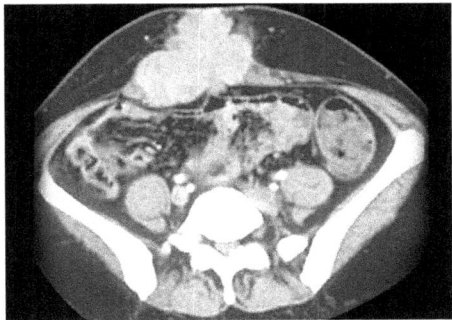

Fig. 1: Axial CT image showing abdominal wall metastases.

TABLE 2: Differentiating features of commonly seen abdominal wall lesions.

Diseases	Differentiating features	Comments
Hematoma	An elliptical or spindle-shaped mass often in one or more layers of the abdominal wall, obliterating or displacing fat planes with variable appearance depending on the stage of hematoma	• The hematoma shows evolution with time • It is usually seen within the rectus sheath • Rectus sheath hematoma crosses the midline, if it is below the level of the arcuate line
Inflammation/ infection	• There is evidence of fat stranding with loss of normal intermuscular fat planes • Thickening and ill-defined hypodensity of abdominal wall muscles • In late stages, there is formation of localized masses of varying density corresponding to abscess that dissect along the fascial planes • A typical abscess appears as a low attenuation lesion with thick, enhancing peripheral wall. Occasional septa, calcification, and air may be seen	
Endometriosis	• A well-defined, cystic mass of variable attenuation usually at the umbilical region • A surgical scar may also be the site of the lesion	

Contd...

Abdomen

Contd...

Diseases	Differentiating features	Comments
Lipoma	• These are well-defined, homogeneous fat attenuation masses • They may sometimes contain soft tissue septa and vessels	Presence of the solid, enhancing, soft tissue masses within the lipoma is suggestive of liposarcoma
Tumoral ossification	It is seen as multifocal, conglomerate, calcified masses in the soft tissues anywhere in the body	Anterior abdominal wall is an uncommon site
Desmoid (Figs. 2 and 3)	• It is seen as an ill-defined, soft tissue, moderately to intensely enhancing mass arising in the anterior abdominal wall muscle • The tumor may grow into the adjacent fat and even invade the peritoneum to become adherent to the bowel loops	• It is usually seen in the rectus abdominis and internal oblique muscle • It occurs predominantly in women of child-bearing age
Urachal cyst	• It is seen as a well-defined, thin-walled, cystic, midline, extraperitoneal mass in the infra-umbilical region. • The contents show fluid attenuation, except in cases of hemorrhage and infection where the density of the fluid may increase	It lies anywhere in the tract between the dome of the bladder to the umbilicus in the median umbilical ligament
Sebaceous cyst	It is seen as a well-defined, nonenhancing, cystic mass in the subcutaneous fat	The attenuation values of the internal contents are variable depending upon the nature of contents

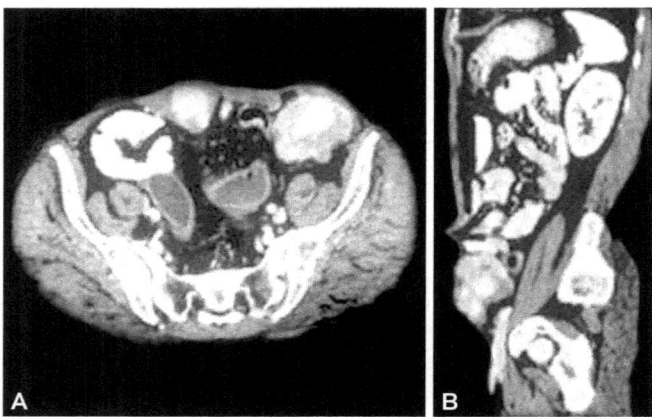

Figs. 2A and B: Axial and sagittal CT images showing abdominal wall desmoid.

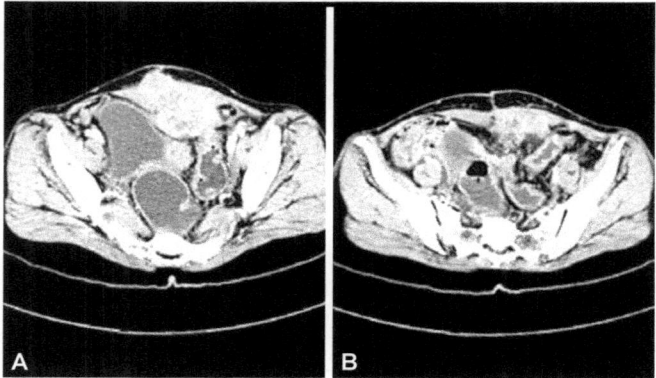

Figs. 3A and B: Axial CT images showing desmoid with invasion of the mesentery.

HERNIAS THROUGH ABDOMINAL WALL (TABLE 3)

TABLE 3: Characteristic features of various types of hernia through abdominal wall.

Types of hernia	Characteristic features	Comments
Ventral hernia (umbilical, paraumbilical, epigastric, incisional) (Figs. 4 and 5)	The peritoneal/mesenteric fat or bowel herniate anteriorly through the defect in the anterior abdominal wall	It is produced when the linea alba of the anterior abdominal wall is disrupted
Spigelian hernia	<ul><li>It is seen as herniation of the peritoneal contents through the linea semilunaris at the arcuate line located between the umbilicus and the pubic symphysis</li><li>The contents are seen beneath the intact external oblique muscle with a defect in the internal oblique muscle</li><li>The hernia has a very narrow neck</li></ul>	<ul><li>It results from weakness in the internal oblique and transversus aponeurosis</li><li>Strangulation is common</li></ul>
Lumbar hernia	<ul><li>It occurs at two sites in the posterolateral (Figs. 6A and B) abdominal wall</li><li>The inferior site is called the inferior lumbar triangle, or Petit's triangle, lies between external oblique, latissimus dorsi muscles, and iliac crest</li><li>The larger superior site is called the superior lumbar triangle or Grynfeltt-Lesshaft triangle, which is bounded by the twelfth rib, the serratus posterior muscle, the internal oblique muscle, and the erector spinae muscle</li></ul>	<ul><li>These are uncommon hernia seen usually in the elderly age</li><li>The contents of the hernia include fat, bowel or even kidney</li></ul>

Contd...

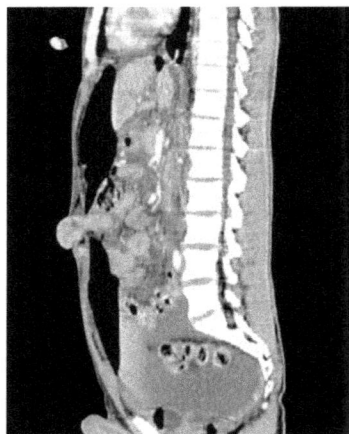

Fig. 4: Sagittal CT image showing a traumatic ventral hernia through the anterior abdominal wall.

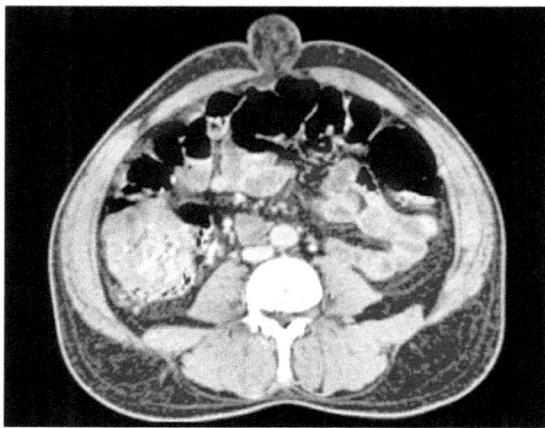

Fig. 5: Axial CT image showing an umbilical hernia in a patient with ascending colon mass.

Abdomen

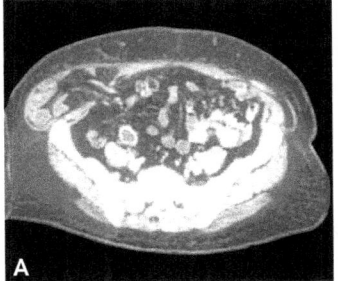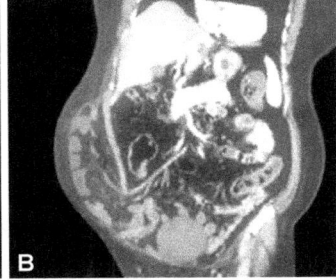

Figs. 6A and B: Axial and oblique coronal CT images showing a large lumbar hernia on right side.

Contd...

Types of hernia	Characteristic features	Comments
Femoral hernia	• In this type, the peritoneal contents enter the femoral canal adjacent to the femoral artery and femoral vein • The sac protrudes lateral to the inguinal canal between the external oblique muscle insertion on the superior pubic ramus and the superior pubic ramus itself	• It is a rare type of hernia, usually seen in females • It has a narrow neck and has a higher incidence of strangulation • In the Richter hernia, only one wall of the bowel is incarcerated and strangulates and perforates
Obturator hernia	It results when intraperitoneal or extraperitoneal contents protrude through the obturator canal and may extend up to the thigh	The contents of the sac can lie between the pectineus and obturator externus or between the superior and middle fascicles of the obturator externus or between the obturator externus and internus

Contd...

Contd...

Types of hernia	Characteristic features	Comments
Direct inguinal hernia	It is seen as protrusion of the intraperitoneal contents medial to the inferior epigastric artery in the inguinal region	It is wide-mouthed and rarely strangulates
Indirect inguinal hernia	• It is seen as protrusion of the intraperitoneal contents lateral to the inferior epigastric artery in the inguinal region through the deep inguinal ring • The sac may extend up to the ipsilateral scrotal sac in males	• This is the most common hernia • It has a narrow neck and may strangulate
Sciatic hernia	• They are seen as the protrusion of the intra- or extraperitoneal contents through the greater or lesser sciatic foramen seen posterior to the ischial tuberosity • The contents of the hernia may include bowel, bladder, ureter, ovary, etc	These are the rarest of all the hernias

HEPATOBILIARY LESIONS

Hepatic Lesions

Focal Hepatic Lesions (Table 4)

TABLE 4: Common causes of focal hepatic lesions.

Cystic	Solid/complex	Calcified	Fat	Air
Benign: • Simple cyst • Cystic hepatic disease • Autosomal dominant polycystic kidney disease • Parasitic cyst (echinococcal cyst) • Caroli disease • Choledochal cyst • Pancreatic pseudocyst • Abscess • Biloma • Chronic hematoma and laceration • Intrahepatic fluid collection • Periportal edema • Biliary cystadenoma	Malignant: • Hepatocellular carcinoma • Fibrolamellar carcinoma • Peripheral cholangiocarcinoma • Metastases • Hepatic sarcoma (angiosarcoma, Kaposi's sarcoma, fibrosarcoma) • Lymphoma • Hepatoblastoma Benign: • Hemangioma • Focal nodular hyperplasia • Adenoma (hepatocellular, biliary)	• Infectious lesions (tuberculosis, histoplasmosis, old abscess, echinococcal cyst) • Vascular lesions (hepatic artery aneurysm, venous thrombus, hematoma) • Biliary calculi • Benign neoplasms (simple cyst, hemangioma, regenerating nodules, hemangioendothelioma • Malignant lesions (hepatoblastoma, cholangiocarcinoma, metastases from carcinoma of colon, breast, stomach, ovary, etc.)	• Focal fatty infiltration • Myelolipoma • Angiomyolipoma • Teratoma • Hepatoma	• Portal venous gas • Pneumobilia • Abscess • Ischemic necrosis • Radionecrosis of neoplasm

Contd...

Contd...

Cystic	Solid/complex	Calcified	Fat	Air
• Mesenchymal hamartoma • Lymphangioma *Malignant:* • Biliary cystadenocarcinoma • Embryonal sarcoma • Malignant mesenchymoma • Cystic metastases (ovarian, gastric) • Necrotic neoplasm	• Nodular regenerating hyperplasia • Leiomyoma • Peliosis hepatis • Sarcoidosis • Hematoma/infarction • Mesothelioma • Infantile hemangioendothelioma • Pancreatic/adrenal rests			

Solitary	Multiple
Benign: • Simple/echinococcal cyst • Cavernous hemangioma • Abscess (amebic) • Hematoma • Focal nodular hyperplasia • Focal fatty change *Malignant:* • Hepatoma • Peripheral cholangiocarcinoma	*Benign:* • Echinococcal cysts • Cystic hepatic disease/ autosomal-dominant polycystic kidney disease (ADPKD) • Caroli disease • Cavernous hemangioma • Abscess (pyogenic, fungal) • Adenoma • Regenerating hepatic nodules • Sarcoidosis *Malignant:* • Metastases • Multifocal hepatoma • Lymphoma

Differential Diagnosis of Hepatic Lesions (Tables 5 and 6)

TABLE 5: Common causes of hepatic tumors with vascular scars.

- Fibrolamellar hepatocellular carcinoma
- Focal nodular hyperplasia
- Giant cavernous hemangioma
- Well-differentiated hepatocellular carcinoma
- Hepatic adenoma
- Hepatic cholangiocarcinoma
- Hypervascular metastases

Diseases	CT findings	Comments
Malignant tumors		
Hepatocellular carcinoma	Focal, multinodular or diffuse. Low attenuation more than high or isodense. May contain fatty tissue, necrosis and calcification. Irregular arterial enhancement is common. Portal vein invasion occurs often (25–40%), hepatic veins are invaded less often (15%)	Most common primary liver tumor
Fibrolamellar hepatocellular carcinoma (HCC)	• Solitary slightly hypodense mass • Central calcification seen in one-third of patients contrast enhancement patterns may be similar to HCC or adenoma	Very uncommon form of hepatocellular carcinoma. Involves young population and is unrelated to cirrhosis. Less malignant than HCC
Metastasis	Low attenuated areas within enhancing liver tissue. May have irregular margins and central necrosis. Vascular metastases may become isodense after contrast administration	More than 20 times more common than primary liver tumors. Usually multiple and involving both lobes. Pre- and postcontrast scans recommended to depict the maximum number of metastasis

Contd...

Contd...

Diseases	CT findings	Comments
Benign tumors		
Hemangioma	Discrete and homogeneous area of decreased attenuation. Contrast enhancement starts as nodular peripheral densities which progress toward the center. Large hemangiomas may contain central fibrotic cleft of low density. Isodense with the blood at a later phase after contrast administration	Most common hepatic neoplasm seen in >7% of the population. May grow from childhood to adulthood, more rapidly during pregnancy. May spontaneously regress
Focal nodular hyperplasia (FNH)	Noncontrast-enhanced CT (NECT) hypodense or isodense compared to the liver. If there is a scar, it is hypodense. Contrast enhancement is variable, early enhancement of the scar or entire lesion is common. May displace normal hepatic vessels	Rare benign tumor most often seen in women between 20 years and 50 years. Usually incidental. Multiple in 7–20% of cases. Central scars also seen in atypical HCC, fibrolamellar hepatoma, hepatic adenoma, and giant hemangioma
Adenoma	Hypodense or isodense lesion with a diameter of 8–15 cm in precontrast scans. Central increased density represents hemorrhage. Contrast enhancement is variable differentiation from HCC is difficult on CT	Typically seen in young women using oral contraceptives. May undergo spontaneous hemorrhage. Internal hemorrhage or necrosis is common (36%)
Hepatic adenomatosis	Multiple focal lesions which have an appearance of multiple adenomas	Rare entity distinct from hepatic adenoma or FNH

Contd...

Contd...

Diseases	CT findings	Comments
Nodular regenerative hyperplasia	Multiple hypodense lesions without significant contrast enhancement. Simulates metastases	Diffuse involvement of liver by hyperplastic nodules composed of normal hepatocytes. Distinct from cirrhosis and FNH
Mesenchymal hamartoma	Usually, a cystic low density lesion, may occasionally be solid. Solid tumor enhances strongly and may mimic a cavernous hemangioma	Rare a mixture of bile ducts and mesenchymal tissue. May be associated with polycystic liver disease
Lipoma	Discrete area of fat attenuation. Sometimes fine septa of soft tissue density are present.	Rare seen mostly but not exclusively in patients with renal angiomyolipoma
Biliary cystadenoma	Cystic mass in the liver parenchyma with septated multilocular appearance	Rare lesion, primarily in middle-aged women may develop into a malignant cystadenocarcinoma

Cysts

Diseases	CT findings	Comments
Hepatic cyst	Sharply delineated, round or oval lesion, near water attenuation may be multiple. No contrast enhancement of the walls or contents	If septations or irregular inner margins are seen, cystic neoplasm should be considered
Echinococcal cyst	May resemble simple cyst. A mature cyst may contain daughter vesicles, calcification, and membrane detachments	Rupture into the biliary tree is a common complication

Contd...

Contd...

Diseases	CT findings	Comments
Caroli disease	Multiple low attenuating cystic masses in the liver associated with a dilated biliary tree	Rare condition characterized by multiple saccular dilatations of the intrahepatic bile ducts throughout the liver. Medullary sponge kidney is associated in 80% of cases
Choledochal cyst	Cystic dilatation of the common bile duct (CBD) and or its tributaries within the liver	Associated with localized constriction of the distal CBD
Infection/Inflammation		
Pyogenic abscess	Sharply defined lesion, denser than water but less dense than liver. Capsule enhances but the central portion does not. May contain septations or mural projections. 20–30% contain gas, but gas fluid level is rare immature abscess may not be cystic	Necrotic metastases from sarcoma and ovarian carcinoma need to be distinguished from pyogenic abscess
Amebic abscess	CT appearance is similar to that of pyogenic abscesses, well-demarcated round or oval low density lesions with enhancing rims and low density centers. Septations are rare	Associated with amebiasis of the cecum and ascending colon
Trauma		
Biloma (bile pseudocyst)	Water-density, usually crescent or ovoid mass within or immediately adjacent to the liver	Intra- or extrahepatic collection of bile after traumatic rupture or surgery of the biliary tree

Contd...

Contd...

Diseases	CT findings	Comments
Laceration	Irregular cleft or low attenuation area that often extends to the periphery of the liver. A stellate or radiating pattern may be seen	Small hyperdense blood clots may be detected within the laceration
Intrahepatic hematoma	Acute hematoma is a hyperdense (70–80 HU), round, oval or irregular lesion in non-contrast scans. By 10–30 days the hematoma will become hypodense (20–25 HU)	Usually secondary to penetrating or blunt trauma, rarely due to adenoma, metastasis or arteriovenous (AV) malformation. A biloma is always hypodense
Subcapsular hematoma	Well-marginated, crescenting or lenticular fluid collection beneath the hepatic capsule. Attenuation high during the first few days and diminishes gradually over several weeks	Result of trauma, surgery, biopsy or biliary drainage procedure

Others

Focal fatty infiltration	Can vary from a small oval focus, typically adjacent to the intersegmental fissure. Margination is usually unsharp. There is no mass effect, contour change or vascular displacement	Regional reversible accumulation of triglycerides within hepatocytes that can simulate neoplasia. Lesion may disappear within weeks. Associated with obesity, alcoholism, chemotherapy, Cushing's syndrome, etc.

Contd...

Contd...

Diseases	CT findings	Comments
Hepatic venous occlusion (Budd-Chiari syndrome)	Hepatomegaly. Regional attenuation differences are characteristic. Ascites is common. NCCT demonstrates peripheral low attenuation of the liver with higher attenuation in the caudate lobe and central portions of the left lobe. Early contrast images demonstrate peripheral enhancement. Later images may show the reverse of this pattern or persistent central enhancement. Hepatic veins are not usually visualized	Rare clinical entity of obstruction of the hepatic venous outflow. Associated with hypercoagulopathy, OCPs, pregnancy, etc
Liver infarction	Wedge-shaped, low attenuation lesion on contrast-enhanced images. A round and central low-density lesion is another pattern. Initially infarcts are poorly marginated but become discrete and have lower attenuation in the later phase	Rare. Due to very low incidence of hepatic artery occlusion. Atherosclerosis, embolism, thrombosis
Radiation injury	Sharply defined band of diminished density in the liver corresponding to the radiation port	May develop days to months after a radiation dose of 35 Gy or more

TABLE 6: Common causes of hyperperfusive hepatic abnormalities.

Early enhancing lesions in left hepatic lobe:	Diffusely heterogeneous:	Segmental:	Subcapsular unknown origin	Subsegmental:
• Capsular vein • Cystic vein • Gastric vein	• Cirrhosis (Fig. 7)	• Cirrhosis with arterioportal shunt • Obstruction of the portal vein by thrombus, neoplasm or iatrogenic ligation		• Acute cholecystitis • Peripheral portal branches obstruction • Percutaneous needle biopsy or ethanol ablation of the lesion

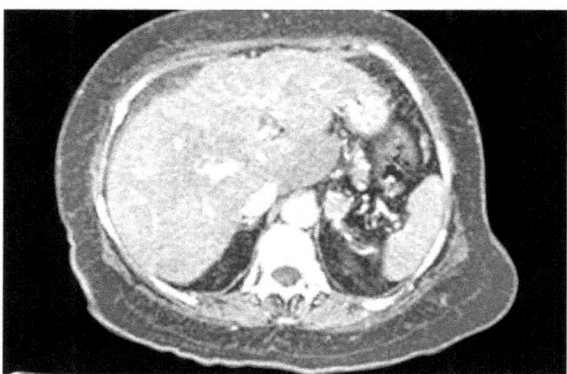

Fig. 7: Axial CT image in a case of cirrhosis of liver.

Hepatocellular Carcinoma (Figs. 8A and B)

- Most common primary hepatic malignancy in adults.
- CT appearance is variable: Focal, single or multinodular; diffuse. May present as a dominant mass with satellite nodules.
- Usually, hypoattenuating and occasionally with hypodense rim surrounding the lesion.
- CT reveals enhancement during the hepatic arterial phase, hypodense on portal phase scans and isodense on delayed scans.
- Perfusion defects due to portal and hepatic venous invasion.

Fibrolamellar Hepatocellular Carcinoma (Figs. 9A and B)

- Very uncommon form of HCC seen in young adults and is less malignant and unrelated to cirrhosis.
- CT reveals a large solitary hypodense mass with central stellate or trabecular calcification in approximately one-third to one-half of patients and prominent fibrous scar in approximately 50% of the patients.

Abdomen

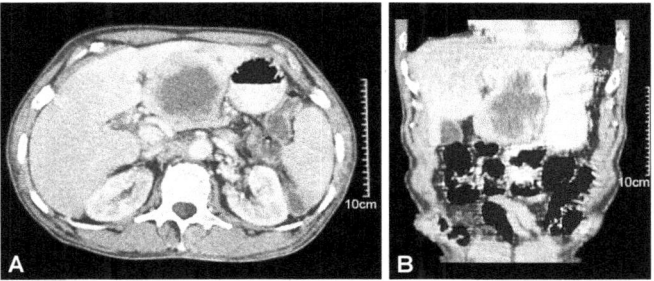

Figs. 8A and B: Axial contrast-enhanced computed tomography (CECT) images of abdomen showing exophytic peripherally enhancing lesion with centrally necrotic area arising from left lobe of liver in case of hepatocellular carcinoma.

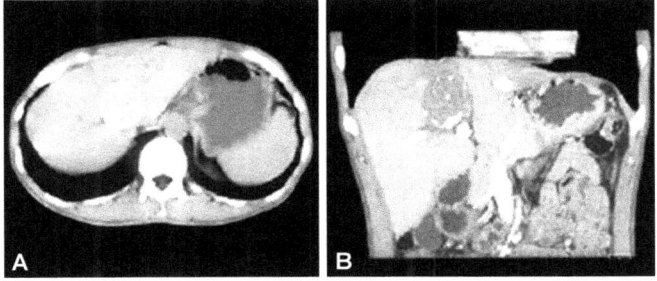

Figs. 9A and B: Axial and coronal CT images showing a case of fibrolamellar hepatocellular carcinoma.

Metastases (Fig. 10)

- Most common hepatic malignancy.
- Usually seen as focal, hypodense, multiple lesions involving both lobes.

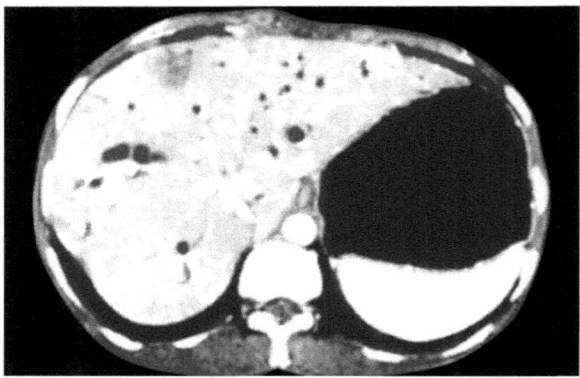

Fig. 10: Axial CT image showing a focal hepatic metastasis with intrahepatic biliary radicals dilatation.

- These show circumferential bead or band-like enhancement during arterial phase with peripheral washout on delayed images.
- Different types of metastases are tabulated in Table 7.

TABLE 7: Common causes of different types of metastases.

Calcified	Hypervascular	Hemorrhagic	Cystic
• Mucinous carcinoma from gastrointestinal tract (GIT), pancreas, ovary • Breast carcinoma • Testicular carcinoma • Renal cell carcinoma	• Carcinoid tumor • Choriocarcinoma • Renal cell carcinoma • Pancreatic islet cell tumors • Ovarian cystadenocarcinoma • Pheochromocytoma	• Breast carcinoma • Choriocarcinoma • Colon carcinoma • Melanoma • Renal cell carcinoma • Thyroid carcinoma	• Bronchogenic carcinoma • Carcinoid tumor • Colon carcinoma • Melanoma • Mucinous ovarian cystadenocarcinoma • Sarcoma

Contd...

Contd...

Calcified	Hypervascular	Hemorrhagic	Cystic
• Thyroid carcinoma • Neuroblastoma • Mesothelioma • Osteosarcoma, melanoma • Lymphoma • Bronchogenic carcinoma	• Breast carcinoma • Melanoma • Colonic carcinoma		

Hepatoblastoma (Figs. 11A and B)

- It is the most common primary hepatic malignancy in children, usually seen in the right lobe.
- CT reveals a hypodense mass with peripheral rim enhancement.

Biliary Cystadenoma/Cystadenocarcinoma

- It appears as a multilocular, cystic mass with nodular and papillary excrescences from the septations of the cyst wall.
- Distinction between adenoma and adenocarcinoma is unimportant since both are treated by surgical resection.

Hemangioma (Figs. 12A and B)

- It is most common hepatic neoplasm.
- They often grow gradually through childhood to adulthood and may regress spontaneously as well; Grow more rapidly during pregnancy.
- On NECT, it appears as a well-circumscribed spherical or oval hypodense mass.

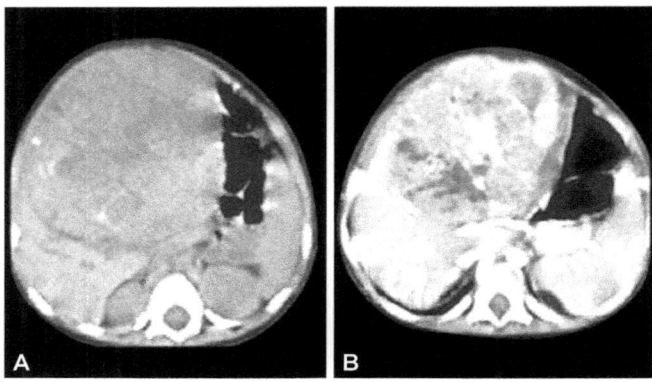

Figs. 11A and B: Axial CT images showing a case of hepatoblastoma.

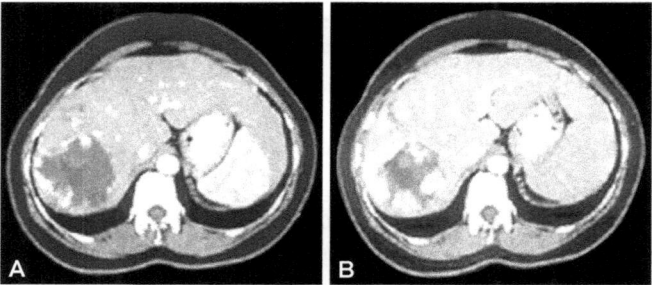

Figs. 12A and B: Axial CT images showing a typical hepatic hemangioma.

- On CECT, it shows usually peripheral, nodular enhancement in early phase that progresses centripetally to give an isodense mass in the delayed images that may require up to 3–30 minutes. However, central or diffuse dense enhancement may also be visualized in up to 20% cases. Partial or no filling in of the mass may be seen in up to 25%.
- Large hemangiomas may contain a central fibrous cleft of low density.

Focal Nodular Hyperplasia

- It is a rare, benign, hepatic tumor usually detected incidentally in women between 20 years and 50 years of age.
- NECT images show a hypodense mass if there is a fibrous central scar, else it is isodense to the hepatic parenchyma.
- It shows transient intense contrast enhancement followed by isodensity.
- Hypodense central scar with septations corresponding to small traversing vessels is seen up to portal venous phase. On delayed images, the scar becomes hyperdense to the lesion and the hepatic parenchyma.

Hepatic Adenoma

- It is typically seen in young females on oral contraceptives. Males also develop these lesions following long-term androgen or anabolic steroid therapy.
- These lesions can undergo spontaneous hemorrhage or necrosis.
- Hyperdensity may be seen in case of hemorrhage in precontrast scans.
- They enhance transiently on arterial phase and become iso- or hypodense on delayed images.

Mesenchymal Hamartoma

- It is a rare cystic hepatic tumor seen at 1–2 years of age.
- It is seen as cystic mass in majority of the patients, but may be solid in which case the tumor enhances strongly and may even mimic cavernous hemangioma.

Hepatic Cyst (Figs. 13 and 14)

- It is seen as a sharply marginated, round to oval, water-attenuating lesion that does not show any contrast enhancement of the wall or its contents on postcontrast images.

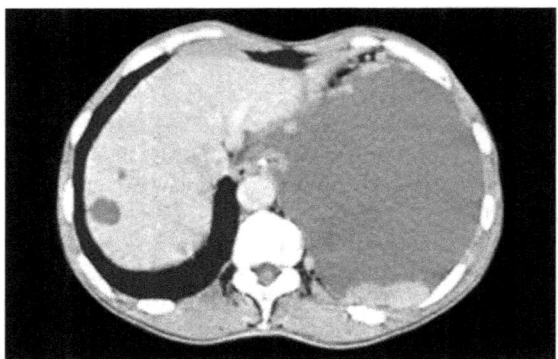

Fig. 13: Axial CT image showing hepatic cysts in right lobe.

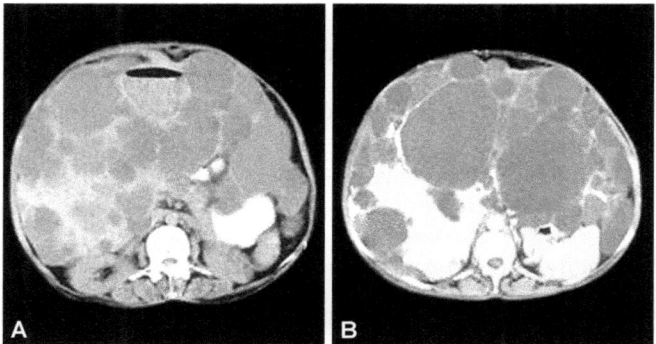

Figs. 14A and B: Axial CT images showing a case of polycystic liver disease.

- Multiple such lesions are frequent especially with von Hippel-Lindau disease or adult polycystic kidney disease.
- Presence of septations or irregularity of the inner wall suggests cystic neoplasm rather than a simple cyst.

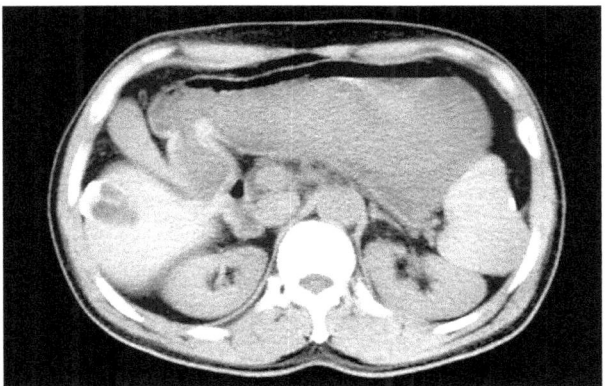

Fig. 15: Transaxial CT image shows healing hydatid cyst of liver.

Hydatid Cyst (Fig. 15)

- These may be indistinguishable from simple cyst.
- A mature cyst may contain daughter cysts, calcification, and detached membranes.
- Fluid-fluid or air-fluid levels may be seen.
- Cyst may rupture through the capsule of liver to cause peritoneal dissemination or may rupture into the biliary tree with biliary obstruction.

Caroli Disease

- It is a rare condition characterized by saccular dilatation of multiple intrahepatic biliary ducts throughout the hepatic parenchyma seen as multiple cystic lesions converging toward the porta hepatis and extending toward the periphery of the liver.
- Portal radicles completely surround the ducts giving rise to *central dot sign*.
- Calculi or sludge may be seen in the dilated ducts.
- Medullary sponge kidneys are associated in the majority.

Abscess (Figs. 16 and 17)

- It is seen as sharply-defined, heterogeneous, hypodense, unilocular or multilocular lesion with ring enhancement on the postcontrast images.

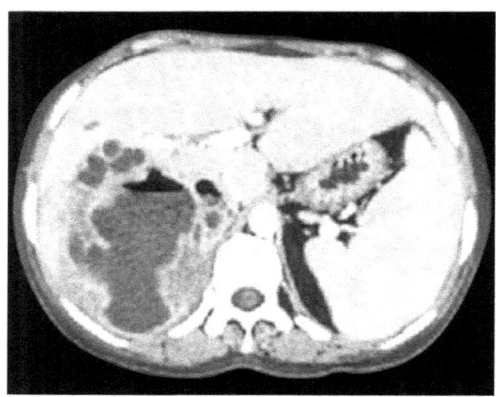

Fig. 16: Axial CT image showing a large hepatic abscess in the right lobe.

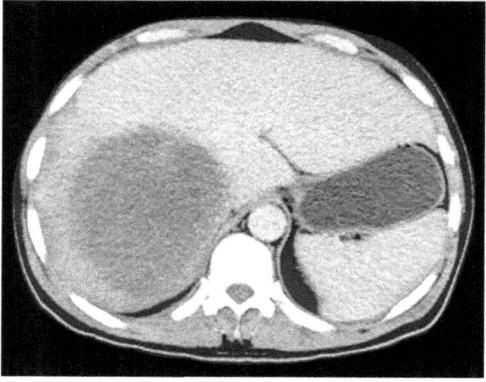

Fig. 17: Transaxial CT image shows amebic hepatic abscess.

- *Double-target sign* may be seen due to the presence of wall enhancement and surrounding hypodense zone.
- *Cluster sign* refers to the cluster-shape arising due to coalescing lesions and is typical of pyogenic abscess.
- May contain air, mural nodules or septations but air-fluid level is rare.

Biloma (Biliary Pseudocyst)

- It is seen as an intra- or extrahepatic (immediately adjacent to the liver), crescentic or ovoid, cystic collection of varying size.
- Traumatic rupture or surgical interventions of the biliary tree are usually associated.

Laceration (Figs. 18A and B)

- It is seen as sharply delineated, irregular, hypodense, nonenhancing, cleft in the hepatic parenchyma that may often contain hyperdense clots.
- These lesions evolve into indistinguishable areas after several weeks of insult to the hepatic parenchyma.

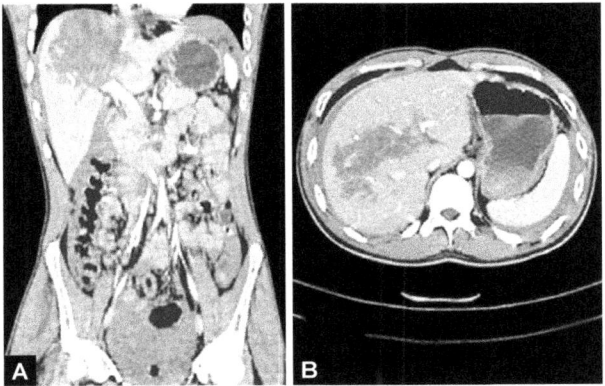

Figs. 18A and B: Coronal CT images showing a large intrahepatic hematoma and laceration with hemoperitoneum.

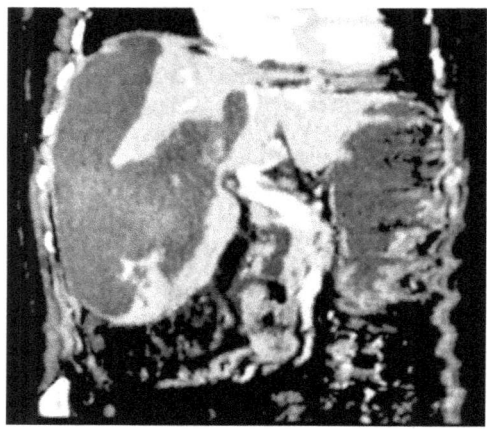

Fig. 19: Coronal CT image showing a large hepatic laceration with a large subcapsular and intrahepatic hematoma.

Intrahepatic/Subcapsular Hematoma (Fig. 19)

- Acute hematoma is hyperdense on noncontrast scans and becomes isodense on contrast scans, as they do not enhance. Over a period of several weeks, clot lysis occurs and chronic hematoma results that is cystic with attenuation values closer to the water.
- Intrahepatic hematoma is surrounded by the hepatic parenchyma and is usually ill-marginated while subcapsular hematoma is seen as a crescentic or lenticular, well-marginated collection pushing the liver away from its capsule.

Periportal Edema

- It is seen as a hypodense, nonenhancing collection that surrounds the branches of the portal vein.
- It is a common postoperative finding in hepatic transplantation but is also seen secondary to hepatic trauma.

Focal Fatty Infiltration

- It is seen as a focal, ovoid, fatty focus in subcapsular location typically adjacent to the fissure for ligamentum teres but may also be seen in a geographic distribution.
- The lesions may fail to reveal a fatty density if they are very small due to volume averaging, hence the appearance and location are more specific than density alone in diagnosing the condition.
- The lesions are usually unsharp on noncontrast images but become very conspicuous on postcontrast images.
- The lesions have imperceptible walls with no mass effect, contour abnormality or vascular displacement.

Hepatic Infarct

- It is seen as a characteristic, wedge-shaped, hypoattenuating lesion best visualized on postcontrast images. A round or oval lesion is another pattern.
- In the beginning, the lesions are poorly delineated; but later on, it becomes discrete and relatively more hypodense.
- In the chronic stage, the lesion is usually cystic with associated atrophy of the involved segment.

Diffuse Liver Disease (Table 8 and Fig. 20)

TABLE 8: Common causes of diffuse liver diseases.

Hyperdense on NECT	Hypodense on NECT
<ul><li>*Diffuse iron deposition disease*:<ul><li>Hemochromatosis</li><li>Bantu siderosis</li><li>Transfusional iron overload</li></ul></li><li>Diffuse copper deposition disease (Wilson's disease)</li><li>Diffuse iodine deposition disease (long-term amiodarone therapy)</li><li>Diffuse gold deposition following long-term gold therapy for rheumatoid arthritis</li><li>Acute massive protein deposition</li><li>Glycogen storage disease</li></ul>	<ul><li>Diffuse fatty infiltration</li><li>Portal vein thrombosis (acute phase)</li><li>Amyloidosis</li><li>Sarcoidosis</li><li>Diffuse hepatocellular carcinoma</li><li>Diffuse lymphoma</li><li>Diffuse metastatic disease</li></ul>

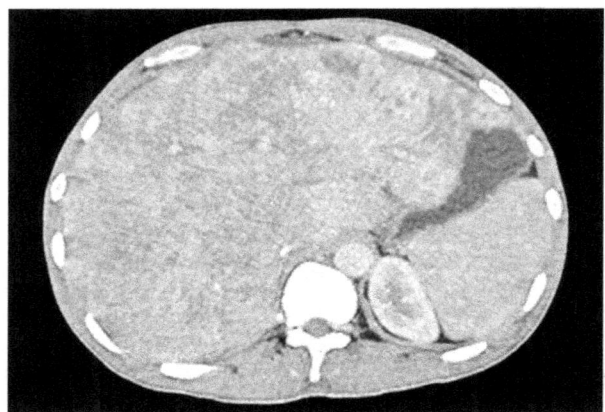

Fig. 20: Axial CT image in a case of diffuse hepatic disease.

Hemochromatosis

- The attenuation values of the hepatic parenchyma are in the range of 75–130 HU depending upon the degree of iron accumulation.
- It may be associated with changes consistent with cirrhosis.

Diffuse Fatty Infiltration (Fig. 21)

- Hepatic parenchyma has lower attenuation than portal vein or inferior vena cava on NECT.
- There is reversal of liver–spleen CT-density relationship on NECT (spleen is normally 6–10 HU lower than liver).
- Intrahepatic vascular structures appear hyperdense on NECT scans.
- There is poor enhancement of the hepatic parenchyma on CECT scans.

Acute Portal Vein Thrombosis (Fig. 22)

- The portal vein is enlarged and isodense with unopacified blood.
- The walls of the portal vein may enhance but not the thrombus.
- Infection, trauma, cirrhosis, and neoplasm are some of the common causes.

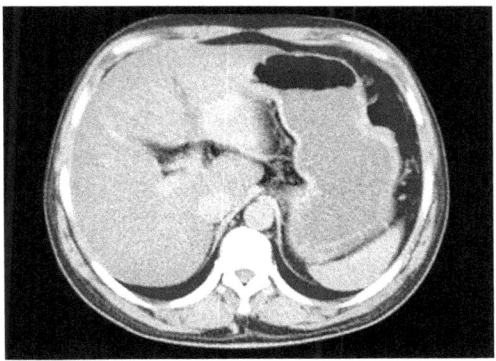

Fig. 21: Transaxial CT image shows diffuse fatty infiltration of liver.

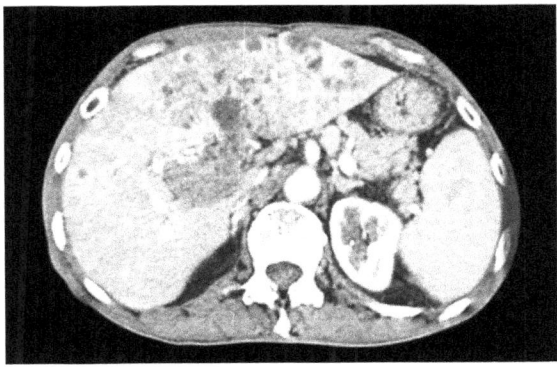

Fig. 22: Axial CECT image of abdomen showing infiltrating mass in liver with tumor thrombus involving the portal vein.

Amyloidosis, Sarcoidosis

- There is nonspecific hepatosplenomegaly in sarcoidosis and hepatomegaly in amyloidosis.
- Delayed poor contrast enhancement is present.

Diffuse HCC

- It is characterized by diffuse, inhomogeneous, hypoattenuating hepatic parenchyma with variable degree of contrast enhancement.
- Cirrhosis is often an overlapping finding.

Diffuse Metastatic Disease (Fig. 23)

- There is diffuse hepatomegaly with variable contrast enhancement and mass effect on the adjacent vascular structures and hepatic parenchyma.
- Presence of the known primary helps in the diagnosis.

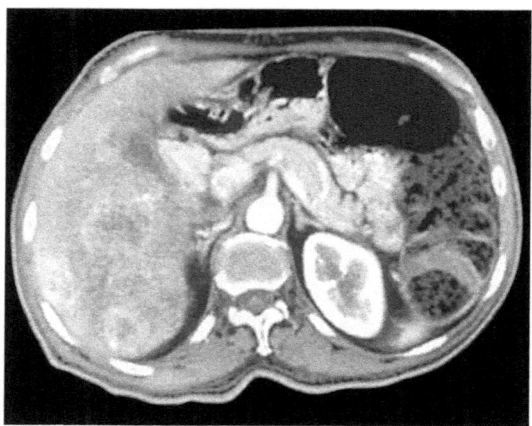

Fig. 23: Axial CT image shows metastatic disease of liver.

Diffuse Lymphoma

- There is nonspecific hepatomegaly with multiple, poorly-delineated, poorly-enhancing lesions involving the hepatic parenchyma.
- Associated extensive adenopathy and splenomegaly with focal lesions clicks the diagnosis.

Differential Diagnosis of Diffuse Hepatic Lesions (Table 9)

TABLE 9: Differential diagnosis of diffuse hepatic lesions.

Diseases	CT findings	Comments
Cirrhosis	In early cirrhosis, the right lobe appears normal while the caudate lobe and left lobe appear enlarged. In the later phase all lobes may appear atrophic. The intrahepatic fissure appears enlarged and the contour is lobulated. Regenerative nodules and HCC may be present	Micronodular (<3 mm) due to alcoholic cirrhosis most commonly. Macronodular (>3 mm) due to viral hepatitis. Splenomegaly, ascites, collateral veins, colonic interposition, and small bowel edema are associated findings
Portal vein thrombosis	• *Acute phase*: Portal vein is enlarged and isodense with unopacified blood. The walls of the portal vein may enhance, the thrombus may not. There may be segmental differences in the contrast enhancement of adjacent liver parenchyma • *Chronic phase*: Portal vein thrombosis shoes recanalization or formation of enlarged collaterals termed cavernous transformation	May be caused by neoplasm, infection, cirrhosis, trauma, hypercoagulable states or hepatic venous obstruction

Contd...

Contd...

Diseases	CT findings	Comments
Fatty liver	Liver attenuation is 10 HU or more below that of the spleen. Can be uniform, multifocal and focal	Occurs after hepatocellular injury or toxicity such as alcohol, obesity, diabetes, steroid treatment
Wilson's disease	Increased attenuation of the liver and cirrhotic changes	Toxic levels of copper accumulate in the liver, brain, cornea secondary to impaired biliary excretion
Hemochromatosis	Diffuse increase in the attenuation of the liver (75–130 HU). Associated changes consistent with cirrhosis are common	Primary hemochromatosis due to iron deposition in the liver, pancreas, myocardium, joints, skin, AR disorder; Secondary hemochromatosis due to iron overload and deposition in the reticuloendothelial system
Schistosomiasis	*Schistosoma japonicum* causes a "tortoise shell" appearance of the liver with calcified septations. *S mansoni* causes low density periportal changes in precontrast images. Marked contrast enhancement takes place, but no calcification is present	Results from granulomatous reaction to the parasite and subsequent periportal fibrosis
Sarcoidosis	Nonspecific hepatosplenomegaly	Noncaseating granulomas are more apparent in the portal triad regions than in the liver parenchyma

Contd...

Contd...

Diseases	CT findings	Comments
Amyloidosis	Nonspecific hepatomegaly. Focal low attenuation area correspond to involved areas. Delayed contrast enhancement may be present	Deposition of fibrils of light chain immunoglobulins in perivascular distribution and in the space of Disse
Diffuse hepatocellular carcinoma	Diffuse irregular low-density changes, variable degree of contrast enhancement	Liver cirrhosis is an overlaying finding
Diffuse metastatic disease	Precontrast scan can be normal or can show diffuse hepatomegaly due to diffuse low-contrast lesions. Contrast enhancement usually shows subtle displacement of normal liver parenchyma with diffuse metastatic involvement	
Diffuse lymphoma	Multiple hypodense, poorly-delineated lesions are better seen after contrast enhancement	Adenopathy and splenomegaly are common

Contour Abnormalities (Table 10)

TABLE 10: Common causes of contour abnormalities of liver.

Focal	Diffuse
Focal subcapsular lesions	• Cirrhosis (Figs. 24A and B) • Diffuse hepatocellular carcinoma

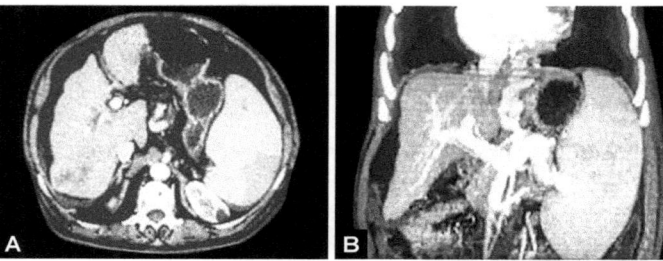

Figs. 24A and B: Axial and coronal CT images showing contour abnormality in a case of cirrhosis complicated with portal hypertension.

GALLBLADDER AND BILIARY TRACT LESIONS

Biliary Lesions (Table 11)

TABLE 11: Common causes of biliary lesions.			
Cystic	*Soft tissue*	*Calcified*	*Fatty*
• Choledochocele • Choledochal cyst • CBD diverticulum • Caroli disease • Biloma • Cholangitis	• Worm infestation • Adenomyomatosis • Carcinoma • Local invasion (hepatic) or distant metastatic deposits	• Cholelithiasis (Fig. 25) • Cholecystolithiasis • Choledocholithiasis (Figs. 26A to C)	Cholelithiasis

Hyperdense Bile

- Limy bile
- Hemobilia
- Contrast excretion in bile, e.g. following urographic studies or contrast studies of the biliary tree as percutaneous transhepatic cholangiography (PTC) or endoscopic retrograde cholangiopancreatography (ERCP).

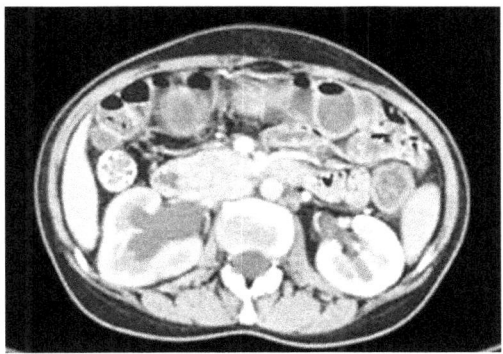

Fig. 25: Axial CT image showing incidental calcified gallbladder calculi in a patient of hydronephrosis on right side.

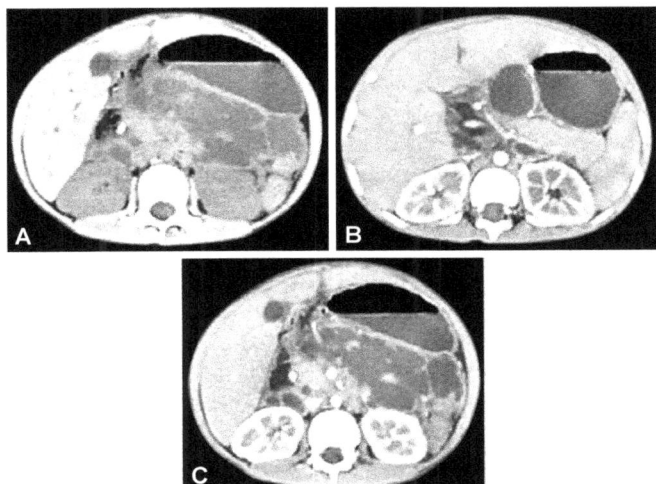

Figs. 26A to C: Choledocholithiasis with secondary common bile duct rupture with collection in the lesser sac.

Biliary Lesions Associated with Wall Thickening (Table 12)

TABLE 12: Common causes of biliary lesions associated with wall thickening.

Diffuse	Focal
• Physiological contracted gallbladder (GB)	• Polyps (inflammatory, cholesterol)
• Cholecystitis (acute and chronic)	• Intramural parasitic granuloma/cyst/calculus
• Cholesterolosis	• Benign tumor (adenoma, papilloma)
• Perforation	
• Cholangiopathy especially AIDS	• Malignant (carcinoma, metastases)
• Cholangitis	
• Benign causes of ascites	• Heterotopic mucosa (gastric, pancreatic)
• Varices (GB)	
• Carcinoma	

Choledochal cyst (Figs. 27A and B):
- It is contiguous with the biliary tree.
- It fills with the biliary contrast media.
- Type III is also known as choledochocele that is seen within the wall or lumen of the duodenum contiguous with the distal CBD, which may show focal dilatation.
- Diverticular processes can also arise from the CBD itself.

Caroli disease:
- It is characterized by multiple intrahepatic cysts contiguous with the biliary tree as confirmed by their filling by biliary contrast media.
- Intrahepatic biliary calculi are commonly associated.
- Polycystic disease of the kidney is also a common association.

Cholangitis:
- Infective and inflammatory variety are associated with smooth, thickened, and enhancing walls with hyperdense bile and diffuse dilatation of the biliary tree with stricture formation in the late chronic stages. Air may be seen in the suppurative type and calculus may be associated in the chronic type.

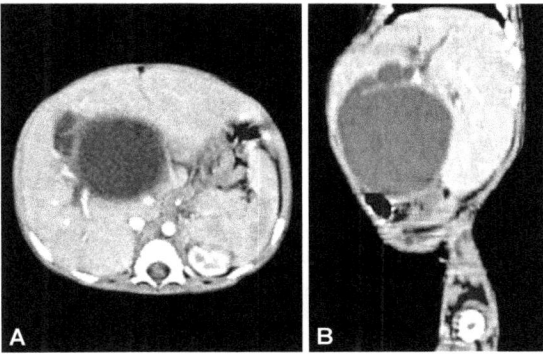

Figs. 27A and B: Axial and coronal CT images showing a large choledochal cyst.

- Sclerosing type is characterized by focal, scattered dilatation of the peripheral part of biliary tree with no demonstrable contiguity with the central ducts. The dilated ducts show nodular wall thickening and wall enhancement.

Carcinoma:
- Gallbladder carcinoma can occur as polypoidal intraluminal enhancing soft tissue mass or as focal or diffusely enhancing, GB wall thickening (Figs. 28 and 29).
- Cholangiocarcinoma usually occurs as focal or diffusely enhancing, wall thickening with short, irregular stricture and sometimes as polypoidal intraluminal mass (Figs. 30A and B).
- Biliary duct dilatation is more common with cholangiocarcinoma, while gallstones and hepatic metastases favor GB carcinoma (Figs. 31A and B).

Cholecystitis (Fig. 32):
- Pericholecystic fluid and hypoattenuating, nonenhancing rim within the GB wall are characteristic features especially in the presence of the cholelithiasis.
- Air within the lumen can be a feature of *emphysematous cholecystitis* if iatrogenic factors and fistulization with the bowel can be excluded.

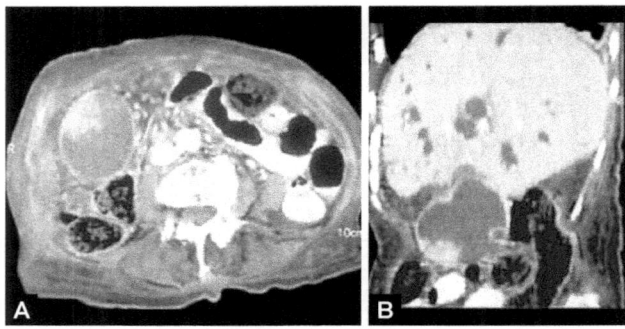

Figs. 28A and B: Axial and oblique coronal CT images showing a polypoidal mass in the fundus of gallbladder.

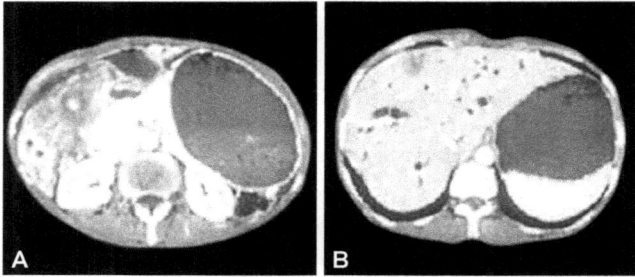

Figs. 29A and B: Axial CT images showing infiltrating GB mass with hepatic metastases and intrahepatic biliary dilation.

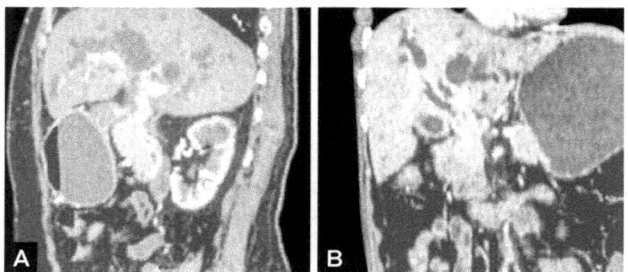

Figs. 30A and B: Oblique coronal CT images showing a diffusely infiltrating cholangiocarcinoma of the CBD with proximal biliary tract dilatation.

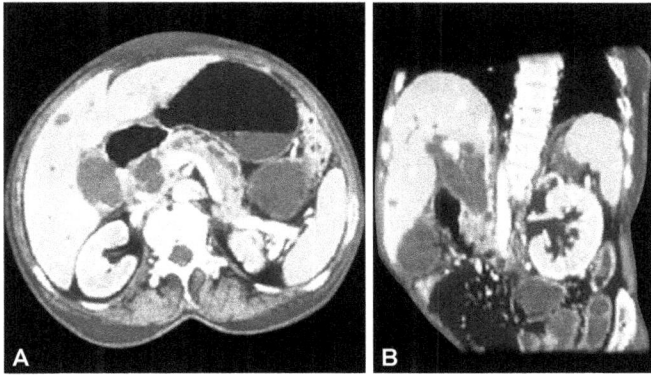

Figs. 31A and B: Axial and coronal CT images showing a mass at distal end of CBD with proximal biliary dilatation.

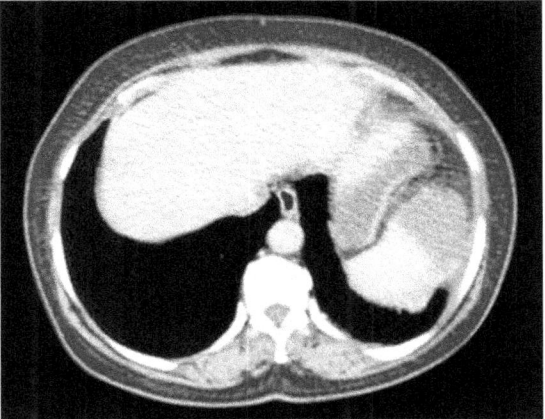

Fig. 32: Transaxial CT image shows cholelithiasis with acute cholecystitis.

SPLENIC AND PANCREATIC LESIONS

Splenic Lesions (Table 13)

TABLE 13: Common causes of lesions of spleen.

Cystic	Solid	Calcified
• Congenital cyst/ epidermoid cyst/true cyst • Chronic hematoma/ post-traumatic pseudocyst • Echinococcal cyst • Pancreatic pseudocyst • Abscess • Chronic splenic infarct • Cavernous hemangioma • Lymphangioma • Angiosarcoma • Cystic metastases	• Hematoma (Figs. 33A and B) • Sarcoidosis • Granulomatous infections (tuberculosis, histoplasmosis) (Fig. 34) • Splenic infarct • Hamartoma • Gaucher's disease • Angiosarcoma • Leukemia and lymphoma • Metastases	• Diffuse distribution (healed granuloma, visceral angiomatosis) • Focal (abscess, infarct, hematoma) • Vascular (arterial, aneurysmal) • Cyst wall

Diffusely Hyperdense Spleen

- Sickle cell anemia
- Hemochromatosis
- Multiple blood transfusions
- Previous history of thorotrast exposure or lymphangiography.

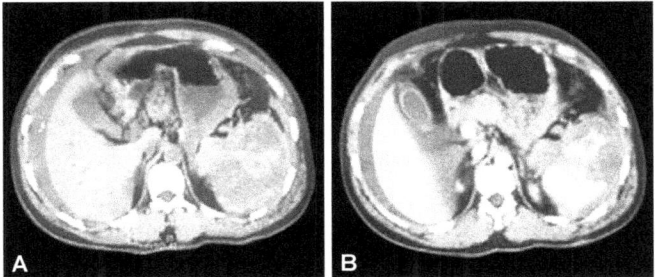

Figs. 33A and B: Axial CT images showing a large splenic hematoma and laceration.

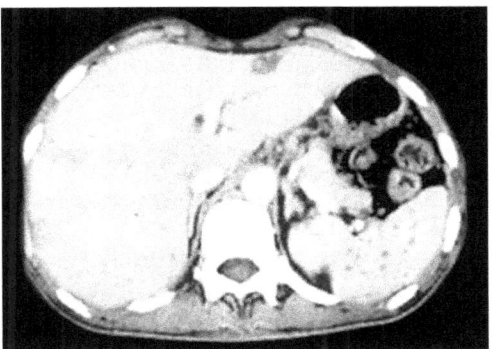

Fig. 34: Axial CT image showing tuberculosis of spleen.

Congenital cyst:
- It is seen as a unilocular, homogeneous, round to ovoid, cystic mass with imperceptible walls.
- Occasional mural calcification may be seen.

Post-traumatic pseudocyst:
- CT findings are similar to congenital cyst but have relatively thicker walls.
- History of old trauma may be suggestive.
- Hemorrhagic cyst may show calcification.

Pancreatic pseudocyst:
- It is seen as a unilocular or multilocular cystic lesion of variable shapes and sizes, often with multiple septations and thick enhancing walls.
- History or imaging evidence of the pancreatic disease highly suggestive.

Echinococcal cyst:
- It is seen as a round to oval, uni- or multilocular cystic mass with sharp enhancing walls that may show calcification in the wall or its lumen.
- Presence of a similar lesion in the liver is highly suggestive.

Abscess (Fig. 35):
- It is seen as a cystic or complex mass with relatively ill-defined and thick enhancing wall.
- Presence of edema in the adjacent parenchyma is characteristic.
- Presence of air suggests necrosis in the absence of any iatrogenic event.

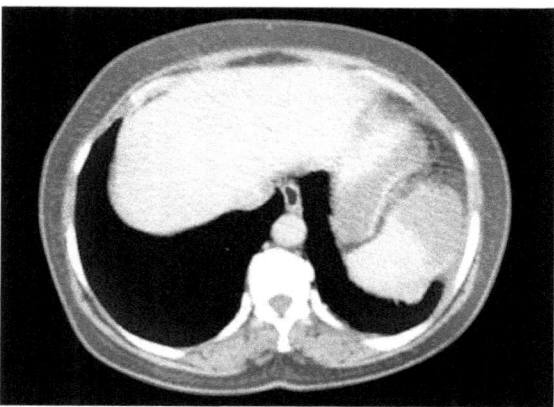

Fig. 35: Transaxial CT image shows abscess in spleen.

Abdomen

Cavernous hemangioma:
- It is seen as a cystic lesion with speckled calcification.
- Nodular peripheral contrast enhancement progressing centripetally is characteristic.
- It may be seen as part of Klippel-Trenaunay syndrome (cutaneous, bowel and soft tissue hemangioma; superficial venous varicosities; unilateral bone hypertrophy of the extremity).

Lymphangioma:
- It is seen as a multicystic, multiseptate, lobulated mass with thin, nonenhancing septae and walls.
- Septal and mural enhancement may be seen in cases of secondary infection.
- Curvilinear calcification may be seen in the wall.

Angiosarcoma:
- It is seen usually as a nonhomogeneous, heterogeneously enhancing cystic mass with solid components.
- It shows rapid growth with early metastases.

Splenic infarct (Fig. 36):
- It is usually seen as a wedge-shaped, hypodense, nonenhancing lesion along the peripheral parenchyma abutting the capsule with the apex facing the hilum.
- Capsular rim enhancement and calcification may be seen.

Sarcoidosis:
- It is usually characterized by multiple, small, hypodense, nonenhancing lesions distributed diffusely in the splenic parenchyma.
- It is invariably associated with pulmonary sarcoidosis and with splenomegaly in up to half of the cases.

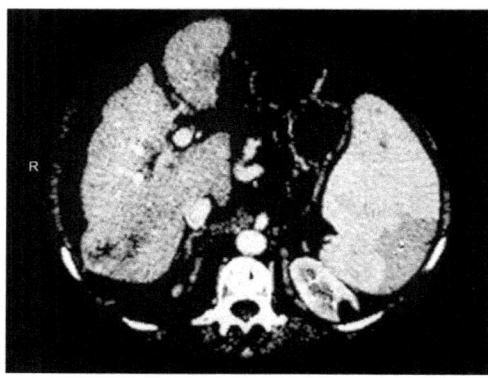

Fig. 36: Axial CT image showing a splenic infarct in a case of cirrhosis with portal hypertension.

Leukemia/lymphoma:
- These are characterized by splenomegaly with multiple, nodular, hypodense, nonenhancing lesions diffusely distributed in the parenchyma.
- Presence of lymphadenopathy elsewhere in the body is suggestive.

Pancreatic Lesions (Table 14)

\	\	\
TABLE 14: Common causes of pancreatic lesions.		
Cystic	Solid	Calcified
• Pancreatic cyst • Pancreatic pseudocyst • Abscess • Mucinous/ Serous cystic tumor	• Carcinoma • Islet cell tumor • Metastases • Lymphoma	• Chronic pancreatitis (alcoholic, biliary, hyperparathyroidism, cystic fibrosis, kwashiorkor) (Figs. 37A to D) • Neoplasm (microcystic, macrocystic, carcinoma, hemangioma) • Old hematoma/abscess/ infarct • Hemochromatosis

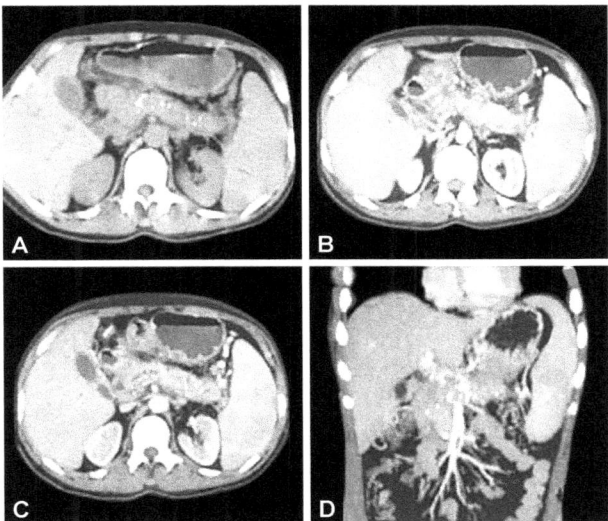

Figs. 37A to D: Axial and coronal CT images showing chronic calcific pancreatitis with mild pancreatic atrophy.

Fatty and Atrophic Pancreas (Fig. 38)

- Old age
- Obesity
- Diabetes mellitus
- Chronic pancreatitis
- Obstructed main pancreatic duct
- Cystic fibrosis
- Hemochromatosis
- Malnutrition
- Sequelae of severe viral infection.

Hypervascular pancreatic lesions:
- *Primary tumors*: Islet cell tumor, hemangioma.
- *Metastatic tumor*: Angiosarcoma, renal cell carcinoma, and thyroid carcinoma.

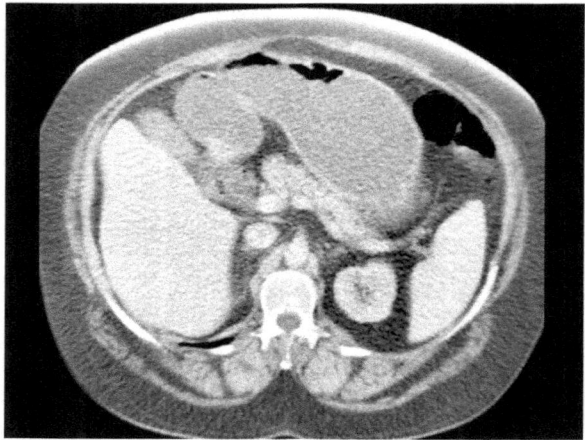

Fig. 38: Transaxial CT image shows atrophic fatty pancreas.

Pancreatic cyst:
- It is seen as a well-defined, nonenhancing, cystic lesion with imperceptible walls with occasional mural calcification.
- These can be seen either as solitary lesions or as part of the adult polycystic kidney disease or von Hippel-Lindau disease.

Pancreatic pseudocyst (Figs. 39A to C):
- It is characterized by a relatively well-defined, cystic lesion with thick, enhancing walls.
- The intracystic contents may be hemorrhagic or necrotic with presence of multiple septa or air.
- The walls of the cyst may calcify.
- The intramural nodule is typically absent though the wall may be occasionally nodular in cases of immature cysts.
- Presence of similar lesions elsewhere in the abdomen and chest and imaging evidence of pancreatic pathology may be highly suggestive.

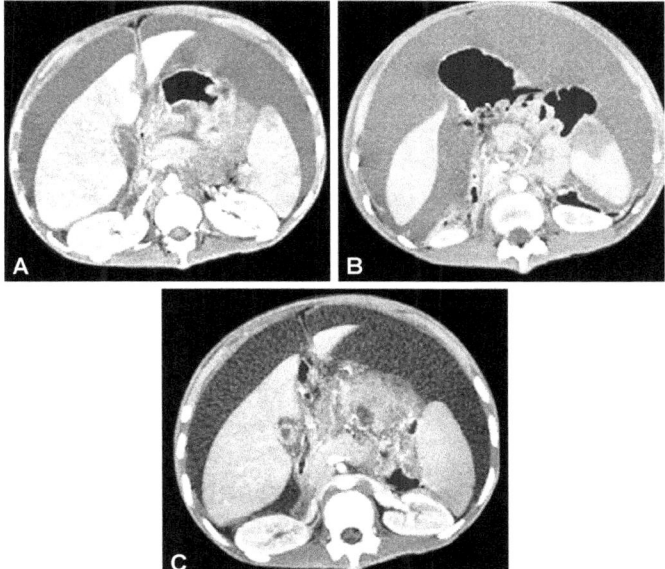

Figs. 39A to C: Axial CT images showing acute pancreatitis with ascites and splenic pseudocyst.

Pancreatic abscess:
- The CT appearance is similar to the abscesses seen elsewhere.
- Presence of gas in the abscess may be secondary to infection or fistulous communication with gastrointestinal tract.

Pancreatic adenocarcinoma:
- It is characterized by solid, ill-defined, hypodense, heterogeneously but moderately enhancing lesions.
- Presence of peripancreatic extension, vascular invasion, regional lymphadenopathy, and distant metastases are highly suggestive of the diagnosis.

- Main pancreatic duct dilatation is commonly associated sometimes with common bile duct dilatation.
- Presence of necrosis may simulate pseudocyst and necrotic pancreatic carcinoma is known as pseudocyst of pancreas. The latter has greater attenuation of the intracystic contents with relatively thickened and enhancing walls.

Pancreatic islet cell tumor:
- No specific feature to differentiate it from carcinoma.
- There detection depends upon their size and vascularity. Usually, they are hypervascular and are usually detected on dynamic contrast studies.
- Presence of calcification makes a diagnosis of islet cell tumor more likely than carcinoma.

Mucinous (macrocystic)/serous (microcystic) tumor:
- *Macrocystic tumor*:
  - Appears as uni- or multilocular cystic mass of >2 cm usually located in the body and tail of the pancreas.
  - There are usually <10 cysts.
  - The walls are well-defined, thick and enhancing.
  - Calcification is seen in up to third of cases and is of amorphous peripheral type.
- *Microcystic tumor*:
  - Appear as cystic mass of <2 cm often with some solid component.
  - There are usually >10 cysts with a honeycomb appearance.
  - The walls are well-defined with thin walls.
  - Calcification is seen in up to half of cases and is in central sunburst pattern.

Lymphoma:
- These are usually seen as solid, homogeneous, and moderately enhancing masses.
- Presence of peripancreatic lymphadenopathy and lesions elsewhere in the body are suggestive.

GASTROINTESTINAL LESIONS

Gastric Lesions (Table 15)

TABLE 15: Common causes of gastric lesions.

Cystic	Solid	Fatty
• Duplication cyst • Diverticulum	• Carcinoma • Polyp (inflammatory, adenomatous, hamartomatous retention) • Leiomyoma • Ectopic pancreas (simulating or gastric lesion due to its ectopic location) • Lymphoma • Leiomyosarcoma • Bezoars • Metastases	• Lipoma • Teratoma

Gastric Lesions Associated with Wall Thickening

- Carcinoma (focal or diffuse)
- Leiomyoma (focal)
- Lymphoma (diffuse)
- Pancreatitis (usually along the posterior wall)
- Eosinophilic gastritis
- Emphysematous gastritis (intramural aeroceles are characteristic)
- Ménétrier's disease
- Gastric varices.

Gastric duplication cyst:
- It is usually seen as a paragastric, spherical, cystic mass that indents along the greater curvature of the stomach with two layers seen on dynamic enhanced studies.
- It seldom communicates with the lumen of the stomach.
- Ectopic pancreatic tissue may be seen in up to 40% of the cases.

Gastric diverticulum:
- It is seen as a tubular, cystic mass communicating with lumen of the stomach at one end with enhancing walls that are contiguous with the gastric wall.
- The most common site is the juxtacardiac position along the posterior wall followed by the prepyloric region.
- The diverticulum lies in close proximity to the Gerota's fascia and left adrenal gland.
- It is often associated with aberrant pancreas in the antral region.

Gastric carcinoma (Figs. 40 and 41):
- It presents in variable forms: polypoidal intraluminal mass; focal wall thickening with or without ulcer and diffuse wall thickening (linitis plastica).
- All forms show moderate-to-intense postcontrast enhancement.
- Features highly suggestive of carcinoma include extragastric spread of tumor locally, to the regional and distant lymph nodes (especially retrocrural group) or distant organs as liver.

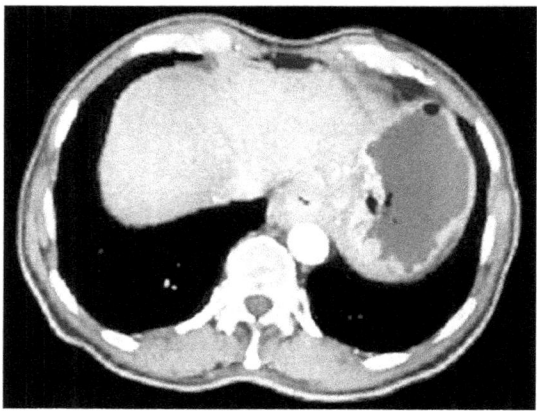

Fig. 40: Axial CT image showing a gastroesophageal junction mass.

Abdomen

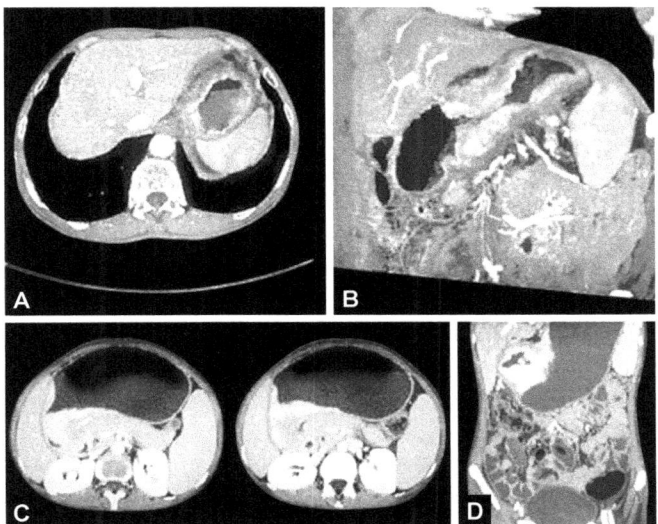

Figs. 41A to D: Axial and coronal CT images showing gastric adenocarcinoma in two different cases.

Adenomatous polyp:
- It is usually seen as a solitary, pedunculated, intraluminal mass with smooth, lobulated contour with no adjacent mural thickening.
- The most common site is antrum and it usually measures >2 cm.

Inflammatory/Hyperplastic/Regenerative polyp:
- CT features are indistinguishable from the adenomatous polyp.
- They are much more commonly encountered than adenomatous polyps and are usually less than 2 cm in diameter.
- They are usually multiple and randomly distributed within the stomach.

Leiomyoma:
- It is seen as a solid, well-defined, homogeneously enhancing mass producing a smooth, focal thickening in the gastric wall.

- It is commonly seen in the antrum and body of the stomach.
- The inner surface of the tumor may be ulcerated and even calcified.
- The tumor is localized to the gastric wall only.

Leiomyosarcoma:
- These are seen as large, exophytic, heterogeneously enhancing soft tissue masses with lobulated, irregular outlines.
- Areas of necrosis and ulceration and calcification are common.
- Distant metastases to the liver are seen relatively early in the disease.

Ectopic pancreas:
- This is seen as smooth, submucosal mass usually located along the greater curvature in the antral and pyloric region of the stomach.
- There is characteristic central umbilication that represents the aberrant pancreatic duct.

Lymphoma (Fig. 42):
- It is usually seen as diffuse gastric wall thickening in centimeters involving more than half of the gastric circumference.
- There is luminal irregularity and narrowing and hyper-rugosity.
- Periaortic lymphadenopathy is common.

Lipoma:
It is seen as a well-defined, intramural mass of fat attenuation usually in antral location.

Teratoma:
- It is seen as a well-circumscribed, intramural mass with cystic and solid components with areas of fat attenuation and calcification.
- It is a rare tumor and seen mainly in children.

Eosinophilic gastritis:
- It is almost always limited to the antral region.
- It can be mucosal type that is characterized by enlarged rugal folds or cobblestone mucosa or intraluminal, polypoidal lesions.

Abdomen

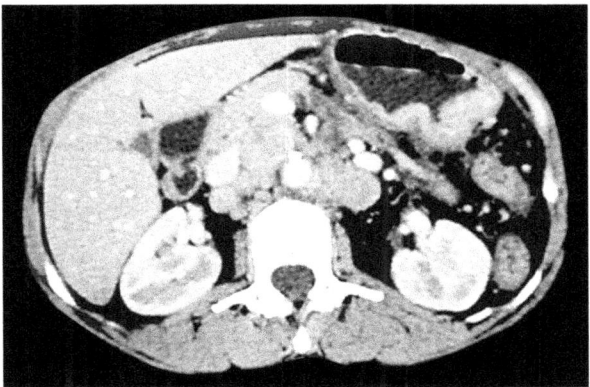

Fig. 42: Transaxial CT image shows diffuse lymphoma of stomach.

- The muscular type is associated with thickened, rigid walls with narrowed gastric antrum or a large, intraluminal, polypoidal mass.

Ménétrier's disease/Giant hypertrophic gastritis/Hyperplastic gastropathy:

- It is characterized by thickening of the stomach wall usually in the fundal and cardiac region especially along the greater curvature with sparing of the antrum.
- The gastric rugae are markedly symmetrically enlarged, nodular, and tortuous.
- There is abrupt transition between the normal and abnormal area of the gastric mucosa.

Gastric varices:

- These are seen as dilated, tortuous, vascular channels that fill with contrast on CECT studies.
- They are usually seen as clusters along the posterior or posteromedial wall of the stomach, especially along the circumference of the fundus of the stomach.
- Evidence of dilated venous channels elsewhere in the abdomen especially in the retroperitoneum and peripancreatic region with

cavernous transformation of the portal vein are highly suggestive of the gastric varices secondary to portal hypertension.

Gastric bezoar (Fig. 43):
- These are seen as a nonenhancing, intraluminal complex masses containing air and food particles in the interstices of the mass.
- Mobility of the mass may at times be demonstrated with changes in posture demonstrating that the mass is nonadherent to the wall.

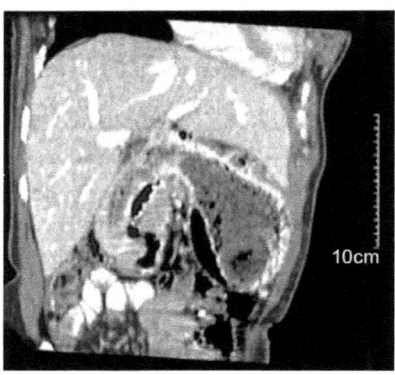

Fig. 43: Oblique coronal CT image showing a trichobezoar in the stomach with extension into the duodenum.

Small Bowel Lesions (Table 16)

TABLE 16: Common causes of small bowel lesions.		
Cystic	*Solid*	*Fatty*
• Duplication cyst • Diverticulum	• Leiomyoma • Polyp • Leiomyosarcoma • Carcinoma • Lymphoma • Carcinoid • Neurogenic tumor • Metastases	Lipoma

Small Bowel Lesions Associated with Wall Thickening

- Crohn's disease
- Tuberculosis
- Hypoproteinemia
- Mural hematoma
- Ischemia
- Graft versus host reaction
- Vasculitis.

Duplication cyst:
- It is seen as a spherical or tubular, cystic lesion with thin, enhancing walls and nonenhancing center lying contiguous and parallel to the bowel loop. Dynamic CT may show typical *Gut wall signature*.
- Sometimes, it is seen as a small intramural cyst.
- They commonly communicate with the lumen of the bowel.
- In the duodenum, it lies on the mesenteric side of the anterior wall of the first and second part of the duodenum in the concavity of the C-loop causing it anterosuperior displacement.
- Small bowel is the most common site for the duplication cyst and one-third are symptomatic in the neonatal period and majority by 2 years of life.
- Aspiration of the cyst material or injection of contrast into the cyst cavity is diagnostic.
- Spinal anomalies are commonly associated.
- Common complications include bowel obstruction, intussusception, and intracystic hemorrhage due to ectopic pancreatic or gastric mucosa.

Diverticulum (Fig. 44):
- It is seen as a cystic, tubular structure with enhancing walls that are contiguous with the bowel wall.
- True diverticulum shows mucosal pattern similar to that of the parent bowel from which it is originating.
- True diverticulum has to be differentiated from pseudo-diverticulum. The latter represents mucosal outpouching into the muscle layer of the bowel wall.

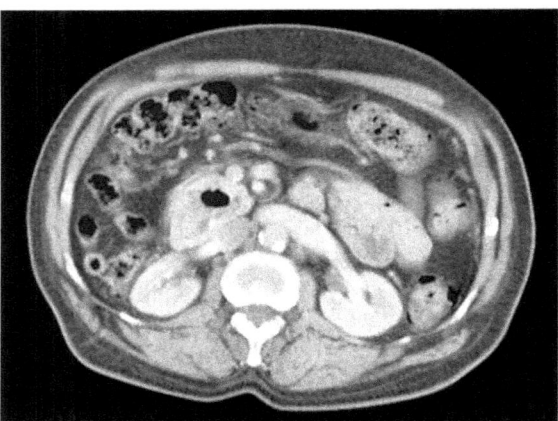

Fig. 44: Transaxial CT image shows duodenal diverticulum.

- An enhancing soft tissue mass with edema in the adjacent mesentery with or without gas indicates diverticulitis.
- Duodenal diverticulum most commonly arises from the 2nd part in and around the region of the ampulla of Vater.

Leiomyoma/Leiomyosarcoma:
- Leiomyoma is most common in jejunum, while leiomyosarcoma is most common in the ileum.
- They are seen as lobulated, soft tissue; enhancing masses present either intraluminally or extraluminally. The latter are more common.
- The core of the tumor may show cystic necrosis with ulceration and calcification.
- They may act as lead points of intussusception.
- Radiologically, it is difficult to differentiate them but leiomyomas are usually less than 5 cm in diameter as against the leiomyosarcomas that are usually more than 6 cm in diameter.

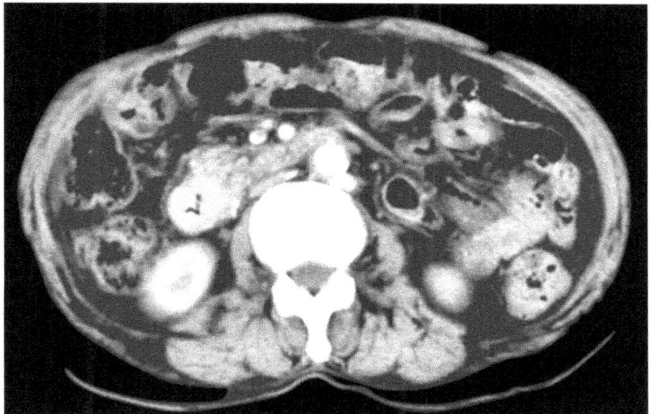

Fig. 45: Transaxial CT image shows adenocarcinoma of duodenum.

Polyps:
- They can be adenomatous or hamartomatous and are most common in the ileum followed by jejunum and duodenum.
- Hamartomatous polyps are most common and half of them are multiple and one-third are associated with Peutz-Jeghers syndrome.
- On CT, they are seen as small, soft tissue masses arising from the small bowel wall with variable diameter and enhancement.
- When these lesions are seen as part of polyposis syndrome, then they are usually smaller than 5 mm and are better picked up on CT enteroscopy.

Carcinoma (Fig. 45):
- Most common are adenocarcinoma, most common in the duodenum near the ampulla of Vater, followed by jejunum and ileum.
- It is usually seen as annular thickening of the wall with luminal narrowing and proximal obstruction.

- It can also be seen as a lobulated or ovoid, moderately enhancing soft tissue mass with ulceration and intussusception in some cases.

Lymphoma:
- It is the most common malignant small bowel tumor occurring most commonly in the ileum followed by jejunum and duodenum.
- It is the most common cause of intussusception after 6 years of age.
- *It may occur in several forms*:
    - Infiltrative form is seen as thickening of walls and mucosal folds with aneurysmally dilated bowel loop due to invasion and destruction of the mural nerve plexus with associated desmoplastic response.
    - Polypoidal mucosal form is characterized by multiple mucosal nodules of variable sizes and number with occasional ulceration and intussusception.
    - Endoexoenteric form is characterized by large soft tissue mass with larger exophytic component and small intraluminal mass with ulceration and aneurysmal dilatation of the bowel loop.
- It is commonly associated with mesenteric and retroperitoneal adenopathy with solitary or conglomerate masses, at times producing a sandwich configuration, whereby the nodal masses are separated by mesenteric fat and vessels.

Carcinoid:
- The most common site is ileum (>90%) followed by jejunum and duodenum.
- It is seen as a soft tissue, moderate to intensely enhancing, mesenteric mass with spiculated margins and retraction of the bowel loops.
- There is beaded appearance of the mesentery with retraction and narrowing and calcification in some cases.
- Associated adenopathy and hepatic metastases are common.

Neurogenic tumor:
- No characteristic feature to differentiate it from other common tumor.
- These tumors are commonly associated with neurofibromatosis.

Lipoma:
It is usually visualized as solitary fat attenuation mass lying either intraluminally or intramurally.

Crohn's disease (Fig. 46):
- It is characterized by circumferential thickening of bowel wall with narrowing of the lumen occurring at multiple sites with intervening normal bowel loops.
- There is fibrofatty proliferation producing a mesenteric mass that shows moderate enhancement and is higher in attenuation than the normal mesenteric fat.
- Abscesses in the mesentery and fistulas are characteristic.

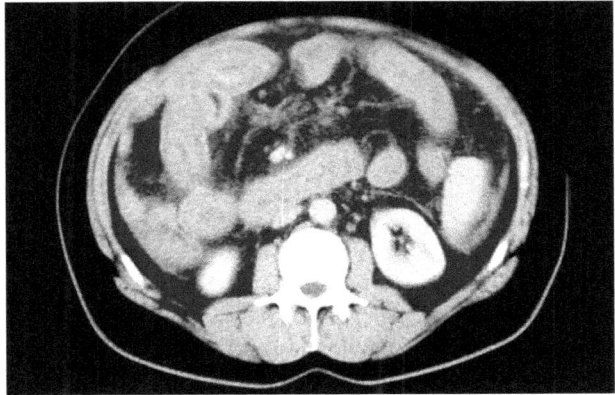

Fig. 46: Transaxial CT image shows Crohn's disease of small bowel.

Tuberculosis:
- It is characterized by bowel wall thickening which may be circumferential or eccentric with proximal obstruction.
- It may be multifocal and the most common is the terminal loops of the ileum and ileocecal region.
- Necrotic lymph nodes with rim enhancement are characteristic and may be seen in the mesentery or porta hepatis or retroperitoneum. The nodes may form conglomerate masses.
- Presence of high density ascites, mesenteric and omental masses favors the diagnosis.

Hypoproteinemia:
- It is characterized by diffuse thickening of the bowel loops with mesenteric infiltration.
- The mesenteric vessels especially the veins become inconspicuous.
- There is sparing of the retroperitoneal fat.

Ischemia:
- It is characterized by thickened bowel loops and mucosal folds with dilatation fluid-filled bowel loops.
- The affected loops show subnormal or no enhancement on postcontrast images.
- Thrombosis of mesenteric artery or vein may be evident.
- Presence of portal vein, mesenteric vascular or intramural air suggests the onset of bowel necrosis following ischemia.

Intramural hematoma:
- It is usually the result of blunt trauma to the abdomen but anticoagulation therapy and pancreatic disease are other important causes.
- It is seen as a focal area of wall thickening that is hyperattenuating with thickening of adjacent mucosal folds.
- Occasionally, a cystic mass with fluid-fluid level may be seen within the wall, especially in cases secondary to anticoagulation therapy.

Colonic Lesions (Table 17)

TABLE 17: Common causes of colonic lesions.		
Cystic	*Solid*	*Fatty*
• Colitis cystica profunda • Pneumatosis cystoides coli • Diverticulum • Mucocele of the appendix • Duplication (Fig. 47)	• Polyp • Leiomyoma • Condyloma acuminatum • Neurogenic tumor • Carcinoid • Carcinoma (Fig. 48) • Lymphoma • Metastases	Lipoma

Lesions Associated with Colonic Wall Thickening

- Intramural hematoma
- Inflammatory bowel disease
- Ischemia

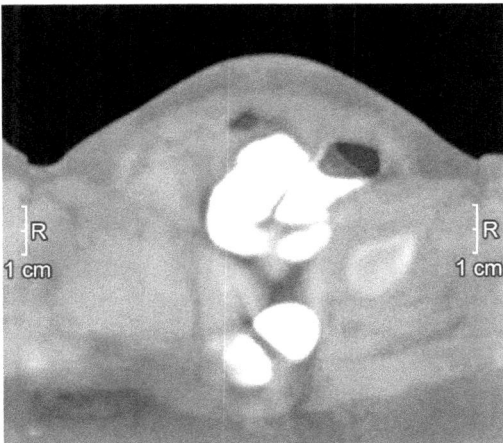

Fig. 47: Axial CT image showing rectal duplication.

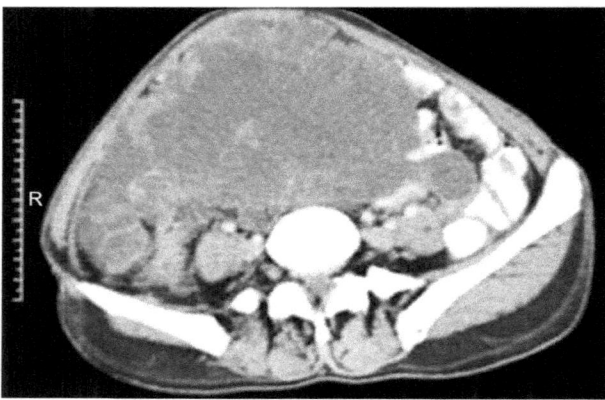

Fig. 48: Axial CECT image of abdomen shows heterogeneously enhancing lobulated solid mass lesion in right iliac fossa in a case of carcinoma cecum.

- Radiation colitis
- Graft-versus-host disease
- Typhlitis
- Pseudomembranous colitis
- Amebic colitis
- Granulomatous colitis (tuberculosis, schistosomiasis, actinomycosis)
- Appendicitis
- Diverticulitis
- Carcinoma (Figs. 49 and 50)
- Lymphoma.

Colitis cystica profunda:
- It is characterized by multiple, intramural, cystic lesions resulting in a polypoidal or nodular appearance of the bowel wall.
- The cysts are usually smaller than 2 cm in diameter and contain fluid.
- The condition is most common in the rectum followed by pelvic colon.

Abdomen

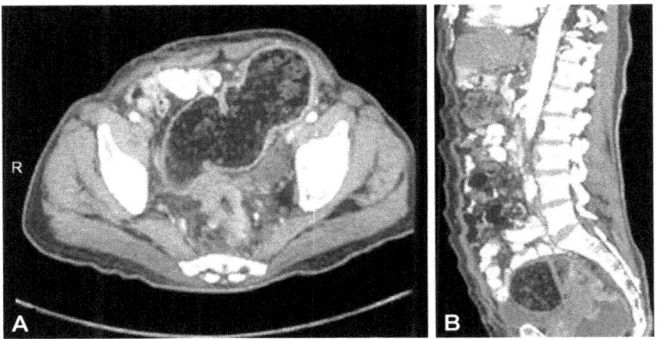

Figs. 49A and B: Axial and sagittal CT images showing rectosigmoid carcinoma.

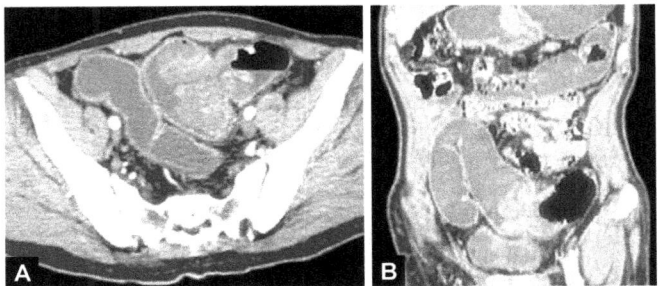

Figs. 50A and B: Axial and coronal CT images showing sigmoid adenocarcinoma.

Pneumatosis cystoides coli:

- It is characterized by cluster of aeroceles within the colonic wall, especially along the mesenteric side.
- It may be associated with segmental mucosal nodularity, pneumoperitoneum, and air within the portal or mesenteric vein.

Diverticulum:
- It is seen as a blind, tubular or saccular, outpouching from the colonic wall that may be filled with air or fluid or fecal matter or admixture of any of the above mentioned.
- These are most common in the sigmoid colon.
- When diverticulum is associated with mural thickening and pericolic fat stranding, it is termed as diverticulitis.
- Diverticulitis may be complicated with pericolic abscess, fistula, and ureteral obstruction.

Lipoma:
- It is the most common submucosal tumor in the colon and is seen as a well-defined, submucosal, and fat attenuating lesion.
- The most common site is cecum and appendix.

Crohn's colitis:
- It is characterized by diffuse wall thickening of homogeneous attenuation frequently affecting the right side of the colon with sparing of the rectum and sigmoid.
- Wall shows typical *double-halo* appearance due to the hypodense, inner layer of edematous mucosa and the hypodense, outer layer of thickened muscularis and serosa.
- The wall thickness usually averages 2 cm.
- Skip areas of unaffected normal mucosa are characteristic.
- Proliferation of fat is seen in the mesentery in approximately half of the patients with separation of the bowel loops. This is termed as *creeping fat*.
- Mesenteric adenopathy is usually associated.
- Late complications include pericolic and mesenteric abscesses, stricture, fistula formation, etc.

Ulcerative colitis (Fig. 51):
- It is characterized by mild wall thickening, usually less than 1 cm with inhomogeneous attenuation almost always affecting the rectum with proximal progression.
- It is a mucosal disease affecting the colon in contiguity without skip lesions with a typical target appearance of the mucosa

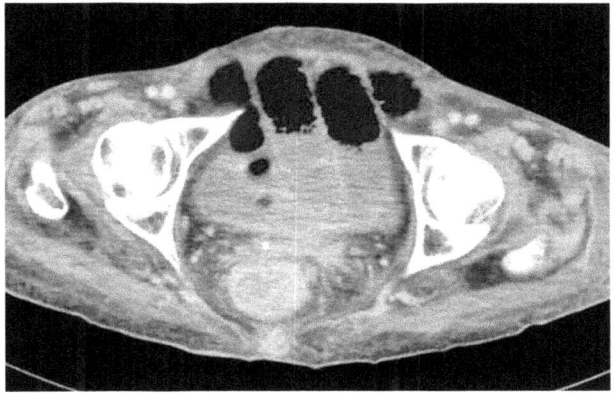

Fig. 51: Transaxial CT image shows ulcerative proctitis.

with inner and outer enhancing mucosal and muscularis layer, respectively.
- There is pseudopolyposis and proliferation of the perirectal and presacral fat.
- Late complications include strictures, backwash ileitis, toxic megacolon, perforation, and adenocarcinoma formation.

Typhlitis:
- There is inhomogeneous, circumferential, thickening of the wall of the cecum and the ascending colon (>3 mm).
- There may be signs of inflammation in the terminal ileum and the pericecal fat.
- Pneumatosis and pericecal/pericolic abscess are common.
- It is commonly seen with severe neutropenia, leukemia, and infection.

Mucocele of the appendix (Fig. 52):
It is seen as a cystic, tubular mass arising from the medial wall of the cecum in the usual position of the appendix.

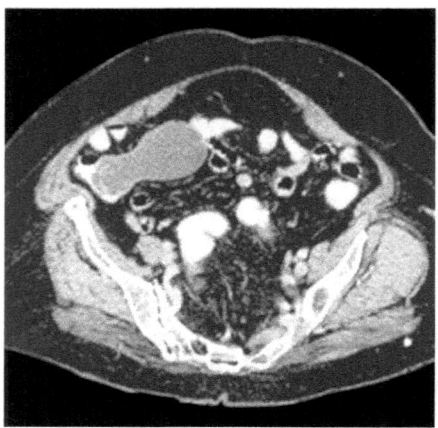

Fig. 52: Axial CT image showing mucocele of the appendix.

Pseudomembranous colitis:
- It is characterized by smooth, circumferential, wall thickening with homogeneous enhancement on postcontrast images.
- Wall thickening is usually in the range of 1–1.5 cm and can be sometimes nodular as well.
- Haustral folds are also thickened and separate the intraluminal contrast medium resulting in *accordion sign*.
- Usually seen in the right-sided colon and may be associated with pericolic fat stranding.

Tuberculous colitis (Figs. 53A and B):
- There is segmental right colonic involvement with irregular wall thickening with spiculations.
- There is narrowing and fibrosis of the cecum that becomes contracted and high positioned with ulcerations and pseudopolyp formation.

Abdomen

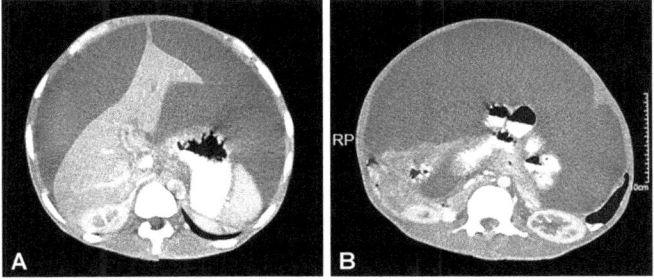

Figs. 53A and B: Axial CECT images of abdomen showing ascites with scalloping of liver surface in case of pseudomyxoma peritonei.

- Characteristic hypodense lymph nodes with rim enhancement are seen in the pericolic region with omental thickening and high density ascites.

Schwannoma:
- These are characterized by multifocal, sessile, moderately enhancing submucosal, soft tissue masses on the mesenteric side of the colon.
- They are commonly associated with neurofibromatosis type I.

Villous adenoma:
- They are commonly seen in the rectosigmoid region.
- They are seen as frond or cauliflower-like soft tissue masses with fluid attenuation occupying nearly half of its volume.

Anorectal condyloma acuminatum/ Buschke-Löwenstein tumor:
- These are seen as giant, cauliflower-like, infiltrating, soft tissue masses in the anorectal region with minimal-to-mild enhancement on postcontrast images.
- They may infiltrate into the adjacent tissue of the ischiorectal fossa, perirectal fat, and subcutaneous tissue.

PERITONEAL AND MESENTERIC/OMENTAL LESIONS (TABLE 18)

TABLE 18: Common causes of peritoneal and mesenteric/omental lesions.

Cystic	Solid	Fatty	Calcified
• Loculated ascites • Peritoneal abscess • Chronic hematoma • Biloma • Pseudomyxoma peritonei • Pancreatic pseudocyst • Mesenteric cyst • Enteric cyst • Lymphangioma	• Acute/subacute hematoma • Inflammatory masses • Lymphadenopathy • Fibrosing mesenteritis/fibromatosis • Leiomyoma • Leiomyosarcoma (Figs. 54A and B) • Castleman's disease • Neurofibroma • Splenosis • Lymphoma • Metastases • Mesothelioma	• Lipoma • Liposarcoma	Peritoneal calcinosis (Figs. 55A and B)

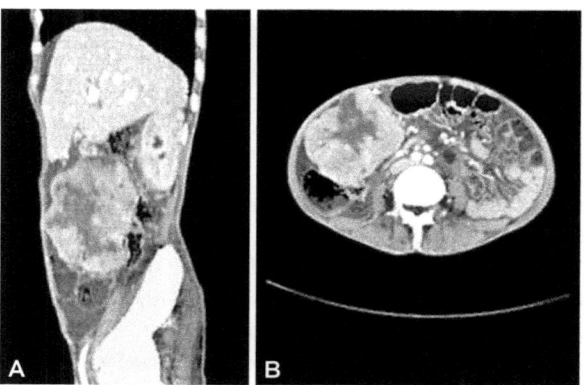

Figs. 54A and B: Sagittal and axial CT images showing a large mesenteric mass.

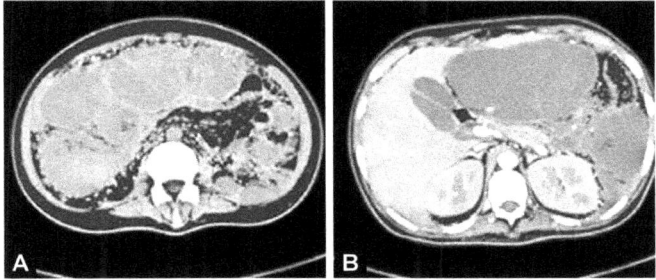

Figs. 55A and B: Axial CT images show peritoneal calcinosis secondary to acute pancreatitis.

Lipoma

- It is seen as a well-defined, fat attenuation mass with thin, smooth walls displacing the adjacent bowel loops with no evidence of soft tissue nodules or septae within the tumor matrix.
- It is the second most common tumor of the mesentery.

Liposarcoma

- The most common site is the lower extremity followed by mesentery and retroperitoneum.
- It has a variegated pattern on CT ranging from solid to cystic pattern.
- Solid type is characterized by an inhomogeneous, infiltrating, soft tissue attenuating, mildly to moderately enhancing mass with mass effect and poorly delineated walls.
- Pseudocystic type is characterized by near homogeneous, water attenuating mass due to averaging of fatty and soft tissue elements.
- Mixed type is characterized by areas of fatty elements and enhancing soft tissue elements.

Enteric Cyst

- It is seen as a smooth, thin-walled, cystic lesion located in the mesentery.
- It is usually unilocular in nature; but occasionally, septations may be seen.

Mesenteric/Omental/Mesothelial Cyst (Figs. 56A and B)

- It is seen as a thin, smooth-walled, usually unilocular cystic mass commonly in the small bowel mesentery but may also be seen in the mesocolon.
- Presence of the fat-fluid level is characteristic.

Lymphangioma

- It is seen as a large, multiseptated, thin-walled, cystic mass in the mesentery with contents ranging from water to fat attenuation.
- It may be associated with partial bowel obstruction.

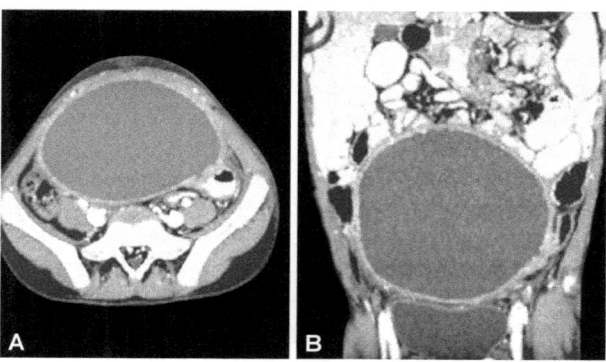

Figs. 56A and B: Axial and coronal CT image showing a mesenteric cyst.

Pseudomyxoma Peritonei (Figs. 57A and B)

- It is seen usually as a low attenuation, multiloculated, none to mildly enhancing mass in the form of layers that displaces the bowel loops. The latter appears to be displaced (posteriorly) rather than floating in the abdominal cavity.
- Uncommonly, it may have soft tissue attenuation.
- Presence of peritoneal/omental thickening or isolated cystic masses, annular calcification, and scalloped hepatic margins are highly suggestive of the diagnosis.

Retractile Mesenteritis/Chronic Fibrosing Mesenteritis/Weber Christian Disease/ Mesenteric Panniculitis (Figs. 58 and 59)

- It is seen as a poorly delineated, soft tissue, moderately enhancing mass interspersed with fatty elements located in the mesentery with fine, stellate pattern.

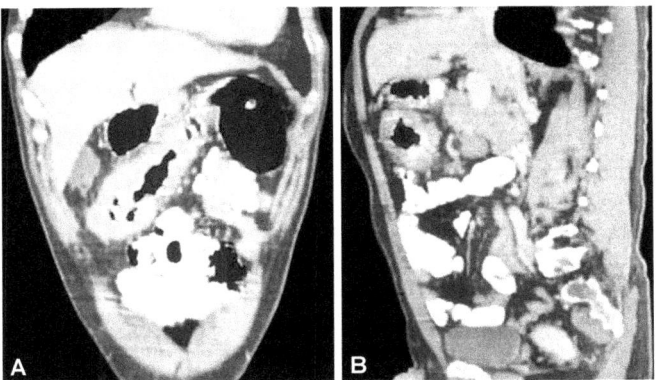

Figs. 57A and B: Sagittal and coronal CECT MPR images of abdomen show enhancing circumferential thickening of hepatic flexure and transverse colon pseudomyxoma in a case of colonic tuberculosis.

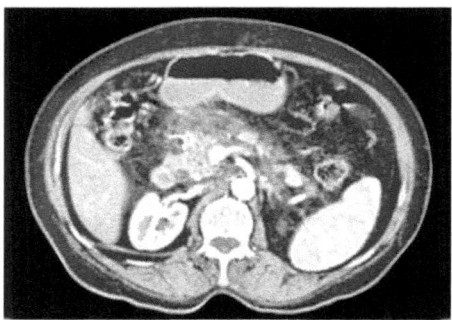

Fig. 58: Axial CT image showing mesenteric fat stranding.

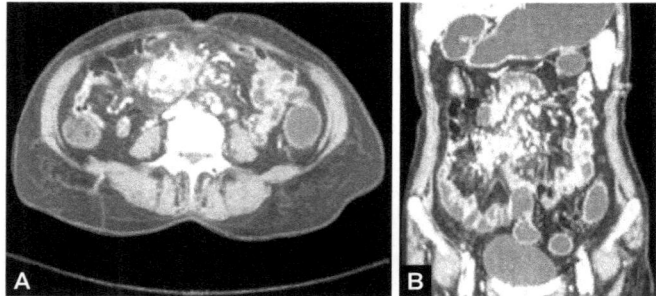

Figs. 59A and B: Axial and coronal CT images showing retractile mesenteritis.

- There is associated mesenteric thickening, kinking and angulation of the bowel loops.
- Calcification is seen commonly.
- When single, well-defined, homogeneous, soft tissue mass is seen in the mesentery, it is termed as the fibroma.
- When above lesions are multiple, the condition is termed as fibromatosis.
- This condition is associated with fibrosing mediastinitis and Gardner's syndrome.

Mesothelioma

- This tumor is commonly seen in the elderly males with variable appearances on CT.
- It may be seen as nodular, irregular, thickening of the peritoneal surfaces or as localized masses or as infiltrating sheets of tissue.
- Postcontrast images show moderate-to-intense enhancement.
- Associated features as foci of calcification, ascites, and stellate configuration of the neurovascular bundles give a clue to the diagnosis.
- Cystic mesothelioma is seen as a uni- or multilocular, thin-walled cystic lesion without calcification arising from the peritoneum and omentum, usually in the pelvis.
- Mesothelioma is associated with asbestos exposure except the cystic variety.

Peritoneal Carcinomatosis (Figs. 60 and 61)

- It is seen in different forms as hyperdense, mesenteric fat stranding; small, enhancing, nodular soft tissue masses on the peritoneal surfaces; thickening of the omentum (omental caking) and lobulated, enhancing, soft tissue attenuating masses in the pouch of Douglas.
- Massive ascites is the usual accompanying feature.
- Calcified implants are seen in cases of metastases of the ovary.

Splenosis

- It is characterized by multiple, small, encapsulated nodular masses on the serosal surfaces of the small bowel, greater omentum, and parietal peritoneum.
- The nodules have attenuation value similar to the splenic parenchyma both on noncontrast and postcontrast scans.
- The condition arises due to autotransplantation of the splenic tissue following splenic trauma.

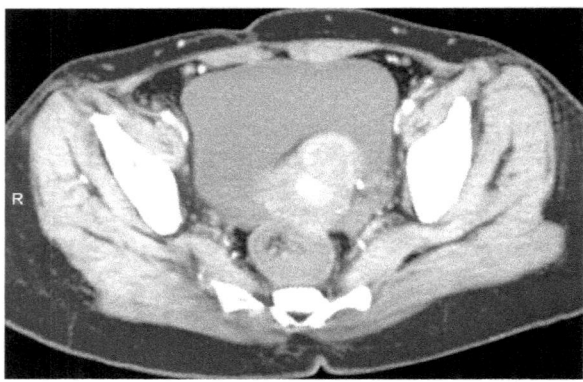

Fig. 60: Axial CT image showing peritoneal metastases in the pouch of Douglas.

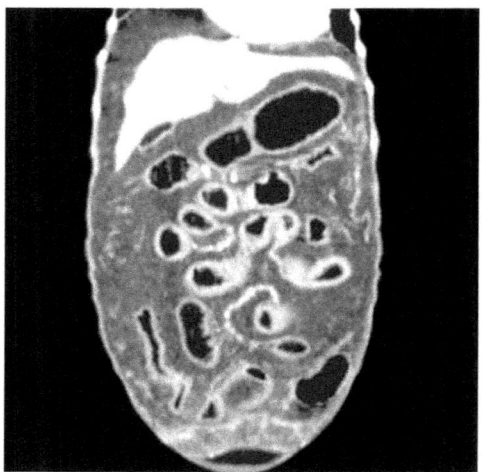

Fig. 61: Coronal MPR image showing massive ascites with floating bowel loops.

Abdomen

RETROPERITONEAL LESIONS (TABLE 19)

TABLE 19: Common causes of retroperitoneal lesions.

Cystic	Solid	Fatty	Vascular
• Chronic hematoma/abscess (Figs. 62 and 63) • Pancreatic pseudocyst • Urinoma • Seroma • Lymphocele • Lymphangiectasia (Fig. 64) • Cystic lymphangioma	• Lymphadenopathy • Hematoma • Mesenchymal tumors (malignant fibrous histiocytoma, fibrosarcoma, leiomyosarcoma, malignant mesenchymoma) • Neurogenic tumors • Undescended testis • Retroperitoneal fibrosis	• Lipoma • Liposarcoma	• Atherosclerosis • Aortic aneurysm • Aortic dissection • Thrombosis of IVC

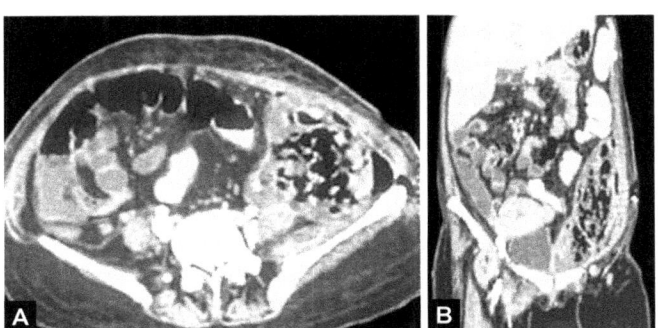

Figs. 62A and B: Axial and oblique coronal CT images showing a large retroperitoneal abscess.

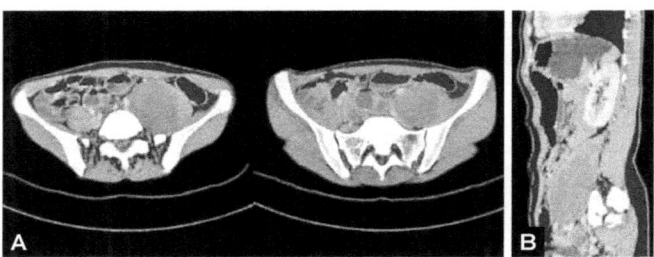

Figs. 63A and B: Axial and sagittal CT images showing psoas abscess on the left side.

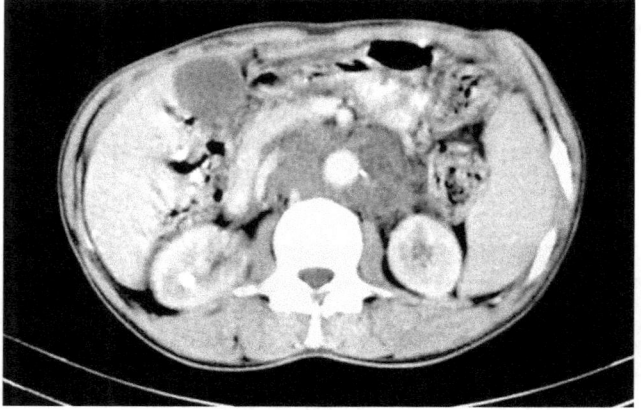

Fig. 64: Axial CECT image of abdomen show hypoattenuating retroperitoneal irregular lesion, displacing the aorta anteriorly in a case of retroperitoneal lymphectasia.

Lymphadenopathy

- The appearance of the enlarged lymph nodes in different diseases is variable and many at times is very suggestive of the disease as described here.

- In lymphoma, the enlarged lymph nodes are hyperdense to the muscles and are as discrete or coalescent nodal masses at multiple sites with mild-to-moderate postcontrast enhancement. The aorta is displaced anteriorly referred to as a floating aorta sign. The involvement of the other solid viscera may be seen as liver and spleen (Fig. 65).
- Hypodense, enlarged lymph nodes at the level of renal hilum are a characteristic finding in nodal metastases from testicular neoplasms.
- Hypodense, enlarged, rim enhancing, conglomerate lymph nodes are characteristic of tuberculosis. Presence of mesenteric and portal adenopathy, intestinal and pulmonary involvement is further suggestive.
- Fatty, nonenhancing, enlarged lymph nodes are characteristic of Whipple's disease but may also be seen in Crohn's disease and metastases.
- Discrete, moderately but homogeneously enhancing lymph nodes associated with hepatosplenomegaly and pulmonary involvement is very suggestive of sarcoidosis.

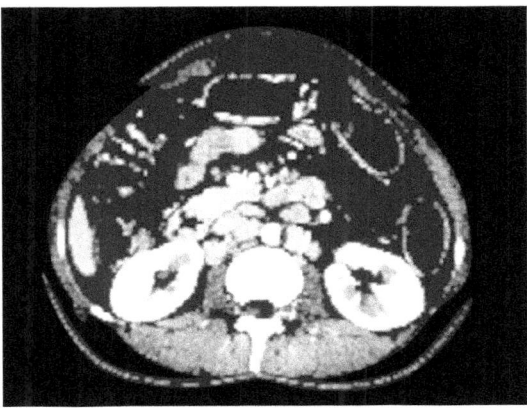

Fig. 65: Axial CT image shows a lymphomatous adenopathy in the retroperitoneum.

- Discrete, homogeneously and intensely enhancing, enlarged lymph nodes associated with middle and posterior mediastinal adenopathy of similar nature are suggestive of Castleman's disease.

Seroma

- It is seen as a water dense collection with imperceptible walls at the operative site usually seen within days to a week following the procedure.
- It may get infected and turn into an abscess.

Retroperitoneal Mesenchymal Tumors (Figs. 66 and 67)

- This group includes large numbers of common and rare tumors, but the most common ones are liposarcoma, malignant fibrous histiocytoma (Figs. 68A and B) and fibrosarcoma.
- Except for the liposarcoma, that has fatty elements within; other tumors cannot be differentiated from each other on imaging.

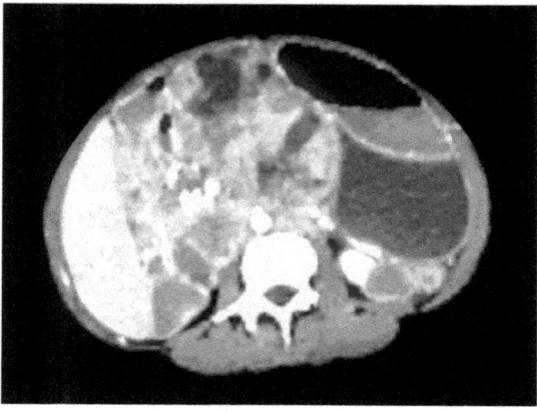

Fig. 66: Axial CT image shows a large retroperitoneal sarcoma.

Abdomen

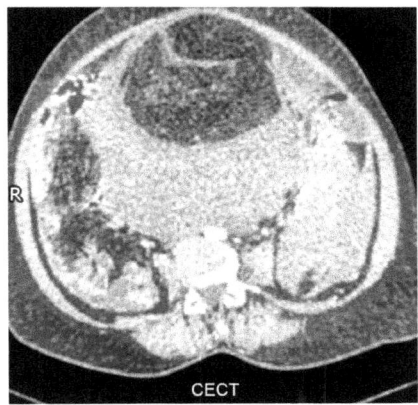

Fig. 67: Axial CT image shows a large retroperitoneal liposarcoma.

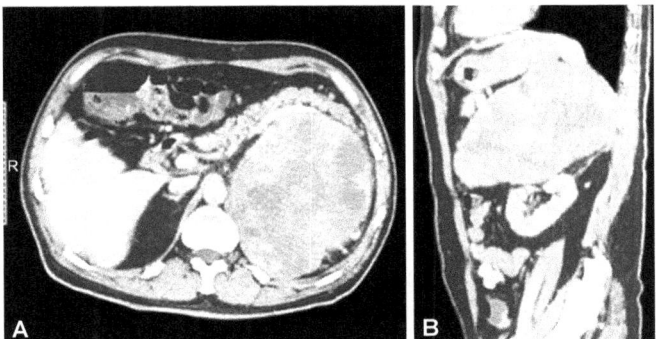

Figs. 68A and B: Axial and sagittal CECT images of abdomen show heterogeneously enhancing, well-defined solid retroperitoneal mass lesion, displacing the pancreas anteriorly and kidney inferiorly a case of histopathologically proven malignant fibrous histiocytoma.

Neurogenic Tumors

- This group also includes a wide variety of tumors with variegated appearance on CT. Common ones include ganglioneuroma,

pheochromocytoma, neurofibroma, and neuroblastoma and they usually occur under 30 years of age.
- These cannot be differentiated with confidence on imaging and majority occurs as hypodense lesions relative to the muscle with mild-to-moderate postcontrast enhancement near or along the course of nerve or chain.

Undescended Testis

- It is seen as a round to oval, well-defined, soft tissue density mass with minimal or mild, homogeneous postcontrast enhancement located anywhere along the course of the gonadal vein that is from the inguinal region to the renal vein.
- Irregular, moderate-to-intense heterogeneous enhancement in the suspected undescended testis suggests malignancy.

Retroperitoneal Fibrosis/Ormond's Disease (Fig. 69)

- It is seen as a thick, sheet of enhancing soft tissue mass in the lower retroperitoneum that is anywhere from the level of the renal hilum to the sacrum. The anterior margins are well-defined while the posterior margins are not so well-delineated.

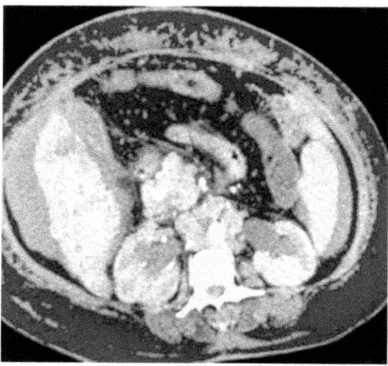

Fig. 69: Axial CT image showing malignant retroperitoneal fibrosis with bilateral hydronephrosis, hepatic metastases, ascites, and subcutaneous edema.

- It encases all the retroperitoneal vessels and the ureters. It can even surround the kidney.
- It pulls the ureters medially toward the spine on both the sides.

Atherosclerosis of Aorta
- It is characterized by dilatation, tortuosity, intimal calcification, and atheromatous plaques in the abdominal aorta.
- The most common portion to be involved is the infrarenal part of the aorta.

Aortic Aneurysm
- It is seen as a focal area of fusiform or saccular aortic dilatation with the diameter exceeding 3 cm.
- A thick mantle of enhancing perianeurysmal tissue may be present.
- Discontinuity in the wall of the aneurysm and obscured adjacent fat planes suggest a contained rupture, while the extravasation of the contrast outside the lumen on postcontrast images suggest active leak and rupture.

Aortic Dissection
- It is seen as double, contrast-filled lumens on postcontrast images that are separated by an intimal flap giving a twisted tape configuration.
- True and false lumens are identified by their different rates and timings of opacification. The true lumen fills faster and earlier than the false and the opacification also fades in the same sequence.
- Intraluminal thrombus, aneurysmal dilatation, and irregular contours of the aorta are associated features.

Thrombosis of the Inferior Vena Cava
- It is seen as a filling defect in the opacified vein with focal dilatation of the vein at the site of the thrombus.

- Dilatation of vein downstream and diminution of the vein size upstream with multiple collaterals in the abdomen are very suggestive of the thrombus formation, even if it is equivocally seen.
- Presence of air densities within the thrombus matrix suggests a septic thrombus.

ADRENAL LESIONS (TABLE 20)

TABLE 20: Common causes of adrenal lesions.

Cystic	Solid	Fatty	Calcified
• True cyst • Pseudocyst (chronic hematoma and infarction) • Hemangioma/lymphangioma • Parasitic cyst (hydatid) • Cystic degeneration in tumor pheochromocytoma • Cortical adenoma	• Abscess • Hematoma • Hemangioma • Cortical adenoma • Neuroblastoma/ganglio neuroma • Pheochromocytoma • Carcinoma • Metastases (Figs. 70A and B)	Myelolipoma	• Infection (tuberculosis, histoplasmosis) • Tumoral (neuroblastoma, carcinoma, dermoid) • Miscellaneous (old hematoma, Addison's and Wolman's disease)

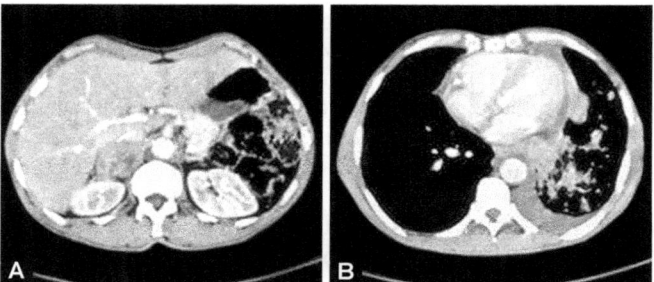

Figs. 70A and B: Axial CT images showing adrenal metastases on the right side secondary to bronchogenic carcinoma.

Causes of Bilateral Adrenal Enlargement

- Hemorrhage
- Hyperplasia
- Granulomatous infection (histoplasmosis, tuberculosis)
- Pheochromocytoma
- Metastases
- Lymphoma.

Adrenal Cyst

- It is usually seen as a solitary, well-defined, uni- or multilocular, water attenuating, nonenhancing lesion with thin (<3 mm), smooth, nonenhancing walls. The cyst usually measures less than 5 cm in diameter.
- Higher attenuation of contents is seen in cases of hemorrhage and infection.
- Calcification is rare except in cases of echinococcal cyst or hemorrhagic cyst.

Adrenal Hemorrhage

- Unilateral involvement is most common and frequently results from blunt abdominal trauma and the right side being the most common to be involved.
- It is seen as a high-attenuation mass evolving with time that is becoming smaller and lower in attenuation as the time progresses.
- It may be seen as uniform enlargement of the adrenal gland or as a focal mass.
- Associated features include periadrenal hemorrhage, ill-defined adrenal margins, periadrenal fat stranding, and thickening of the diaphragmatic crux.
- Calcification may be seen after a week.

Adrenal Adenoma (Fig. 71)

- It is seen as a well-defined, sharply-delineated, soft tissue or water attenuating, focal mass, usually <5 cm in diameter with variable postcontrast enhancement.
- Attenuation values of <10 HU on noncontrast scans and values <35 HU on 15-min postcontrast scans are diagnostic.
- The contralateral adrenal may be atrophic in cases of functioning adenoma.
- Calcification is rare.

Adrenal Carcinoma

- It is seen as a heterogeneous, ill-marginated, hypoattenuating mass, usually >5 cm in diameter showing heterogeneous postcontrast enhancement.
- Calcification, hemorrhage, and necrosis are common.
- Vascular invasion, metastatic adenopathy, and distant metastases are reliable signs of malignancy.
- Contralateral adrenal atrophy may be seen in functioning tumors.

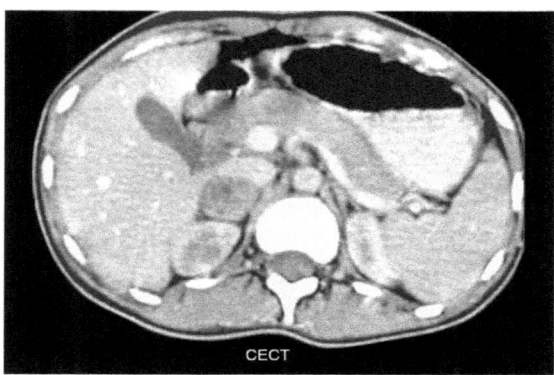

Fig. 71: Axial CT image showing adrenal adenoma on the right side.

Adrenal Hyperplasia

- It is characterized by bilateral, diffuse enlargement of the adrenal glands with preservation of the morphology.
- The glands usually have smooth outlines but may be nodular. The latter may be micronodular or macronodular (>2.5 cm in diameter).
- The glands may even be normal in size in up to 30% of the patients despite clinical signs of hyperfunctioning adrenal.

Myelolipoma

- It is characterized by a well-defined mass of predominantly fat attenuation interspersed with areas of soft tissue attenuation.
- They are usually very large in size at the time of presentation (>10 cm).
- Calcification is seen in up to one-fifth of the cases.
- Hemorrhage and necrosis may also occur.

Neuroblastoma (Fig. 72)

- It is usually seen in children less than 3 years of age as a heterogeneous, lobulated soft tissue mass with heterogeneous postcontrast enhancement.

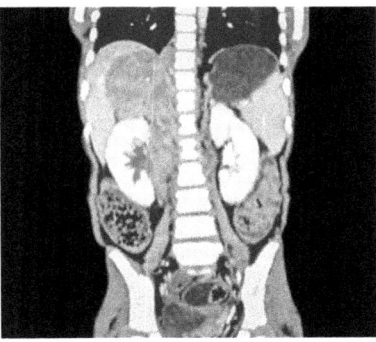

Fig. 72: Coronal MPR CT image shows neuroblastoma arising from right adrenal with retroperitoneal metastases.

- Calcification, hemorrhage, and necrosis are very common.
- Invasion of the kidney and vessels with encasement of the latter is very common.
- It may extend into spinal canal or may cross the midline.
- Retroperitoneal adenopathy and bony, hepatic or pulmonary metastases are other signs of malignancy.

Pheochromocytoma/Adrenal Paraganglioma

- It is seen as a discrete, round to oval, solid, cystic or complex mass with variable postcontrast enhancement, usually intense in the solid areas.
- Hemorrhage and necrosis are common.
- Hypertensive crisis occurring during the intravenous examination of the contrast material is characteristic.

GENITOURINARY LESIONS

Renal Lesions (Table 21)

TABLE 21: Common causes of renal lesions.

Cystic	Solid	Fatty
• Simple cyst • Parapelvic cyst • Pyelocalyceal diverticulum • Focal caliectasis • Chronic abscess/hematoma/infarct • Polycystic kidney disease • Multicystic dysplastic kidney • Multilocular cystic nephroma • Medullary cystic disease • Acquired cystic disease of dialysis • VHL disease • Pancreatic pseudocyst (simulating as renal lesion)	• Acute focal nephritis • Abscess • Hematoma • Infarct • Xanthogranulomatous pyelonephritis • Pseudotumor • Nephroblastomatosis • Adenoma • Oncocytoma • Arteriovenous malformation • Renal cell carcinoma • Transitional cell carcinoma • Wilms' tumor • Mesoblastic nephroma • Lymphoma	• Xanthogranulomatous pyelonephritis • Lipomatosis • Fibrolipomatosis • Lipoma • Teratoma • Angiomyolipoma • Oncocytoma • Liposarcoma • Renal cell carcinoma

Hyperdense Renal Lesion on NECT

- Complicated renal cyst (hemorrhagic, gelatinous/mucinous, calcified) (Fig. 73)
- Thrombus in a renal vein
- Lipoma
- Angiomyolipoma
- Renal cell carcinoma
- Metastatic deposits from thyroid carcinoma.

Bilateral Renal Lesions

- Benign neoplasms—angiomyolipoma, nephroblastomatosis.
- Malignant neoplasms—Wilms' tumor, renal cell carcinoma, lymphoma, metastases.
- Cystic disease—polycystic kidney disease, acquired cystic disease, etc.

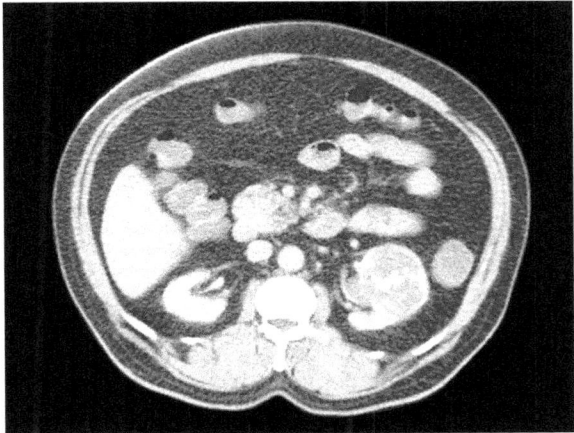

Fig. 73: Transaxial CT image shows calcification in renal cyst.

Renal Lesions Presenting in Neonatal Period

- Hydronephrosis
- Renal vein thrombosis
- Multicystic dysplastic kidney
- Polycystic kidney disease
- Nephroblastomatosis
- Mesoblastic nephroma
- Wilms' tumor.

Renal Lesions Presenting in Childhood Period

- Hydronephrosis
- Cyst and abscess
- Polycystic kidney disease
- Angiomyolipoma
- Teratoma
- Nephroblastomatosis
- Wilms' tumor
- Multilocular cystic nephroma
- Renal cell carcinoma
- Rhabdomyosarcoma
- Clear cell sarcoma of the kidney
- Neuroblastoma
- Lymphoma
- Leukemia.

Renal Sinus Lipomatosis/Fibrolipomatosis

- It is an elderly disease usually seen after 50 years of age.
- It is characterized by excessive fat in the renal sinus with loss of renal parenchymal morphology.
- The fat may encase the pelvicalyceal system giving rise to spider or trumpet-like configuration with no obvious obstruction.
- The kidney may be enlarged and may sometimes show focal pelvicalyceal system abnormality due to focal fat deposition.

Focal Caliectasis

- It is seen as a focal dilatation of the calyx, usually at the upper pole due to infundibular stenosis.
- Postcontrast studies confirm that it is a part of the collecting system.

Pelvicalyceal Cyst/Diverticulum

- It is an outpouching of the collecting system into the corticomedullary region.
- The diverticulum is a smooth-walled, mainly spherical cavity connected by a thin channel to a calyx, typically in the upper or lower pole.
- It is known as a *pyelogenic cyst*, especially if it arises from the renal pelvis.
- Diverticula occasionally develop calculi referred to as *seed calculi*.
- Calyceal diverticula can be easily recognized on CT on postcontrast studies, sometimes a urine-contrast level may be visualized.

Simple Cyst

- Most renal cysts are simple cysts, which can be regarded as part of normal aging.
- Most arise in the renal cortex.
- The CT criteria are round or ovoid, homogeneously, water dense, lesion with imperceptible, nonenhancing walls, and smooth interface with the renal parenchyma.
- It is termed as complicated/complex renal cyst when it has many of the features of a simple cyst but does not completely fulfill all the imaging criteria.
- Cysts may appear complex at imaging because of the presence of septa, hemorrhage, infection or calcification.

- In general, the imaging features of cystic renal lesion must be integrated with the clinical setting and the results of other and prior imaging.

Parapelvic/Peripelvic Cyst/Renal Sinus Cyst/ Parapelvic Lymphangiectasia

- It is seen as an irregular, cystic mass of water attenuation with imperceptible, nonenhancing walls lying in proximation to the renal pelvis.
- It may cause smooth, stretching or deformity of the collecting system.
- It does not communicate with the pelvicalyceal system.

Autosomal Dominant or Adult Polycystic Kidney Disease

- It is characterized by bilateral but asymmetrically enlarged, lobulated kidneys with multiple cystic lesions resembling simple or complicated simple cysts.
- The pelvicalyceal system is elongated, distorted, and attenuated.
- Similar cystic lesions may be seen in liver, pancreas, and lungs.

Autosomal Recessive/Neonatal or Infantile Polycystic Kidney Disease

- It is characterized by dilatation of renal collecting tubules, cystic dilatation of biliary radicles, and periportal fibrosis with varying degrees of renal failure and portal hypertension.
- Renal disease is dominant in the neonatal form; with onset in childhood, liver disease is usually dominant.
- It is characterized by bilateral, grossly enlarged kidneys with increasingly dense nephrogram and prolonged corticomedullary phase on postcontrast images.
- Presence of fetal lobulations in the kidney and striated nephrogram with persistence of contrast in the pelvicalyceal system on delayed images is characteristic.

Multicystic Dysplastic Kidney

- It is more common in males and is seen unilaterally as bilateral condition is usually incompatible with life.
- It is characterized by multiple cysts of varying sizes with a large dominant cyst situated peripherally with no identifiable, functioning renal parenchyma on postcontrast images with distortion of the reniform shape.
- The cysts may increase in size after birth but frequently stabilize, decrease in size, and ultimately disappear.
- Multicystic kidney has associated atresia of the renal artery and proximal ureter.
- There is a 20% incidence of contralateral renal abnormality such as pelvic ureteric junction (PUJ) obstruction and vesicoureteral reflux (VUR).

Multilocular Cystic Nephroma (Fig. 74)

- It is predominantly seen in males under 4 years or females above 4 years of age.

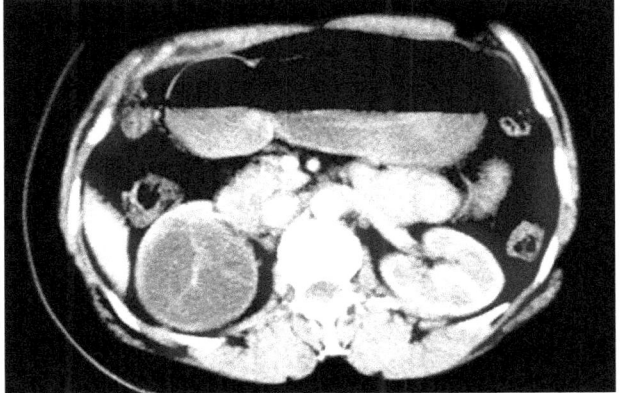

Fig. 74: Transaxial CT image shows multilocular nephroma in right kidney.

- It is seen as a well-circumscribed, multiseptated mass with thick, enhancing capsule and contents of near water density.
- The septa are thick and may show calcification and enhancement on postcontrast images due to tortuous fine vessels running through them.

Medullary Cystic Disease/Nephronophthisis

- It is a bilateral disease characterized by a variable number of small medullary or corticomedullary cysts measuring up to 2 cm with preservation of the renal contour and shape. The kidneys are normal or smaller in size.
- Postcontrast studies show persistent, striated medullary nephrogram with poor opacification of the collecting system.
- Childhood medullary cystic disease is often associated with extrarenal abnormalities, particularly congenital hepatic fibrosis and skeletal dysplasia.
- Renal and retinal dysplasia associated with retinitis pigmentosa.

Acquired Cystic Disease of Dialysis

- It refers to the development of multiple cysts in chronically failed kidneys during long-term dialysis therapy.
- Solid tumors, including oncocytomas and adenocarcinomas, occur with increased frequency in dialysis patients.
- The cysts are often small initially, but with time may enlarge and result in renal enlargement and multifocal distortion of the renal outline.
- CT demonstrates a variable number of cysts of variable size. There may be from five to innumerable cysts, and cyst size may range from microscopic to 3 cm.
- Calcification in the cyst walls and hemorrhage may be seen.

Von Hippel-Lindau Disease

- It is characterized by bilateral, multiple renal cysts, and solid tumors. The latter may include carcinoma, adenoma, and hemangioma.

Abdomen

- The disease involves multiple organs as cerebellum, retina, pancreas, adrenal, and liver.

Renal Pseudotumor

- It refers to focal enlargement of the normal renal parenchyma that mimics a tumor.
- On CT, it has all the characteristic of the normal renal parenchyma.
- *These include*:
  - *Fetal lobulations*: These refer to cortical bulges overlying the calices.
  - *Dromedary hump*: This refers to the splenic bump seen in the midportion of the lateral border of the left kidney resulting in the triangular contour and elongation of the midpolar calyx.
  - *Hypertrophied column of Bertini*: It refers to the hypertrophied septal cortex that appear as mass of <3 cm in diameter, usually between the upper and midpolar region with large indentation at the renal sinus resulting in the deformation of adjacent calyx and infundibulum.
  - *Hilar lip*: It refers to the supra- or infrahilar cortical bulge arising from the medial part of kidney, usually on the left side.
  - *Nodular compensatory hypertrophy*: It refers to the hypertrophied, nodular renal parenchyma in response to the focal destruction of tissue that mimics as a focal mass.

Nephroblastomatosis

- It refers to the presence of the focal or diffuse nephrogenic rests in the renal cortex or the columns that have the potential to form Wilms' tumor.
- These are seen usually as a solitary or multifocal, subcapsular nonenhancing nodules that distort the renal pelvicalyceal system.

- It is associated with nephromegaly and Wilms' tumor.
- Hemihypertrophy, aniridia, trisomy 18, and Beckwith-Wiedemann syndrome may be associated with the disease.

Oncocytoma/Proximal Tubular Adenoma

- It is seen as a well-circumscribed, solid mass with homogeneous low attenuation on noncontrast images.
- Postcontrast images show homogeneous enhancement that is less than normal renal parenchyma with a central stellate scar only in one-third of cases due to central necrosis, hemorrhage or infarction.

Angiomyolipoma/Renal Hamartoma (Figs. 75A and B)

- It is seen as a solitary or multifocal, well-marginated, cortical tumor of fat attenuation on noncontrast images with variable postcontrast enhancement.
- It may sometimes be hyperdense on noncontrast images due to lower fat content.
- It may occur as an isolated lesion in the middle-aged females, but it also has an association with tuberous sclerosis where the tumor can occur bilaterally.

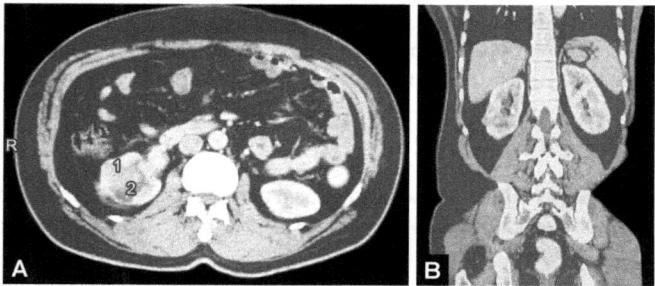

Figs. 75A and B: Axial CECT images of abdomen show heterogeneously enhancing mass lesion at lower pole of right kidney with area of fat density suggestive of angiomyolipoma.

Renal Cell Carcinoma (Figs. 76 and 77)

- It is the most common renal malignancy in adults and is seen as a heterogeneous, lobulated, ill-defined mass causing

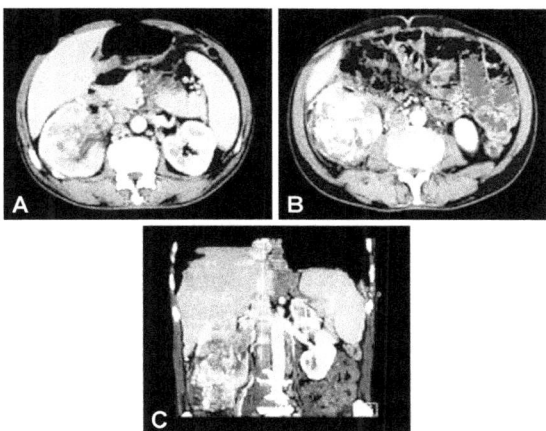

Figs. 76A to C: Axial and coronal CT images showing renal cell carcinoma.

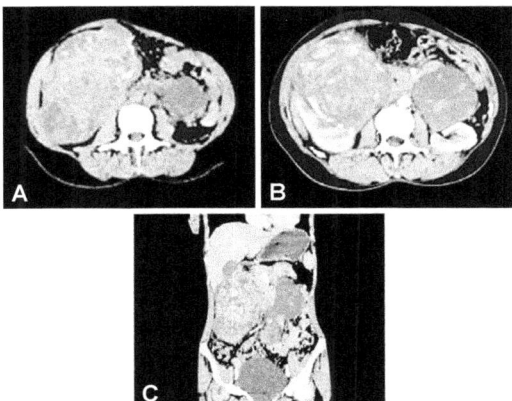

Figs. 77A to C: Axial and coronal CT images showing renal cell carcinoma with cystic metastases in the retroperitoneum.

enlargement of the affected portion of the kidney with variable inhomogeneous postcontrast enhancement.
- The calyceal system in the involved part of the kidney is distorted, displaced, and digested.
- Necrosis, hemorrhage, and stippled calcification are very common.
- Tumor spreads commonly to the perinephric space, renal vein, IVC, lymph nodes, and bone.

Transitional Cell Carcinoma (Figs. 78A and B)

- They are seen as frond or cauliflower-like growth in the renal pelvis with mild-to-moderate contrast enhancement and are seen as filling defect in the opacified pelvicalyceal system.
- They may be seen as subtle thickening and induration of the wall of the collecting system.
- They produce partial or complete obstruction to the outflow of urine resulting in hydronephrosis.
- Renal calculi are commonly associated but calcification is rare.
- The tumor can spread to the peripelvic region or invade into the renal parenchyma or can seed downstream in the urinary tract.

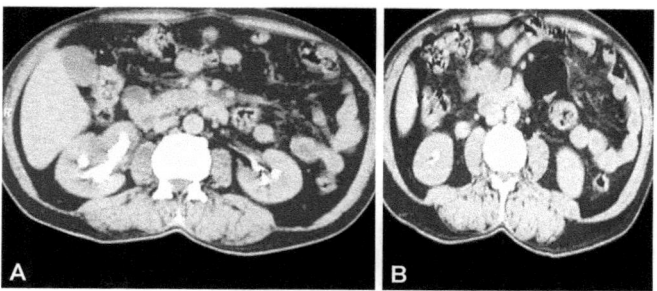

Figs. 78A and B: Axial CECT images of abdomen show an infiltrating mass lesion involving right renal pelvis with evidence of ureteric thickening in a case of transitional cell carcinoma of right renal pelvis and upper ureter.

Wilms' Tumor/Nephroblastoma

- It is seen as a large, lobulated, sharply marginated, inhomogeneous mass with compression of the adjacent renal parenchyma that forms its pseudocapsule. The tumor expands and distorts the involved renal parenchyma with distortion and digestion of the adjacent calices.
- Hemorrhage and necrosis are common but calcification is rare.
- The tumor invades the vessels, adrenal gland, and lymph nodes and displaces the retroperitoneal structures.
- The tumor is often associated with nephroblastomatosis and may cross the midline.

Mesoblastic Nephroma

- It is a benign mass with similar CT characteristics as that of Wilms' tumor.
- The tumor, however, is seen in the neonatal period and is not associated with intravenous invasion.

Leukemia/Lymphoma

- They are characterized by bilateral diffuse enlargement of kidneys or multiple intrarenal focal lesions that are hypodense to renal parenchyma on both noncontrast and postcontrast images.
- The enhancement seen is mild-to-moderate.
- Lymphoma of the retroperitoneum can also spread to the kidney in contiguity.

Renal Leiomyoma/Capsuloma

- It is seen as a well-circumscribed, exophytic, solid, mild to moderately enhancing lesion arising in the subcapsular, capsular or pelvic location.
- Presence of the cleavage between the cortex and the tumor is characteristic.
- Cystic degeneration, hemorrhage or malignant degeneration may be seen.

Lobar Nephronia/Acute Focal Bacterial Nephritis

- It is seen as a focal area of absent or poor postcontrast enhancement with distortion and displacement of the pelvicalyceal system and the renal arteries.
- Renal veins are compressed and the reniform shape of the kidney is preserved with smooth outlines.
- There is poor demarcation of the lesion from the normal renal parenchyma.

Renal Abscess (Fig. 79)

- It is seen as a well-circumscribed mass with thick, enhancing walls with displacement of adjacent intrarenal structures.
- The internal contents are higher in attenuation than urine and may sometimes show aeroceles and thickened, enhancing septae.
- Thickening of the Gerota's fascia and perinephric fat stranding are characteristic.

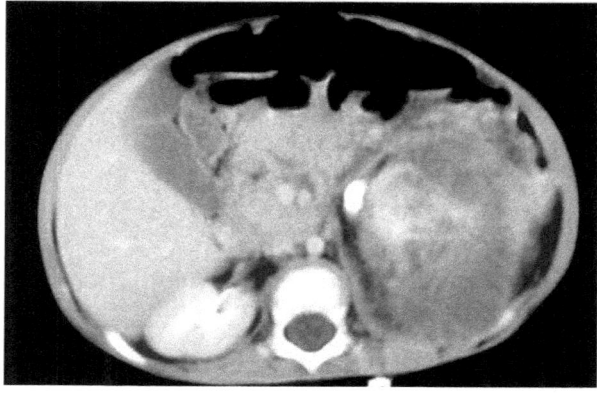

Fig. 79: Transaxial CT image shows renal and perirenal abscess on left side.

Xanthogranulomatous Pyelonephritis

- It is seen either as a globally enlarged kidney or as a focal hypodense mass, often with fatty elements within.
- The contour of the kidney is lobulated with small pelvis and dilated calyceal system.
- The nephrogram may be globally or focally absent on postcontrast studies.
- Centrally obstructing staghorn calculus is seen in three-fourths of the cases.
- Extension of the inflammatory process may be seen into the perinephric space, crux of diaphragm, psoas muscles, Gerota's fascia, and colon and posterior abdominal wall.

Arteriovenous Malformation

- These are seen as well-defined lesions that have attenuation values similar to that of the blood on both pre- and postcontrast images.
- Large tortuous feeding and draining vessels are characteristic.
- Calcification may be seen but is rare.

Perinephric Lesions (Table 22)

TABLE 22: Common causes of perinephric lesions.

Cystic	Solid	Fatty
• Urinoma	• Hematoma	• Lipoma
• Chronic hematoma/ abscess	• Abscess	• Metastases
• Lymphocele	• Fibroma	• Liposarcoma
• Lymphangiomatosis		

Urinoma/Perirenal Pseudocyst (Figs. 80A and B)

- It is seen as an encapsulated, extra-pelvicalyceal collection of urine that forms from urine leakage through a tear in the collecting system or the proximal ureter when ureteric obstruction is present.
- It has a radiological appearance of a water attenuating or soft tissue mass that usually conforms to the cone of renal fascia. Long-standing lesions have well-defined walls.
- Larger lesions displace the kidney superiorly and deviate the lower pole laterally and may extend down as inferiorly as the pelvic inlet.
- Active extravasation of the urine into the lesion may be seen on postcontrast images.
- Blood debris may produce low-level echoes or raise the attenuation values.

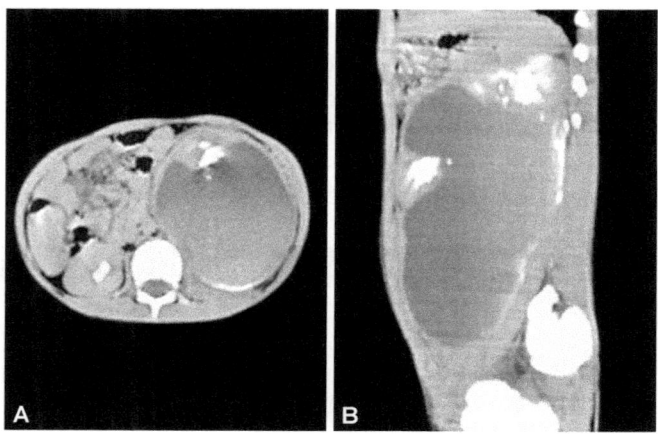

Figs. 80A and B: Axial and sagittal CT images showing urinoma secondary to renal fracture with active excretion of the contrast into the urinoma.

Lymphocele

- It is seen as a pararenal or retroperitoneal fluid collection of water density with thin nonenhancing walls usually occurring weeks to months following the renal surgery or transplantation or retroperitoneal lymphadenectomy.
- Presence of internal debris and thick septae are seen in approximately half of the cases.
- The fluid does not contain creatinine.

Lymphangiomatosis/Lymphangiectasia (Fig. 81)

- Renal lymphangiectasia is a rare disorder characterized by ectatic perirenal, peripelvic, and intrarenal lymphatic vessels.
- Imaging findings include nephromegaly, peripelvic cysts, and perirenal fluid collections.
- Retroperitoneal fluid collections, presumably dilated lymphatic vessels, are a variable finding noted in multiple cases.

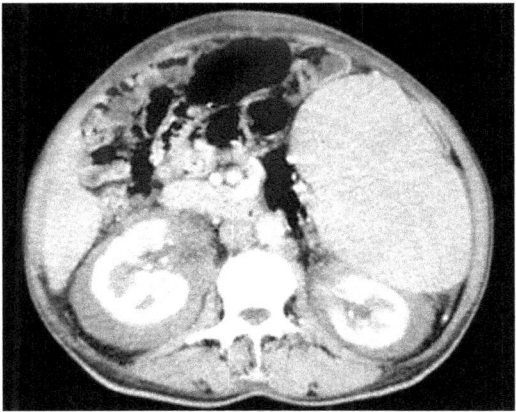

Fig. 81: Transaxial CT image shows bilateral renal lymphangiectasia

Bladder and Pelvic Lesions

Urinary Bladder Lesions

- Duplication anomalies
- Diverticulum
- Urachal anomalies
- Bladder endometriosis
- Bladder calculi
- Inflammatory disease
- Granulomatous cystitis
- Cystitis emphysematosa
- Cystitis cystica
- Fungal ball in bladder
- Malakoplakia
- Mesenchymal bladder tumors
- Bladder carcinoma
- Ureterocele
- Intraluminal pseudomasses of bladder
- Intramural bladder hematoma.

Duplication anomalies:
- A septum may be present within the bladder resulting two cavities.
- It is associated with penile didelphys.

Vesical diverticulum:
- It is seen as an outpouching from the bladder wall that may fill up with contrast in the cystographic phase.
- The diverticulum may be narrow or wide mouthed.

Urachal anomalies:
- It includes a spectrum of findings from patent urachus, urachal diverticulum to urachal cyst.
- Persistent urachus and urachal sinus are small caliber tubular structures that are best evaluated with CT fistulography.
- Urachal cyst and diverticulum are easily identified by CT.

- Urachal diverticulum has a wide communication with bladder dome and empties when the bladder is emptied.
- The urachal cyst appears as a midline thin-walled, fluid-filled mass beneath rectus abdominis muscle. Increased density or heterogeneous fluid content and cyst wall thickening may be seen with infection or hemorrhage. It does not fill with contrast from the bladder lumen.

Bladder endometriosis:
- It is commonly seen along the posterior bladder wall.
- It appears as a focal, irregular, bladder wall thickening with intravesical and/or extravesical component containing solitary or multiple hemorrhagic cysts with blood products of different ages.
- Cystic with fluid-fluid levels with blood products of different ages in the adnexa suggests the possibility.

Bladder calculi:
- They have high attenuation value regardless of their composition.
- A noncontract CT should always precede contrast CT for bladder calculi.

Inflammatory disease:
- Most cases occur in adult female.
- Granulomatous cystitis has a variable appearance depending upon the type as described under:
    - *Type I*: It is usually a complication of chronic granulomatous disease of childhood with irregular indentation of bladder wall that appears as extravesical lesion.
    - *Type II*: It results from direct extension of adjacent granulomatous disease of bowel and appears as a large infiltrating mass with variable enhancement.
    - *Type III*: It is usually secondary to granulomatous prostatitis and involves floor of bladder which may be irregular.
    - *Type IV*: In this, the granulomatous disease is isolated to bladder. Nodular irregularity may be seen with stippled appearance of mucosa in cystographic phase.

Cystitis emphysematosa:
- It is characterized by thickened bladder wall with intramural gas vesicles.
- It is usually secondary to infection, instrumentation or diabetes and noncontrast CT is diagnostic.

Cystitis cystica:
It is characterized by thickened bladder wall with multiple intramural cysts of fluid attenuation imparting a nodular appearance to the bladder wall.

Hemorrhagic cystitis:
- It is characterized by thickened bladder wall with higher attenuation due to submucosal bleed.
- Blood densities may also be seen within the bladder lumen with urine blood levels; sometimes a retracted clot may be seen.

Fungal ball in bladder:
- On noncontrast CT, fungus ball appears as heterogeneous lesion of high attenuation standing out against the urine in the bladder lumen.
- Gas may be present within it or around the fungal ball.
- It may change its position with scanning in prone position and does not show any postcontrast enhancement.

Malakoplakia:
- It is an uncommon granulomatous response to Gram-negative infection, found in diabetics with female predominance.
- Single or multiple focal plaques or nodules less than 3 cm in diameter, preferentially located in bladder floor with central necrosis or cyst formation.

Mesenchymal bladder tumors:
- These tumors are rare and include leiomyoma, rhabdomyoma, neurofibroma, hemangioma, and fibroadenoma.
- They are seen as small, polypoidal or large, often fungating mass lesion with or without wall thickening.

Abdomen

- Bladder pheochromocytoma is usually located at bladder base and characteristically present with sudden episodic hypertension, tachycardia and flushing during micturition are intensely enhancing on postcontrast images.
- Embryonal rhabdomyosarcoma (botryoid sarcoma) is most common bladder tumor in children. On CT, they present as bulky soft tissue sessile/polypoidal masses with variable attenuation and postcontrast enhancement secondary to necrosis and calcification.

Bladder carcinoma (Fig. 82):

- They appear as a sessile or pedunculated soft tissue masses projecting into bladder lumen. These tumors have a density similar to that of bladder wall on enhanced scans and occasionally intraluminal surface is encrusted with calcification.
- Extravesical extension is characterized by poor delineation of outer aspect of bladder wall with increase in density of perivesical fat.

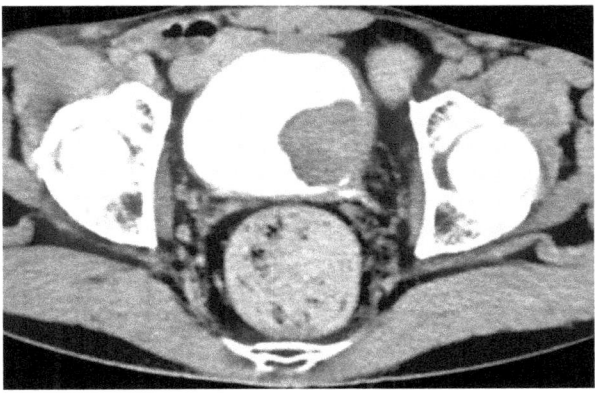

Fig. 82: Axial CECT image of pelvis showing soft tissue mass lesion arising from left lateral wall of urinary bladder in a case bladder carcinoma.

- Tumor invasion of seminal vesicle should be suspected if seminal vesicle is enlarged and shows heterogeneous enhancement or there is obliteration of the angle between the prostate and seminal vesicles.
- Loss of angle may also be seen, if rectum overdistended or if patient is prone.
- CT is also useful in detection lymph node metastases.

Ureterocele:

It is seen as a small, unilateral or bilateral cystic lesion adjacent to the normal ureteral orifice filling up with contrast in the cystographic phase.

Intraluminal pseudomasses of bladder:
- Bladder calculi
- Blood clots
- Fungal balls
- Foreign objects like Foley's bulb or metallic objects.

Intramural bladder hematoma:
- It is seen as focal wall thickening that may be associated with perivesical involvement and intraluminal blood clots.
- In acute stage—high density, subacute stage—isodensity and chronic stage localized bladder wall fibrosis with hypodensity is seen.

Pelvic Lesions

- Pelvic lipomatosis
- Pelvic fibrosis
- Pelvic edema
- Pelvic carcinomatosis
- Pelvic lymphocele
- Pelvic urinoma
- Pelvic hematoma
- Pelvic abscess
- Fistula

- *Colon and rectal lesions*:
  - Colorectal duplication cyst
  - Endometriosis of rectosigmoid
  - Colonic lipoma
  - Carcinoid
  - Colorectal lymphoma and metastasis
  - Colorectal carcinoma
  - Adenoma
  - Diverticulitis
  - Inflammatory bowel disease.

Pelvic lipomatosis:
- It is often an incidental finding occurring at a wide range of age with male predominance.
- It is seen as a noncircumscribed, fat attenuating tissue compressing pelvic organs with no soft tissue nodules.
- Narrowing, elongation, and elevation of the rectosigmoid.
- Similar finding is seen with urinary bladder producing an inverted pear-shaped appearance.

Pelvic fibrosis:
- It may be idiopathic or may be associated with retroperitoneal fibrosis or more commonly with pelvic irradiation, inflammation or hemorrhage.
- It is characterized by ill-defined, soft tissue attenuating mass encasing the pelvic structures without postcontrast enhancement.

Pelvic edema:
- It is seen as soft tissue attenuating, strands in the pelvic fat without any mass effect.
- Often associated with edema of lower leg.

Pelvic carcinomatosis:
- Metastatic and lymphomatous diseases are the most common pelvic malignancy.

- Extensive tumor infiltration with enlargement or invasion of pelvic organs. There is significant heterogeneous and sometimes homogeneous postcontrast enhancement.

Pelvic lymphocele:
- It is seen as a large, cystic fluid collection occurring after lymphadenectomy or renal transplant.
- Internal septations may be seen.
- It is usually seen at the site of surgery often after weeks to months following surgery.

Pelvic urinoma:
- Urine containing pseudocyst secondary to a tear in the distal ureter or bladder presenting as thin-walled homogeneous fluid collection with low density.
- Extravasation of the contrast agent into the lesion is diagnostic.

Pelvic hematoma:
- It is seen as a poorly marginated mass of variable attenuation evolving with time.
- Sedimentation may occur within acute stage causing fluid-fluid levels.

Pelvic abscess:
- It is seen as an irregularly, heterogeneous mass of low density.
- After IV contrast, the abscess wall enhances whereas necrotic center does not.
- Air bubbles within the lesion are highly suggestive of abscess.

Fistula:
- CT fistulogram may show contrast filled tract with internal communication.
- The tract may also be outlined with contrast in cystographic phase of scanning.
- Focal discontinuity of the involved organ wall is seen at sites of fistula penetration.

MALE REPRODUCTIVE SYSTEM LESIONS

Prostatic Lesions (Table 23)

TABLE 23: Common causes of prostatic lesions.

Cystic	Solid
• Simple cyst • Retention cyst • Cavitatory prostatitis • Abscess • Utricular cyst • Ejaculatory duct cyst • Ectopic ureter	• Benign prostatic hyperplasia • Carcinoma prostate • Prostatitis • Prostatic calculi

Prostatic Cyst

- It is the most common cystic lesion in prostate.
- It is the result of cystic degeneration in benign prostatic hyperplasia (BPH).
- The cyst is well-defined, smooth-walled, rounded with imperceptible walls and is located in transition zone of the prostatic parenchyma.

Retention Cyst

It is seen as a well-defined, oblong or oval, cystic lesion with imperceptible walls that arises secondary to the ductal obstruction of the glandular acini.

Cavitary Prostatitis

- There is an irregular, thick-walled cavity with postcontrast enhancement of the wall.
- The internal contents of the cavity have an attenuation value higher than that of urine.
- It is seen in chronic or tuberculous prostatitis.

Prostatic Abscess

- It is seen as an enlarged prostate with a ring enhancing lesion in peripheral zone of gland with edema in the adjacent parenchyma.
- Periprostatic inflammation can be detected based on strands of soft tissue in periprostatic fat.
- Septations can be seen sometimes.

Surgical Defect

- It is seen as a cystic defect continuous with the bladder neck secondary to transurethral resection of prostate (TURP).
- The defect corresponds to the postoperative dilatation of the posterior urethra and may fill with bladder contrast in cystographic phase of scanning.

Utricular Cyst

It is seen as a midline from verumontanum in posterosuperior direction without extension above the prostate.

Müllerian Duct Cyst

It arises from region of verumontanum slightly lateral to midline with cephalad extension above the prostate.

Ejaculatory Duct Cyst

- It is seen as an intraprostatic, well-defined, elongated cystic lesion along expected course of ejaculatory duct due to congenital or acquired obstruction of the latter.
- In cases of hemorrhage and infection high density with or without septations can be seen.

Ectopic Ureter

It can be seen as an elongated, cystic lesion in the prostate that may fill up with contrast in the pyelographic or cystographic phase of scanning.

Benign Prostatic Hyperplasia (Figs. 83A and B)

- There is diffuse prostatic enlargement with smooth surfaces.
- On CT, a prostate is considered to be enlarged if section obtained 1 cm above pubic symphysis shows prostate.
- BPH can only be suggested by CT on the basis of the enlarged size of gland and secondary signs of urinary retention such as dilated and trabeculated bladder, presence of bladder diverticulum, and elevation of bladder floor.

Carcinoma Prostate

- CT is useful in advanced cancer and in particular for evaluation of adenopathy where detection of lymph node metastasis is based on size.
- CT does not illustrate internal architecture of nodes and microinvasion in normal sized nodes (<10 mm) cannot be

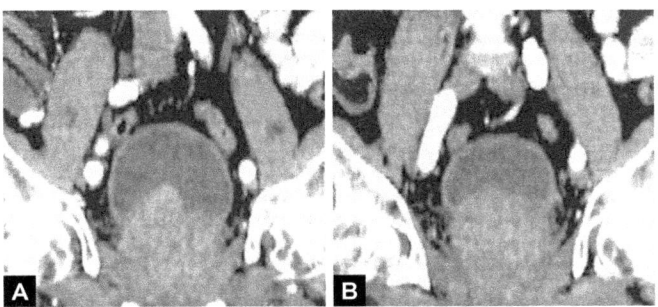

Figs. 83A and B: Coronal CT images showing benign hyperplasia of the prostate.

detected. If no adenopathy is present in the pelvis, a CT examination for staging of prostatic carcinoma need only be carried to aortic bifurcation.

Prostatic Calculi

- It is commonly seen at 40–70 years of age.
- It is seen as punctuate scattered high-density areas in various distribution patterns.
- Calcified foci in periurethral regions are horseshoe-shaped.

Seminal Vesicle Lesions

Seminal Vesicle Cyst

- Congenital is frequently associated with ipsilateral mesonephric duct anomalies including ectopic ureter insertion, renal dysgenesis, and duplication of collecting system.
- Acquired cyst results from infection or tumor obstruction (e.g. prostatic carcinoma).
- Seminal vesicle cyst is seen as unilateral or bilateral, homogeneous cystic mass cephalad to prostate, between bladder and rectum.
- It does not show any central enhancement, but subtle peripheral enhancement can be seen.

Seminal Vesicle Neoplasms

- Metastatic prostate carcinoma is by far the most common malignancy presenting as unilateral or less commonly bilateral enlargement of the seminal vesicles, sometimes associated with cyst due to an obstructing mass.
- There is variable degree of postcontrast enhancement.

Testes

Undescended/Ectopic Testis

- It may occur on unilaterally or bilaterally.
- The normal descent of testis from abdomen to scrotum is interrupted, commonly in inguinal canal (70%); in remainder, testis is found high in scrotum or in abdomen and lower pelvis. There is increased incidence of infertility and malignant changes with ectopic testis.
- CT features of undescended testis are an oval, homogeneously enhancing, soft tissue mass located anywhere along the pathway of testicular descent. It is usually smaller than descended testis. If the testes appear heterogeneous or show nonhomogeneous enhancement, malignant transformation should be suspected.
- In the abdomen and pelvis, the undescended or ectopic testis has to be differentiated from the bowel loops. The oral contrast used to opacify the bowel loops helps in differentiation.

FEMALE REPRODUCTIVE SYSTEM LESIONS

Vagina and Vulva

- Vaginal atresia
- Gartner's duct cyst
- Bartholin's cyst
- Vulvar/vaginal carcinoma
- Vaginal embryonal rhabdomyosarcoma.

Cervix and Uterus

- Nabothian cyst
- Adenomyosis
- Uterine collection
- Uterine leiomyoma
- Lymphoma/metastases

- Endometrial polyp
- Cervical carcinoma
- Uterine cancer
- Gestational trophoblastic disease (GTD)
- Choriocarcinoma
- Leiomyosarcoma.

Adnexa

- Congenital paraovarian cyst
- Simple ovarian cyst
- Complex cystic adnexal mass
- Multiple ovarian cysts
- PCOD (Stein-Leventhal syndrome)
- Endometrioma
- Tubo-ovarian abscess
- Adnexal torsion
- Ectopic pregnancy
- Ovarian cystadenoma
- Dermoid
- Ovarian cancer.

Vaginal Atresia

It is caused by transverse vaginal septum or imperforate hymen, leading to accumulation of fluid (hydrocolpos), blood (hematocolpos) or pus (pyocolpos) within distended, cystic vagina.

Gartner's Duct Cyst

- It is the vestigial remnant of Wolffian duct.
- It is seen as a well-defined, cystic lesion lateral to vaginal and uterine wall.

Bartholin's Cyst

It is seen as a well-defined, cystic lesion measuring up to 5 cm in diameter in the vulvovaginal region.

Vulvar/Vaginal Carcinoma

- It is seen as an ill-defined, soft tissue mass with variable degree of postcontrast enhancement and homogeneity.
- The main role of CT is in staging, detecting invasion of ischiorectal fat and pelvic walls as well as regional lymph node metastases.
- Invasion into the fat is seen as soft tissue stranding with postcontrast enhancement.
- Vaginal endometriosis is difficult to be differentiated from carcinoma.

Vaginal Embryonal Rhabdomyosarcoma

- It is usually in children below 5 years of age.
- It appears as a large, lobulated, soft tissue mass with variable postcontrast enhancement that enlarges the vaginal lumen.
- Signs of local invasion as fat stranding and ill-defined interfaces may be seen.
- Secondary findings include uterine enlargement and fluid collection in endometrial cavity when there is obstruction of cervix by tumor.

Uterus

Congenital Anomalies

- Unicornuate uterus is seen as an elongated banana-like shape uterus. It is usually associated with renal agenesis.
- Bicornuate uterus is seen as two cornua with variable degree of fusion.

- Septate uterus has a convex fundal contour with complete midline septum extending into endocervical canal (recognized on CT only if the endometrial cavity is filled with fluid).
- Didelphys uterus shows two separate uteri and cervices.
- Arcuate uterus may just reveal a fundal notch or indentation.
- Hypoplastic, T-shaped uterus is seen when there is exposure to diethylstibestrol (DES) in the fetal life.

Nabothian Cyst

It is seen as single or multiple, well-defined, fluid-filled structures in the cervical region.

Uterine Collection (Pyometra/Hydrometra) (Fig. 84)

- It is seen as a fluid density collection in the uterine cavity that is nonenhancing on postcontrast studies.
- The common cause in the adults is either cervical or endometrial carcinoma and in young females, imperforate hymen.

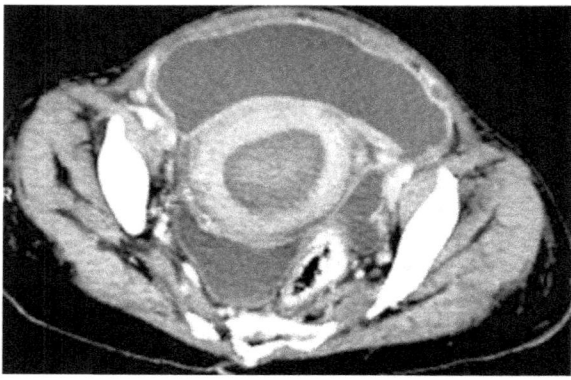

Fig. 84: Axial CT image showing mixed density collection in the uterine cavity suggestive of pyometra.

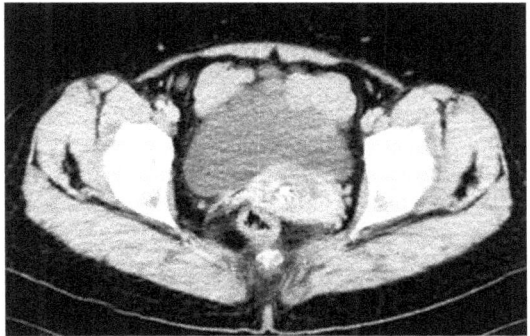

Fig. 85: Transaxial CT image shows fibroid in lower uterine segment and cervical region.

Uterine Leiomyoma (Fig. 85)

- It is seen as homogeneous, soft tissue attenuation masses (florids) causing uterine enlargement and lobulated contours. It may be iso-, hypo- or hyperdense relative to normal myometrium on postcontrast images.
- Calcification though uncommon is the most specific CT sign.
- Presence of necrosis or degeneration can give a low attenuation appearance.

Cervical Carcinoma

- It is usually seen in the childbearing age.
- Main role of CT is in advanced disease.
- Cervix may appear as enlarged with an irregular contour and enhancement may be inhomogeneous with areas of necrosis and ulceration.
- Poorly defined lateral cervical margins, stranding of the parametrial fat, and eccentric parametrial soft tissue mass are signs of local invasion.
- Effacement of fat planes around ureter is more reliable CT sign; occurs in advanced cases.

- CT elegantly demonstrates hydronephrosis and hydroureter.
- Nodal metastases have low attenuation centers reflecting necrosis.

Uterine Cancer

- It usually affects postmenopausal females.
- CT is done in advanced stage disease for demonstrating disease extension to pelvic side walls, pelvic and nodal enlargement.
- Endometrial tumor appears as a hypodense, enhancing mass within uterine cavity or within the myometrium.

Choriocarcinoma

- Uterine invasive mole or choriocarcinoma typically appears as eccentric hypodense foci in myometrium or endometrial cavity with variable enhancement on postcontrast images.
- There may be invasion of the broad ligament, parametrial and pelvic fascia and muscles seen as extension from the tumor mass.
- Theca lutein cysts are demonstrated as multiloculated cysts that are often bilateral.

Adnexa (Table 24)

TABLE 24: Common causes of adnexal lesions.

Cystic	Solid	Complex
• Congenital paraovarian cysts • Simple ovarian • Follicular cysts • Corpus luteal cysts • Chocolate cysts • Abscess • Cystic teratoma • Polycystic ovarian disease (PCOD) • Hydrosalpinx/pyosalpinx • Cystadenoma (serous/mucinous)	• Torsion of the ovary • Fibroma • Thecoma • Germ cell tumors (Fig. 86) • Krukenberg's/metastatic tumor	• Cystadenocarcinoma • Mature teratoma (fat, calcification, soft tissue) • Hemorrhagic/infected cyst • Abscess (air, soft tissue) • Endometrioma

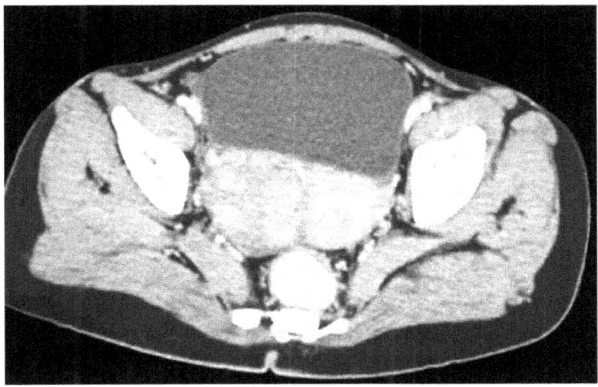

Fig. 86: Axial CECT image of pelvis shows heterogeneously enhancing solid mass lesion in right adnexal region in a young female in a case of germinoma.

Common Hemorrhagic Lesions of the Ovary

- Corpus luteal cyst
- Theca lutein cyst
- Torsion of the ovary
- Chocolate cyst of the ovary.

Congenital Paraovarian Cysts

They are seen as a cystic lesion in suspensory ligament of the ovary between ovary and fallopian tube.

Simple Ovarian/Follicular/Corpus Luteal/ Theca Lutein Cysts

- These are seen as homogeneous, unilocular water density masses with smooth, thin walls.
- They are usually under 5 cm in diameter.

- Hemorrhage may be seen within the cyst, more commonly in the corpus luteal cyst.
- Theca lutein cysts are multiple and bilateral and are commonly associated with gestational trophoblastic disease and may show hemorrhage as well.

Endometrioma

- It has variegated appearance on CT ranging from a purely cystic to hemorrhagic cyst with heterogeneous attenuation values with no or minimal postcontrast enhancement.
- A hyperdense blood clot adhered to the wall of the lesion are suggestive of the diagnosis.
- It is usually bilateral and causes enlargement of the ovaries.
- Associated uterine enlargement and endometrial thickening may also be appreciated on CT in some cases.

PCOD (Stein-Leventhal Syndrome)

- It is characterized by bilaterally, diffuse, enlargement of the ovaries with multiple tiny cystic lesion characteristically arranged at periphery of ovaries.
- The cysts are usually less than 10 mm in diameter but may be smaller than that CT can resolve.
- As the condition progresses, the ovaries assume round shape rather than their oval shape with relative increase in the anteroposterior diameter.

Tubo-ovarian Abscess Complex

- In a typical case, a tubular fluid density mass representing a dilated fallopian tube (hydrosalpinx or pyosalpinx) with septated thick-walled, ring enhancing masses corresponding to ovarian abscess is seen.
- There is loss of fat planes, thickened uterosacral ligaments with adenopathy and soft tissue stranding in the parametrial tissue.

Adnexal Torsion

- It is commonly seen in adolescent females, especially with an ovarian mass (e.g. dermoid).
- The affected ovary is enlarged and hypodense relative to the normal ovary and sometimes hemorrhagic as seen on noncontrast images. Multiple cystic lesions corresponding to the enlarged follicles may be seen arranged at the periphery of the ovary.
- Postcontrast images may reveal variable enhancement depending upon the vascular compromise and whether it is arterial or venous and multiple dilated tortuous vascular channels may be seen around the ovary.
- Complete lack of enhancement denotes infarction.
- Minimal ascites and soft tissue stranding of the paraovarian fat may be seen.

Ovarian Dermoid (Fig. 87)

- It is characterized by well-defined, heterogeneous mass with minimal postcontrast enhancement causing enlargement of the ovary.

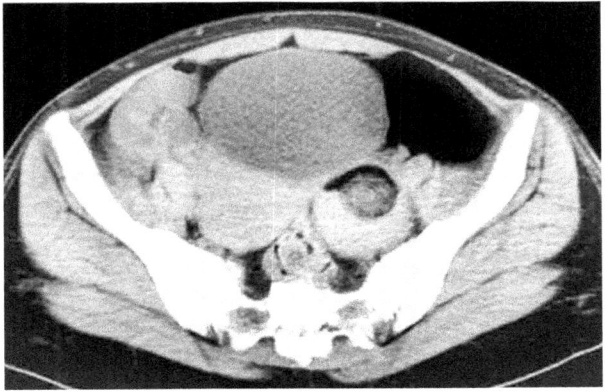

Fig. 87: Transaxial CT image shows ovarian dermoid on left side.

- The attenuation values may range from that of fat to soft tissues and dense calcification.
- Presence of dental elements, fat-fluid level, and dermoid plug is diagnostic.
- Presence of irregular, enhancing, solid component of greater than 10 cm suggests malignant transformation.

Ovarian Cystadenoma/Cystadenocarcinoma (Serous or Mucinous) (Figs. 88 and 89)

- They have variable appearance on CT imaging ranging from purely unilocular, cystic masses to complex multilocular lesions showing varying degrees of wall and septal thickness, enhancement, and nodularity.

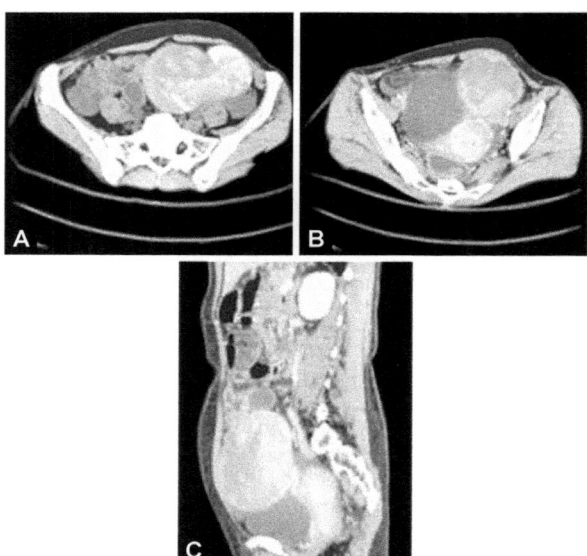

Figs. 88A to C: Axial and sagittal CT images showing a hemorrhagic ovarian mass.

Abdomen

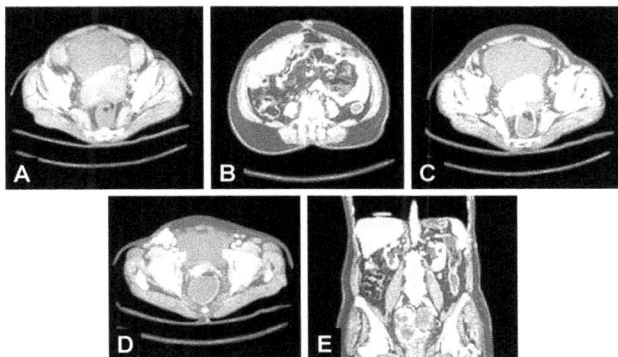

Figs. 89A to E: Axial and coronal CT images showing ovarian mass with peritoneal dissemination and adenopathy.

- Mucinous cystadenoma and cystadenocarcinoma contain high density fluid relative to their serous counterparts but higher density may also result from hemorrhage.
- Calcification may be seen in the wall or the papillary projection within the lesions.
- Thick, irregular wall and septae with enhancing soft tissue nodules, ascites, and pseudomyxoma peritonei should raise the suspicion of malignancy; however, presence of distant visceral and peritoneal/omental metastases is the only specific CT criterion of malignancy.

Metastatic Tumor

- It is seen as multifocal, enhancing, nodular lesions involving both ovaries in a patient with known primary tumor.
- It has wide range of CT appearance from cystic to solid and usually mimics the primary tumor.
- Similar lesions in the peritoneum/omentum/mesentery may be seen.
- Common primary tumors producing metastases to the ovary include breast carcinoma, gastric adenocarcinoma, and pancreatic carcinoma.

Chapter 9

Musculoskeletal System

BONY LESIONS

Well-defined Lytic Lesions (Table 1)

TABLE 1: Common causes of well-defined lytic lesions.

	Unilocular	Multilocular
With expansion	• Unicameral bone cyst • Aneurysmal bone cyst • Enchondroma • Brown tumor of hyperparathyroidism • Juxtacortical chondroma • Plasmacytoma • Chordoma	• Simple bone cyst • Aneurysmal bone cyst • Giant cell tumor • Fibrous dysplasia
No expansion	• Unicameral bone cyst • Fibrous cortical defect • Nonossifying fibroma • Giant cell tumor • Enchondroma • Eosinophilic granuloma • Epidermoid inclusion cyst • Intraosseous ganglion • Hemophilic pseudotumor • Degenerative cyst • Fibrous dysplasia	• Simple bone cyst • Fibrous dysplasia • Aneurysmal bone cyst

Ill-defined Lytic Lesions (Table 2)

TABLE 2: Common causes of ill-defined lytic lesions.

With periosteal reaction	*No periosteal reaction*
• Osteomyelitis • Ewing's sarcoma • Osteosarcoma	*With expansion:* • Chondrosarcoma • Giant cell tumor • Malignant fibrous histiocytoma • Angiosarcoma • Plasmacytoma • Metastasis (renal, thyroid) *No expansion:* • Hemangioma • Eosinophilic granuloma • Multiple myeloma • Metastases

Lytic Lesions with Surrounding Sclerosis

- Osteoblastoma
- Osteoid osteoma
- Tuberculosis
- Chronic osteomyelitis.

Expansile and Hypodense Bony Lesion (Table 3)

TABLE 3: Common causes of expansile and hypodense bony lesions.

Malignant bone neoplasm	Benign bone neoplasm	Non-neoplastic
• Metastasis • Plasmacytoma • Central chondrosarcoma • Lymphoma • Fibrosarcoma • Telangiectatic osteosarcoma	• Aneurysmal bone cyst • Giant cell tumor • Enchondroma	• Fibrous dysplasia • Hemophilic pseudotumor • Brown tumor of hyperparathyroidism • Hydatid cyst

Moth-eaten Lesions in Bone (Table 4)

TABLE 4: Common causes of moth-eaten lesions in bone.

Neoplastic	Infective
<ul><li>Metastasis</li><li>Multiple myeloma</li><li>Leukemia</li><li>*Long-bone sarcomas:*<ul><li>Ewing's sarcoma</li><li>Lymphoma of bone</li><li>Osteosarcoma</li><li>Chondrosarcoma</li><li>Fibrosarcoma and malignant fibrous histiocytoma (MFH)</li></ul></li><li>Langerhans' cell histiocytosis</li></ul>	Osteomyelitis

Lucent Bone Lesions Containing Calcium or Bone (Table 5)

TABLE 5: Common causes of lucent bone lesions containing calcium or bone.

Neoplastic	Miscellaneous
<ul><li>Metastasis</li><li>*Cartilage tumors:*<ul><li>Enchondroma</li><li>Chondroblastoma</li><li>Chondromyxoid fibroma</li><li>Chondrosarcoma</li></ul></li><li>*Osteoid neoplasms:*<ul><li>Osteoid osteoma</li><li>Osteoblastoma</li><li>Osteosarcoma</li></ul></li><li>*Fibrous tissue tumors:*<ul><li>Fibrosarcoma</li><li>Malignant fibrous histiocytoma</li></ul></li></ul>	<ul><li>Fibrous dysplasia</li><li>Paget's disease (osteoporosis circumscripta)</li><li>Bone infarction</li><li>Osteomyelitis with sequestrum</li><li>Eosinophilic granuloma</li><li>Intraosseous lipoma</li></ul>

Sclerotic Bone Disease (Table 6)

TABLE 6: Common causes of sclerotic bone lesions.

Congenital	Neoplastic	Vascular	Infective	Traumatic	Idiopathic
• Bone island • Tuberous sclerosis	• Metastasis • Lymphoma • Osteoma/osteoid osteoma/osteoblastoma • Primary bone sarcoma • Healed or healing bone lesion • Multicentric osteosarcoma	Infarct	Garre's osteomyelitis	Callus	Paget's disease

Bone Sclerosis with a Periosteal Reaction

- *Traumatic*: Healing fracture with callus
- *Neoplastic*:
  - Metastasis
  - Osteoid osteoma/osteoblastoma
  - Lymphoma
  - Osteosarcoma
  - Ewing's sarcoma
  - Chondrosarcoma.
- *Idiopathic*: Infantile cortical hyperostosis (Caffey's disease)
- *Infective*: Osteomyelitis (Garre's osteomyelitis, Brodie abscess).

Solitary Sclerotic Bone Lesion with a Lucent Center

- *Neoplastic*: Osteoid osteoma, osteoblastoma
- *Infective*: Brodie abscess, syphilis, yaws disease, tuberculosis.

Mixed Sclerotic and Lytic Lesions (Table 7)

TABLE 7: Common causes of mixed sclerotic and lytic lesions.

With sequestrum	No sequestrum
• Osteomyelitis • Eosinophilic granuloma	• Osteomyelitis • Tuberculosis • Ewing's sarcoma • Metastasis • Osteosarcoma

Fluid Levels in Bone Tumors

TABLE 8: Fluid levels in benign and malignant tumors.

Benign	Malignant
• Aneurysmal bone cyst • Chondroblastoma • Giant cell tumor • Simple bone cyst • Fibrous dysplasia	• Telangiectatic osteosarcoma • Malignant fibrous histiocytoma • Synovial cell sarcoma • Any necrotic bone tumor

Salient Features of Bone Tumors and Tumor-like Lesions

Actinomycosis

- It is seen as ill-defined areas of osteolysis without new bone formation.
- Vertebral lesion resembles tuberculosis, however, disks are spared.
- Rib lesions show periosteal reaction with irregular thickening and association with cutaneous sinus tracts and pleuritis is diagnostic.
- Common sites of involvement are vertebrae, mandible, and ribs.

Adamantinoma of the Long Bones/Angioblastoma

- It is seen as a large, multiloculated, expansile lytic lesion with or without reactive sclerosis in diaphyseal location.

- It is usually seen in adolescents and young adults.
- The common bones to be involved include tibia (majority), fibula, humerus, ulna, femur, and radius.
- It resembles ameloblastoma of the jaw (Figs. 1 and 2).

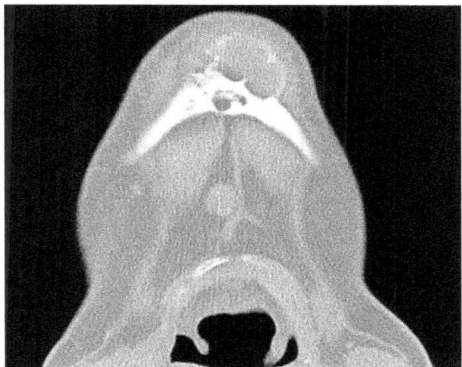

Fig. 1: Transaxial computed tomography (CT) image shows evidence of expansile, osteolytic lesion in the mandible in a case of ameloblastoma.

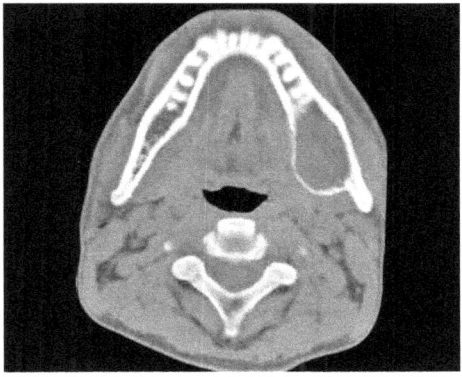

Fig. 2: Transaxial CT image shows unicystic ameloblastoma of mandible on left side.

Aneurysmal Bone Cyst (Figs. 3A to C)

- It is seen as an eccentric, lytic, grossly expansile lesion with cortical thinning involving the metaphysis of long bones.
- The lesions may appear multiloculated with fine trabeculations and occasionally with fluid-fluid levels.
- Occasionally, cortical breach and soft tissue extension may be evident.
- It is commonly seen in the first and second decades of life in the humerus, femur, tibia, vertebra (posterior elements), and innominate bones.
- Secondary aneurysmal bone cyst (ABC) is associated with other skeletal lesions as giant cell tumor (GCT), osteoblastoma, chondroblastoma, osteosarcoma, metastases, fibrous dysplasia, and Paget's disease.

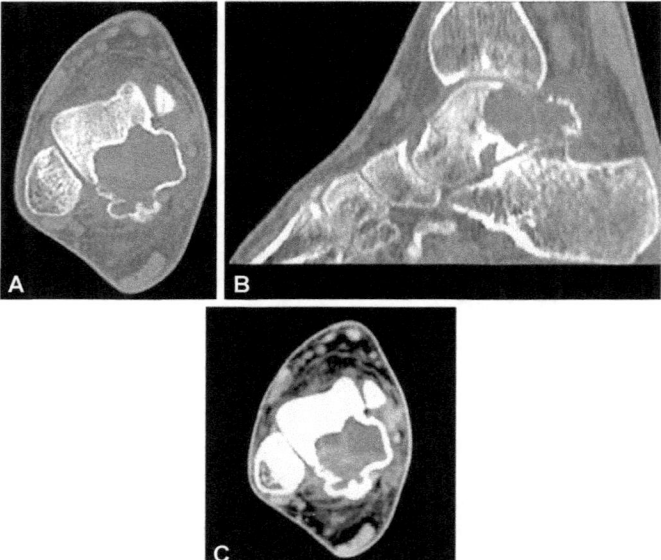

Figs. 3A to C: Axial and sagittal CT images showing aneurysmal bone cyst of the talus.

Angiosarcoma of Bone

- It is characterized by multiple, poor to well-defined, osteolytic lesions occasionally accompanied with sclerosis usually occurring in the metadiaphysis of the long bones.
- It is associated with cortical thinning and mild-to-moderate bone expansion with infrequent periostitis.
- Multifocal involvement within a single bone or involvement of multiple bones in a single extremity is a characteristic finding.
- Commonly involved bones include tibia, femur and humerus, occasionally pelvis, skull and ribs may be affected.

Avascular Necrosis of Bone

- In the long bones, the computed tomography (CT) appearance varies with the site.
- In the epiphysis, avascular necrosis of bone (AVN) is seen as subchondral circular areas of decreased attenuation with patchy areas of lysis and sclerosis in the adjacent bone with resultant collapse. Secondary osteoarthritic changes may be seen in the adjacent joint.
- In the diametaphyseal region, AVN of bone is seen as an irregular, intramedullary lucent lesion with marginal sclerosis and periostitis.
- In the flat bones, tarsal and carpal bones, AVN of bone is seen as patchy lucent and sclerotic areas with bone collapse.
- Multiplanar reformation (MPR) images along the axis of the bone are more helpful as they better delineate the subtle areas of subchondral fracture, buckling and collapse of the articular surface that is indicative of the advanced disease that limits the therapeutic intervention.
- Common sites of affection include femoral head, talus, scaphoid, humeral head, capitate, and vertebral body.

Bone Island/Enostosis

- It is seen as focus of homogeneously dense bone with thorny spicules radiating from the lesion.
- It ranges from few mm to few cm in size.
- The common sites include pelvis and spine.
- Lesions can show a change in size with time.
- Osteoblastic metastases and osteopoikilosis (multiple tiny lesions distributed symmetrically in periarticular location) are important differential diagnosis.

Brodie Abscess (Figs. 4A and B)

- It is seen in localized subacute or chronic osteomyelitis and is characterized by a well-defined, lytic area with thick sclerotic border usually occurring in metaphysis of long bones and occasionally in the diaphysis or epiphysis, flat or irregular bones may be involved.
- Demonstration of a tortuous channel connecting the metaphyseal lesion with the growth plate is diagnostic and is termed as *tunneling*.

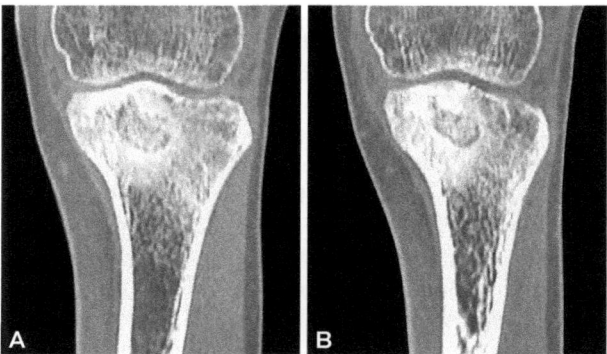

Figs. 4A and B: Coronal and sagittal CT images of right knee showing lytic lesion with sclerotic margins with medullary tunneling involving the metaphysis of right tibia.

Brown Tumors of Hyperparathyroidism

- It is seen as a solitary or multiple, well-defined, lytic, expansile lesion in the axial or appendicular skeleton with endosteal scalloping and no sclerosis.
- Common sites include facial bones, pelvis, ribs, and femur.
- Other manifestation of the hyperparathyroidism seen in the hands and other part of skeleton suggests the diagnosis.

Chondroblastoma/Codman's Tumor

- It is seen as a well-demarcated, eccentric lytic lesion with expansion and cortical thinning involving the epiphysis or apophysis of the long bones with chondroid calcification.
- Linear periosteal reaction is seen in about a third of patients.
- Usual age of presentation is second and third decades of life with male predominance (M:F = 2:1).
- Usual sites of involvement are femur, tibia, and humerus.

Chondromyxoid Fibroma

- It is seen as a sharply defined, eccentric, lytic, intramedullary lesion seen in metaphyseal location.
- The lesion is usually elongated with its long axis parallel to the bone.
- The lesion can extend to the epiphysis after its fusion with the shaft.
- Cortical expansion, exuberant endosteal sclerosis and coarse trabeculations are commonly seen.
- Usual age of presentation is second and third decades of life.
- The common sites of involvement are tibia, femur, fibula, innominate, and small bones of foot.

Chondrosarcoma (Figs. 5 and 6)

The CT features depend upon the type of the chondrosarcoma.

- *Central type* is an expansile, multilocular, osteolytic lesion with endosteal scalloping and erosions.
    - Irregular stippled calcification in the matrix is the hallmark.

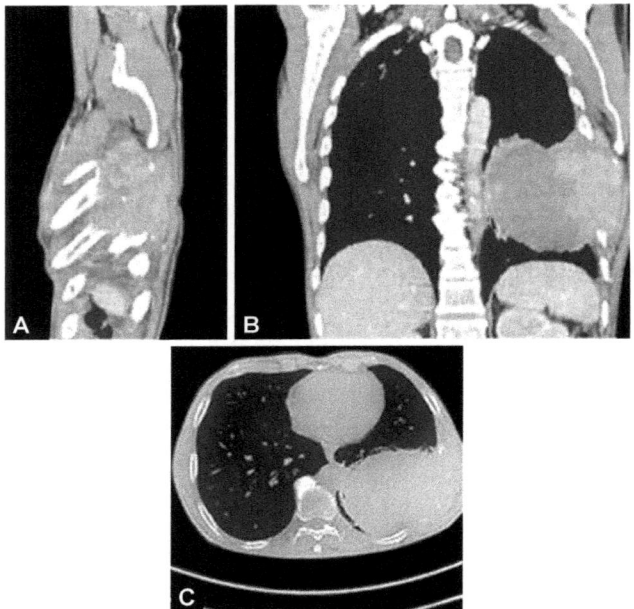

Figs. 5A to C: Sagittal, coronal and axial CT images showing chondrosarcoma of the ribs.

- Cortical breach with a large soft tissue mass is usual (soft tissue mass is out of proportion to the bony elements within the tumor).
- Common sites of involvement are flat bones, pelvis, ribs, and metaphysis of long bones.
- Usual age of presentation is 30-60 years.
- *Mesenchymal type* is radiologically indistinguishable from central type but is more common in mandible and ribs and has a younger age of presentation.
- *Peripheral type* arises from the cartilaginous cap of the osteochondroma. Such lesions are more common in diaphyseal achalasia.

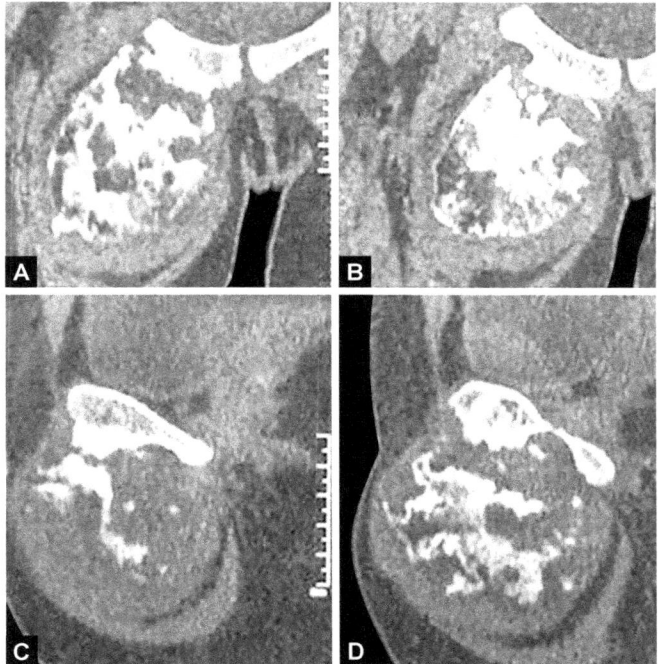

Fig. 6A to D: Coronal multiplanar reformation (MPR) CT images of chondrosarcoma of pubis.

- It is seen as flocculent or streaky calcification within the cap of an osteochondroma extending into the adjacent soft tissues.
- Bony part of the osteochondroma shows osteolysis.
- If the cartilaginous cap measures >2 cm in thickness, malignant is suggested.
- *Clear cell type* is seen as ill- or well-defined, expansile, osteolytic with or without a sclerotic rim involving the epiphysis of the long tubular bones (femur, humerus, and tibia).
    - It is usually seen in third to fifth decades of life.

Chordoma

- It is seen as an expansile, lytic lesion involving the axial skeleton in the midline associated with large soft tissue mass with flocculent calcification.
- Usual age of presentation is fourth to sixth decades of life.
- Common sites of involvement are sacrococcygeal region, sphenooccipital region and other parts of the spine.

Cortical Dermoid

- It is seen as a subperiosteal lesion that develops at the outer margin of the cortex.
- It may shows some cortical new bone formation and scalloping of the cortex.
- Usual age of presentation is first and second decades of life.
- Common sites involved are distal femur.

Desmoplastic Fibroma

- It is seen as a central, lytic lesion with soap bubble pattern and endosteal erosion in the flat bones and the metaphysis of long bones.
- It is usually seen before 30 years of age.
- Usual sites of involvement include mandible, pelvis, and tubular bones.

Enchondroma

- It is seen as a well-circumscribed, lytic lesion with endosteal scalloping with varying degree of chondroid (spotty) calcification.
- It is commonly seen in diaphysis of the short tubular bones of the hand and feet. Other sites include metaphysis of long tubular bones as femur and humerus.
- In long bones, large areas of uncalcified matrix (more than one-third) should raise the suspicion of malignant transformation.

- Multiple enchondromas occur in Ollier disease and Maffucci syndrome.
- Maffucci syndrome also shows multiple soft tissue hemangiomas.
- Ollier disease is also associated with vertical metaphyseal lucent lines.

Epidermoid/Inclusion Cyst

- Well-defined intraosseous lytic lesion with sclerotic margin in terminal phalanx of hand or skull. Rarely metacarpals, tibia, ulna, femur, and sternum involved.
- May be expansile with thinning and destruction of cortex.
- In skull sharp edges of the lesion help in differentiation from metastasis and infections.
- Cysts contain thick waxy material, which has a Hounsfield unit (HU) value of –5 HU to 20 HU.
- Age at presentation is usually second to fourth decades of life.

Ewing's Sarcoma (Figs. 7A and B)

- It is seen as a poorly-defined, permeative or moth-eaten, osteolysis involving the diaphysis of long bones with occasional sclerosis.
- Exuberant periosteal reaction with lamellated onion peel appearance is the hallmark; however, hair on end appearance of the periosteal reaction may also be seen.
- Cortical breach with associated soft tissue mass is commonly encountered.
- Subperiosteal lesion produces saucerization of the outer cortex with a large soft tissue mass.
- In the flat bones, it is seen as an ill-defined lesion with a larger soft tissue mass.
- The age of presentation is usually in the first decade with male predominance.
- Common sites of involvement include femur, ilium, tibia, humerus, fibula, ribs, and the vertebral bodies (in the spine, sacrum is the most common site of affection).

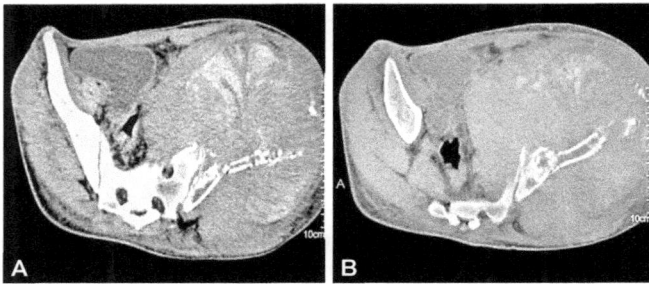

Figs. 7A and B: Axial CT images of pelvis showing large soft tissue mass lesion causing destruction of left iliac blade in a case of Ewing's sarcoma left iliac blade.

Fibrosarcoma

- It is seen as a permeative or moth-eaten lytic lesion without calcification or new bone formation.
- The cortex may be eroded or expanded with extension into the adjacent soft tissue which is small relative to the size of the bony lesion.
- A bone sequestrum within tumor is frequently seen.
- Usual sites involved include metaphyseal region of the distal femur and proximal tibia, humerus, mandible, skull.
- Usual age of presentation is third to fifth decades of life.
- It can be secondary to Paget's disease, chondrosarcoma, infarct, radiation, or osteomyelitis.

Fibrous Cortical Defect

- It is seen as a well-defined, flame-shaped, lytic lesion lying within the metaphyseal cortex of the long bones.
- The lesions are usually 1–2 cm in diameter with its long-axis parallel to bone.
- Commonly seen along posteromedial aspect of femora, tibia, and fibula.
- The lesion usually undergoes spontaneous regression by 8 years of age.

Fibrous Dysplasia

- It may be monostotic (70-80%) or polyostotic (20-30%).
- In the long bones, the lesions are lytic and expansile with ground-glass density, peripheral sclerosis and internal septae or trabeculations in intramedullary and diaphyseal location. Endosteal scalloping and remodeling of the expanded bone (*Shepherd's crook deformity*) are common with occasional pathological fractures.
- In the skull calvarium, the lesions are seen as homogeneous increase in bone density with widened diploic space with an outward expansion of the intact skull table.
- Involved facial bones have a similar appearance and are associated with facial asymmetry. There may be complete obliteration of the sinus cavity secondary to fibrous dysplasia.
- In the spine, the lesions are well-defined, lytic, expansile with internal striations involving the vertebral body and occasionally the pedicle and the arch.
- Age of involvement is second and third decades in monostotic, while first decade in polyostotic form.
- When monostotic, the common sites of involvement include ribs, femur, tibia, mandible, and calvaria. When polyostotic, the sites of involvement include skull and facial bones, spine, and the girdle bones.

Garre's Osteomyelitis

- It is rare type of osteomyelitis characterized by intense sclerosis with cortical thickening without periosteal reaction.
- Areas of frank destruction are rare.
- Children and young adults are mainly affected with predilection for mandible and shafts of long bones.

Geode/Subchondral Cyst

- It is seen as a subarticular solitary or multiple lytic defects with sclerotic borders often communicating with adjacent joint space.

- Associated with osteoarthritis (OA), rheumatoid arthritis (RA), AVN, and pseudogout.

Giant Cell Tumor/Osteoclastoma (Fig. 8)

- It is seen as a fairly well-defined, eccentric, slightly trabeculated, expansile (*soap bubble appearance*), lytic lesion extending to subarticular region of the long bones.
- Cortical breach with soft tissue extension is common.
- Calcification, sclerosis, and periosteal reactions are typically not seen.
- The common age of presentation is second and third decades of life.
- Common sites are distal radius, distal femur, proximal tibia, and humerus. Pelvis and spine can also be involved.
- Multicentric GCT is unusual, where the lesions are metaphyseal and occur most frequently in the small bones of the hand.
- In the skull and facial bones, GCT may be accompanied with Paget's disease.

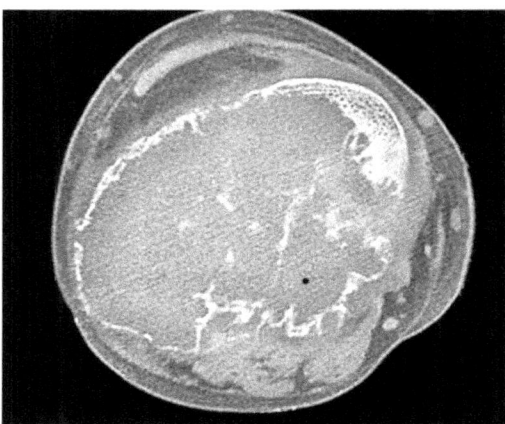

Fig. 8: Axial CT image showing osteoclastoma of the upper end of tibia.

Glomus Tumor

- It is seen as a well-defined, expansile, lytic lesion encased by cortical rim with characteristic absence of calcification.
- It is seen at distal aspect of the terminal phalanx of the digits.
- Soft tissue glomus tumors produce smooth scalloping of the adjacent bone.
- Postcontrast enhancement is intense.

Hemangioma (Fig. 9)

- It is seen an expansile, loculated, coarsely trabeculated, lytic lesion.
- In the flat bones and skull, it presents a typical *sunburst appearance* with thickened, coarse trabeculae perpendicular to the bone.
- In the vertebral body, coarse, vertical trabecular pattern is seen giving a *corduroy appearance* on sagittal scans. On transaxial scans, the lesion show a typical *polka dot appearance*.
- Usual age of presentation is after 40 years of age with female preponderance.

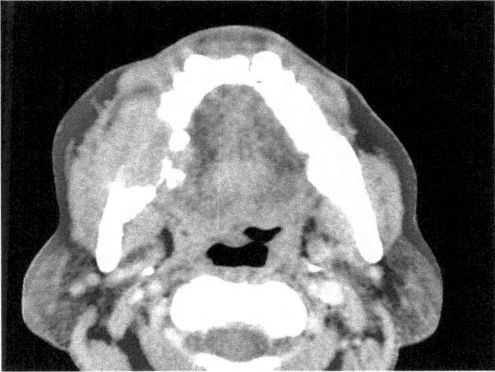

Fig. 9: Transaxial contrast-enhanced computed tomography (CECT) image shows central hemangioma of mandible.

Hemophilic Pseudotumor

- They may be intraosseous or subperiosteal.
- Intraosseous lesions are seen as large, expansile, lytic areas with internal trabeculations and well-defined sclerotic margins in intramedullary location. Cortical breach and periosteal reaction with associated large soft tissue masses may be seen.
- Subperiosteal lesions cause periosteal reaction and adjacent cortical scalloping and often mimics malignant or an infective process.
- Soft tissue pseudotumor commonly encountered in the thigh and gluteal region causes pressure erosion of the adjacent bone. Calcification may be seen in soft tissue masses.
- Associated features of the hemophilic arthropathy suggest the diagnosis.
- It commonly involves femur, pelvis, tibia, and small bones of the hand.

Histiocytosis

There are three major conditions in this category—eosinophilic granuloma (two-third of cases), Hand-Schüller-Christian disease, and Letterer-Siwe disease.

1. *Eosinophilic granuloma* is the most mild form characterized by single or multiple, well-defined, lytic bones lesions with or without marginal sclerosis.
    - In the long bones, endosteal scalloping and periosteal reactions are typical.
    - In the skull vault, lytic lesion may show a central radiodense focus (*button sequestrum*).
    - In the mandible, the lytic lesions may destroy the supporting bone of the teeth leading to *floating teeth appearance*.
    - In the spine, vertebral body is involved and may be completely destroyed (*vertebra plana*).
    - The lesions are commonly seen in children and young adults.
    - Most common sites of involvement are mandible, skull, spine, ribs, pelvis, and long bones.

2. *Hand-Schüller-Christian disease* is characterized by classic triad of diabetes insipidus, unilateral or bilateral exophthalmos and single or multiple bone lesions.
    - Skeletal lesions are similar in appearance to that of eosinophilic granuloma, however, are multiple and more widely disseminated.
    - In the skull, coalescence of multiple lesions gives rise to a typical *geographical or map-like appearance*.
    - Associated cutaneous and visceral organ involvement may be seen.
    - It is predominantly seen in children with two-thirds younger than 5 years.
3. *Letterer-Siwe disease* is an acute syndrome seen in children younger than 3 years of age with extensive and predominant visceral organ and cutaneous involvement with or without skeletal lesions that are similar to that seen in Hand-Schüller-Christian disease.

Hydatid Disease of Bone

- It is characterized by an expansile, multicystic lesion with absence of periosteal reaction or new bone formation.
- It commonly involves the vertebral bodies, pelvis, and sacrum.

Intraosseous Ganglion

- It is seen as a well-defined, mildly expansile, lytic lesion with sclerotic margins in subchondral location.
- It may be unilocular or multilocular.
- Calcification is characteristically absent.
- Preferred locations are medial malleolus, femoral head, distal femur, acetabulum, carpal bones, distal radius, and ulna.
- Occasionally, associated with extraosseous soft tissue ganglion.

Leukemia

The imaging features depend upon the age of presentation and type of the leukemia.

- *Acute leukemia of childhood* is the most common childhood malignancy with peak age of manifestation between 3 years and 5 years with the following varied appearances:
  - Diffuse osteopenia with medullary widening and cortical thinning in tubular bones or vertebral compression.
  - Symmetrical metaphyseal band-like lucencies at sites of rapid bone growth (distal femur and radius, proximal tibia, and humerus).
  - Multiple lytic areas in the metaphyseal region of long bones (*medial cortex of proximal humerus is the characteristic site*) or in skull vault, pelvis, ribs, and shoulder girdle.
  - Prominent symmetrical periosteal reaction and subperiosteal hemorrhages are usual.
  - Sutural diastasis secondary to raised intracranial pressure (ICP) is common in infants.
- *Acute leukemia in adults* is mainly characterized by diffuse osteopenia; though findings seen in childhood leukemia may also be seen with decreased frequency.
- Osseous manifestations in *chronic leukemia* are less common and less severe than in acute leukemia.

Lipoma

- It is seen as an expansile, lytic lesion with small central calcification and thinned out cortex.
- Lobulations or internal osseous ridges are frequently seen.
- Fat attenuation within the lesion is diagnostic.
- Periosteal variety is characterized by fat attenuating mass abutting the external osseous surface of the long bone with associated periostitis and cortical thickening.
- Common sites include calcaneum, skull, ribs, and extremities.

Maduramycosis (Madura Foot)

- It is a form of chronic osteomyelitis caused by fungi or actinomycosis.

- The disease arises in the soft tissue of the foot with secondary osteomyelitis of the adjacent bones.
- Lamellated, periosteal reaction is hallmark of the disease with characteristic absence of osteopenia and sequestrum.
- Multiple bones are involved with osteolytic areas and sclerosis.

Malignant Fibrous Histiocytoma

- It is seen as a moth-eaten or permeative osteolysis with cortical erosion and a soft tissue mass.
- It is usually metaphyseal in location but frequently extends to the epiphysis and diaphysis.
- There is no new bone formation, matrix calcification or significant periosteal reaction.

Metastases (Fig. 10)

- The radiological appearance is highly variable ranging from purely lytic to purely sclerotic.
- Multiplicity of the lesions is the rule, however, solitary lesions may be occasionally encountered.
- The lesions are of variable shape and size.
- The lytic lesions may have variable appearance ranging from well-defined, geographic lesions to poorly defined permeative destruction.
- Marginal sclerosis and periosteal reactions are rare. Occasional sunburst periosteal reaction may be seen in carcinoma prostate, retinoblastoma, neuroblastoma, and gastrointestinal (GI) tumors.
- Sclerotic lesions may be nodular or diffuse in distribution.
- Associated soft tissue mass is usually small except in ribs and pelvis.
- The lesions have special predilection for axial skeleton but no bone is spared.
- In the spine, posterior elements (especially pedicles) of the vertebra are more commonly involved than body.
- In the long bones, the lesions are rarely seen below the elbow and knees.

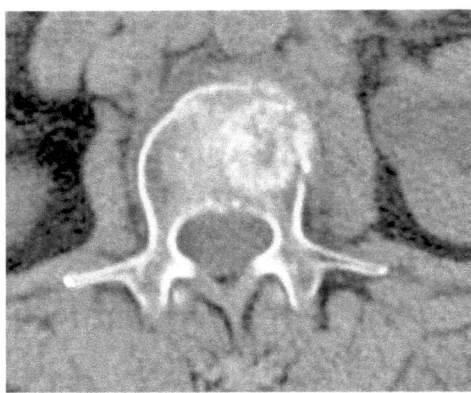

Fig. 10: Transaxial CT image shows mixed metastases from breast carcinoma.

- Majority of the metastatic lesions are seen in the middle-aged and elderly; but skeletal metastases in children can be seen in neuroblastoma, Ewing's sarcoma, osteosarcoma, retinoblastoma, medulloblastoma, and soft tissue tumors.
- Common primary tumors producing purely lytic metastases include lung, breast, thyroid, kidney, GI tract (GIT), and neuroblastoma. Expansile, lytic lesions are characteristics of renal cell carcinoma, thyroid carcinoma, and rarely hepatoma.
- Common primary tumors producing purely sclerotic metastases include prostate, breast, lymphoma, carcinoid, medulloblastoma GIT, urinary bladder, pancreas, and neuroblastoma.
- Common primary tumors producing mixed metastases include prostate, breast, lymphoma, and GIT.

Multiple Myeloma

- It is usually seen in sixth to seventh decades with male preponderance.
- It is characterized by diffuse skeletal osteopenia, multiple punched out, lytic lesions of nearly the same size.

- In the long bones both cortex and medulla are involved; while in the skull, both the tables and the diploic spaces are involved.
- It predominantly involves the axial skeleton [ribs, spine (vertebral body), pelvis and skull] but appendicular may also be involved.
- The closest differential diagnosis is the lytic metastases. Points in favor of multiple myeloma include:
  - Presence of diffuse osteopenia
  - The lesions are nearly similar in shape and size
  - Mandible involvement is common
  - Vertebral body is relatively more affected than the posterior elements
  - Presence of associated large soft tissue mass
  - Multiple rib fractures with exuberant callus formation.

Nonossifying Fibroma

- It is seen as sharply-defined, ovoid, lytic, cortical, metaphyseal lesion with or without sclerotic border.
- The lesion may be occasionally multilocular or may cause expansion of the involved bone.
- The lesion is usually identified after first decade of life.

Osteoblastoma/Giant Osteoid Osteoma

- It is usually seen as a well-demarcated, expansile, lytic, intramedullary bone lesion measuring >1 cm in diameter with variable degree of calcification and reactive sclerosis.
- The lesion may, however, be sclerotic or mixed in nature.
- Usual age of presentation is first and second decades of life.
- Common sites include neural arch of the vertebra, diaphysis of long bones, mandible, and skull.
- It may be seen as a juxtacortical mass with multiple contiguous vertebral involvement.

Osteochondroma (Figs. 11 to 13)

- It is seen as bony protuberance originating from the external surface of the bone with its cortex continuous with the parent bone.
- It has a cartilaginous cap, which appears as a hypodense rim with or without spotty calcification. If the thickness of cap is >1 cm and has disorganized calcification, malignant transformation should be suspected.
- The lesion is metaphyseal in location and points away from the nearby joint.
- The tumor can be pedunculated or may be sessile with broad base.
- The common sites of involvement include around knee joint, humerus, pelvis, and vertebra in the decreasing order of frequency.
- Multiple osteochondromata are usually associated with diaphyseal achalasia, which is a hereditary condition.

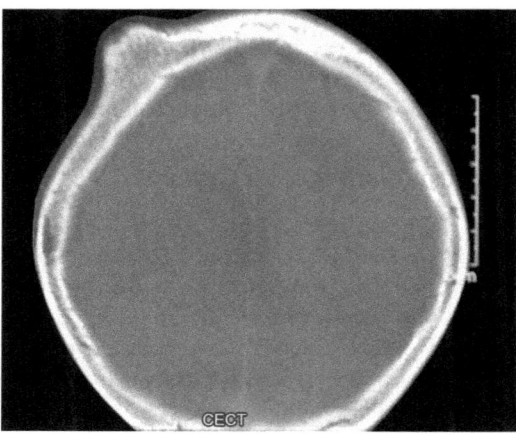

Fig. 11: Axial CT scan showing exostosis arising from the right parietal bone.

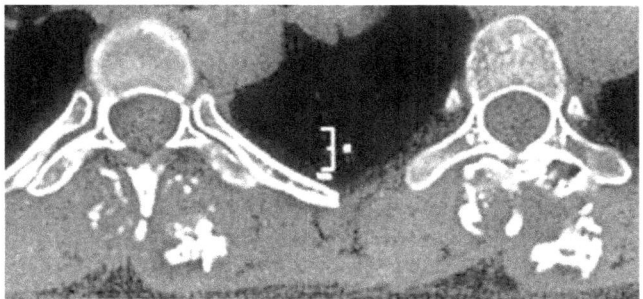

Fig. 12: Transaxial CT images showing osteochondroma arising from posterior elements of vertebra.

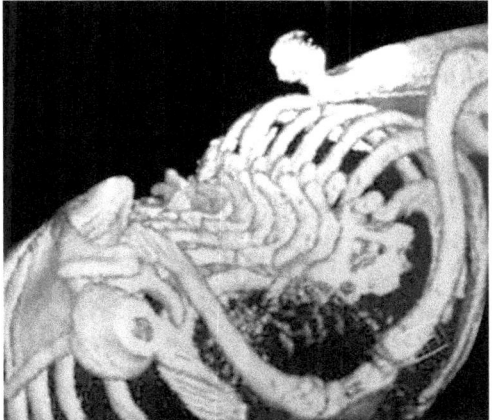

Fig. 13: Surface shaded display (SSD) CT image shows osteochondroma arising from scapula.

- Diaphyseal achalasia is characterized by multiple and bilateral osteochondroma involving the axial skeleton and long tubular bones; widening of the metaphysis with bone deformities; bilateral coxa valga and shortening of the radius (Madelung's deformity).
- Calvaria and mandible are uncommonly involved.

Osteoid Osteoma (Figs. 14A and B)

- It is seen as a dense sclerotic zone of cortical thickening with <1 cm radiolucent nidus, occasionally with central calcific speck. In the diaphysis of the long bones.
- Nidus is highly vascular and enhances after contrast administration.
- Nidus may be intracortical, intramedullary or subperiosteal.
- Approximately 90% are seen under 25 years with M:F = 2:1.
- Common sites include femur, spine (commonly posterior arch), humerus, small bones of hand and foot (especially talus). However, no site is exempted. It is diaphyseal in location, when seen in long bones.
- In carpal or tarsal bones the lesion is completely calcified with no evidence of sclerosis.
- Most common presentation is night pain that is relieved with nonsteroidal anti-inflammatory drugs (NSAIDs) especially aspirin.

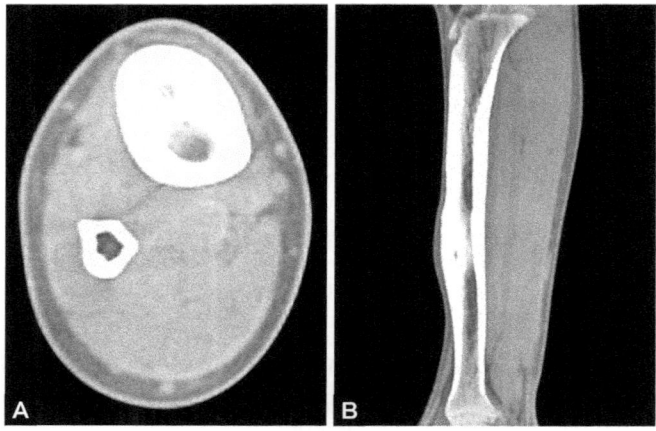

Figs. 14A and B: Axial and sagittal CT images of right tibia showing small nidus with surrounding sclerosis in diaphysis of right tibia suggestive of osteoid osteoma.

Osteoma

- Dense, sclerotic, rounded, well-defined mass often termed as *cortical or ivory osteoma*.
- Occasionally, can have less dense cancellous bone.
- Common sites are the skull, paranasal sinuses, maxilla, mandible, and nasal bones.
- Multiple osteomas are seen in Gardner's syndrome along with colonic polyposis and soft tissue tumors.

Osteomyelitis

Radiological appearances depend upon the type and stage of infection.

Acute Osteomyelitis (Figs. 15 and 16):
- Bony changes are evident after 1–2 weeks of infection.
- In the long bones, metaphyseal involvement is commonly seen with secondary extension into the epiphysis and adjacent joint, especially in infants.
- Soft tissue thickening and stranding, lamellar periostitis and focal lytic areas are the earliest changes.

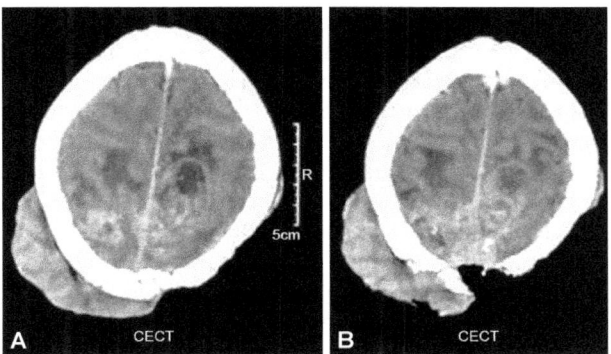

Figs. 15A and B: Axial CT images showing osteomyelitis of calvarium with intracranial extension.

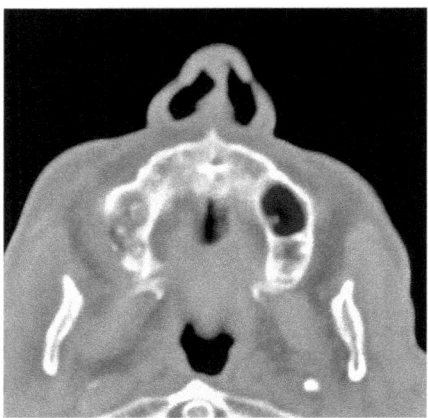

Fig. 16: Transaxial CT image shows osteomyelitis of maxilla.

- Specific signs include permeative cortical destruction, intra-osseous gas, intracortical fissuring, and fat-fluid levels with surrounding osteopenia.
- It affects all ages but is more common in children, diabetics, sickle cell disease, and intravenous drug abusers.

Subacute and Chronic Osteomyelitis (Figs. 17 and 18):
- After 3–4 weeks, hyperdense dead bone (sequestrum), cortical new bone (involucrum), and cloacae are evident.
- Adjacent soft tissues may show abscess formation and sinus tract.
- In chronic stages, multiple lytic areas are seen with adjacent sclerosis.
- Multilaminated, well-organized periosteal reaction is associated with bone remodeling and deformities.
- Signs of remaining activity include change from previous scans, poorly-defined areas of osteolysis, thin periosteal reaction, and demonstration of sinus tracts and abscesses. However, radiological impression regarding activity is often equivocal.

Musculoskeletal System

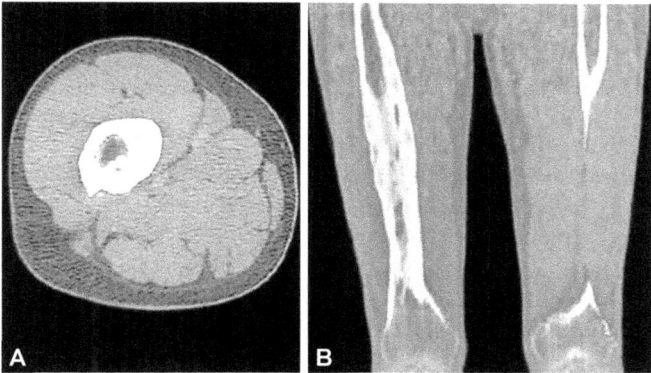

Figs. 17A and B: Axial and coronal CT images showing chronic osteomyelitis of femur on the right side.

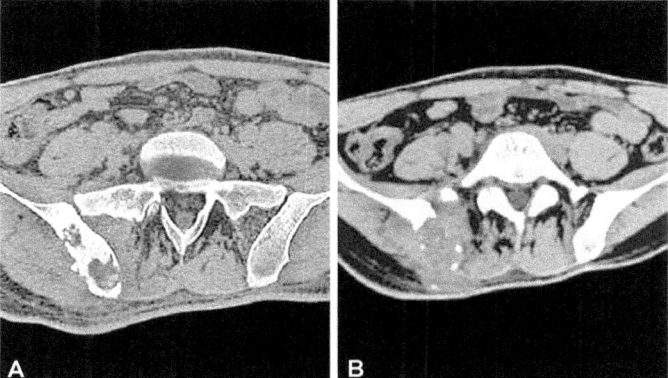

Figs. 18A and B: Axial CT images showing osteomyelitis of ilium on the right side.

- Sequestrum formation is less prominent in flat bones, skull lesions typically do not show sclerosis.

Tubercular Osteomyelitis (Figs. 19 to 22):
- It is characterized by an eccentric, lytic lesion with little or no surrounding sclerosis in the metaphysis of the long bone with surrounding osteopenia.
- Cortical breach, mild periostitis and soft tissue abscess is usual, abscess appearing as rim enhancing hypodense lesion on contrast-enhanced computed tomography.
- Transphyseal spread in children is virtually diagnostic.
- Monoosseous involvement is more common; however, multifocal involvement can occur (multicystic variety in children).
- Usually seen in children and young adults; however, no age is exempted.

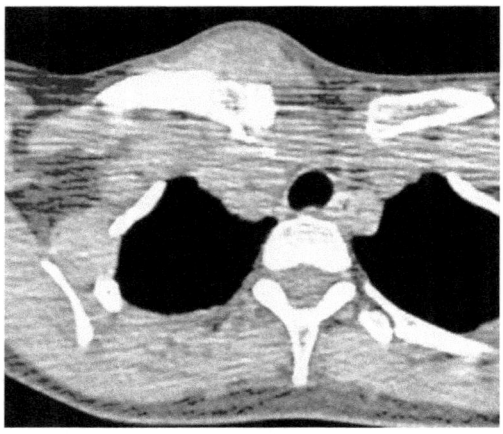

Fig. 19: Axial CT image showing tubercular osteomyelitis of the right clavicle.

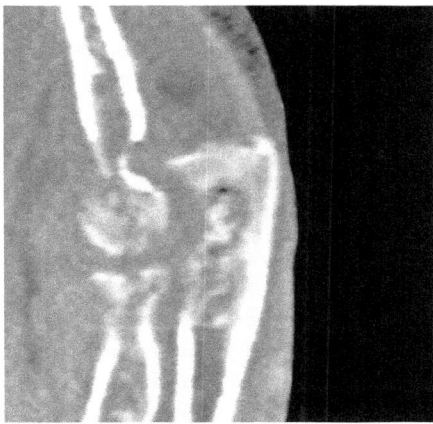

Fig. 20: Sagittal CT image showing tubercular osteomyelitis of the elbow.

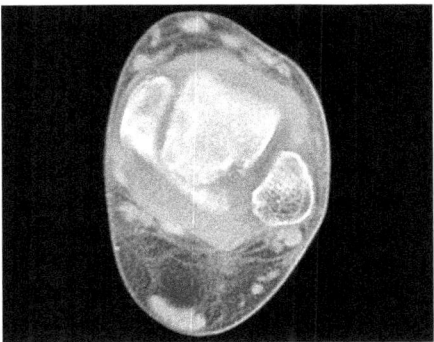

Fig. 21: Transaxial CT image shows tubercular osteomyelitis of talus with ankle joint effusion.

- *Spina ventosa* is the tuberculous involvement of the small bones of the hand and foot and is characterized by an intramedullary, expansile, lytic lesion with cortical thinning with no periosteal reaction.

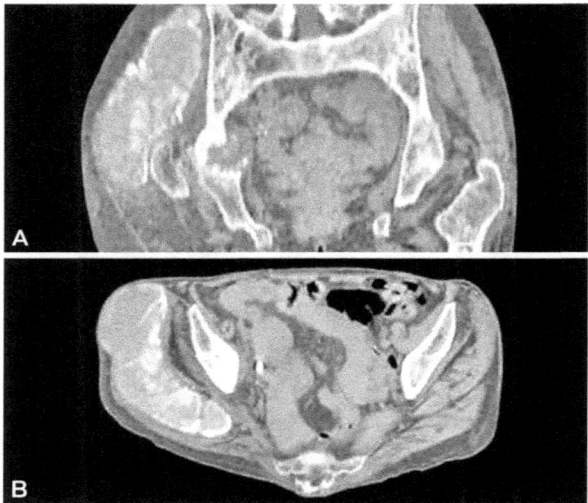

Figs. 22A and B: Coronal and axial CT images of pelvis showing soft tissue lesion with calcified walls involving right thigh in a case of tuberculosis hip with calcified cold abscess.

Osteosarcoma (Figs. 23A and B)

CT appearance depends upon the type of the osteosarcoma.

Conventional/central type is seen as a poorly-defined, intramedullary lesion usually seen at central metaphysis or diaphysis of long bones (distal femur, proximal tibia, proximal humerus, distal radius) and pelvis.

- Varying degrees of osteolysis and osteosclerosis, cortical destruction, and periosteal reaction (*sunburst pattern, Codman's triangle*) are associated with a large soft tissue mass.
- Telangiectatic and clear cell types are purely lytic with no bone formation.
- Intraosseous low-grade type can be purely sclerotic.

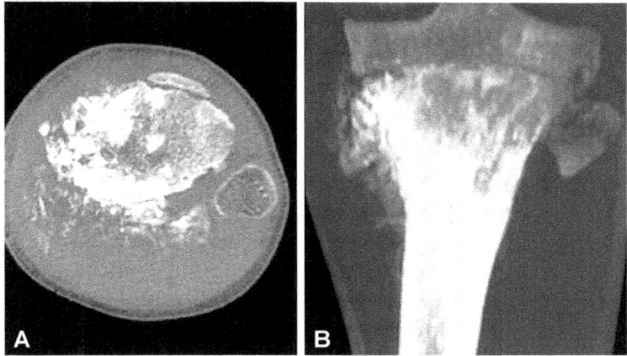

Figs. 23A and B: Axial and coronal CT images showing osteosarcoma of the upper end of the tibia.

- Age of presentation shows two peaks; first at second and third decades and second at fifth decade and later.
- In the second peak flat bone involvement is more common.

Parosteal osteosarcoma is seen as a hyperdense mass lesion with lobulations that wraps the external surface of the parent bone in sessile fashion at metaphyseal location.
- A thin radiolucent line or cleavage plane between cortex of bone and tumor periphery may be seen and is diagnostic.
- Intramedullary extension is uncommon.
- It is commonly seen at second and third decades.
- Common sites of involvement include distal femur, proximal tibia, and humerus.

Periosteal osteosarcoma is seen as a nonhomogeneous mass attached to the cortex with radiating osseous spicules extending into adjacent soft tissues.
- The underlying cortex is thickened and medullary cavity may be involved.
- Diaphysis of long tubular bones is involved, common sites being femur and tibia.

Periosteal/Juxtacortical Chondroma

- It is usually seen as well-defined, soft tissue attenuating mass with spotty calcification of the matrix causing pressure erosion and saucerization of the adjacent cortex.
- Periostitis and buttressing and thickening of the marginal cortex may be seen.
- Common bones to be involved are humerus, tibia, and bone of hands.

Paget's Disease

- It is characterized by polyostotic lesions, asymmetric in distribution.
- The lesions can be purely lytic (osteoporosis circumscripta in skull, V-shaped lytic defect in the long bones) or purely sclerotic (ivory vertebra) or can have a mixed pattern.
- The involved bones are enlarged with cortical thickening and coarse trabeculations; bone softening with resultant deformities (protrusio acetabuli, biconcave vertebra, basilar invagination) may be seen.
- Common age of presentation is fourth and fifth decades and is more common in men.
- Commonly involved bones include skull, vertebra, femur, pelvis, scapula, tibia, and humerus.
- CT is especially useful in detecting the complications, e.g. neurological compromise, articular involvement, and malignant transformation.

Plasmacytoma

- It is seen as a lytic, expansile lesion with thick internal trabeculae.
- Common sites of involvement are the vertebral bodies, pelvis, and ribs.

Primary Lymphoma of Bone/Reticulum Cell Sarcoma

- It is a rare malignant tumor seen in wide range of age groups.
- It is characterized by permeative pattern of bone destruction with skip areas commonly seen in diaphysis of long bones and occasionally in the flat bones.
- Periosteal reaction and soft tissue mass are usually associated.
- Secondary involvement of bone by lymphoma is more common than its primary involvement.

Unicameral/Simple Bone Cyst (Fig. 24)

- It is seen as a large, well-defined, unilocular, intramedullary, expansile, lytic lesion in metaphyseal location of long tubular bones with thinning of the overlying cortex.
- The lesion may show fractured bony fragments within the cyst, often termed as *fallen fragment sign*.
- The lesion grows till the time of epiphyseal fusion.

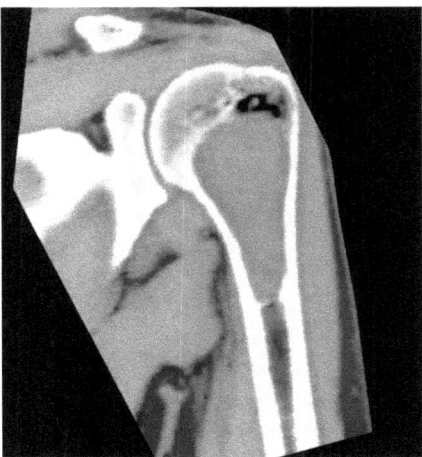

Fig. 24: Coronal CT image showing simple bone cyst in the proximal shaft of humerus.

- The lesions are mostly seen in the first and second decades of life with proximal humerus, femur, and tibia being the common sites. When the lesions present in the older age group, calcaneum and innominate bones are the usual sites.

RIB LESIONS

Lytic Lesions (Table 9)

TABLE 9: Common causes of lytic rib lesions.

Well-defined	Ill-defined

• *Malignant lesions:*
  − Metastases
  − Multiple myeloma
  − Plasmacytoma
  − Giant cell tumor
• *Benign tumors:*
  − Enchondroma
  − Eosinophilic granuloma
  − Hemangioma
  − Giant cell tumor
  − Aneurysmal bone cyst
  − Chondromyxoid fibroma
• *Miscellaneous:*
  − Fibrous dysplasia
  − Brown tumor
	• *Malignant lesions:*
	  − Metastases
	  − Chondrosarcoma
	  − Lymphoma/leukemia
	  − Ewing's sarcoma
	  − Osteosarcoma
	• *Benign tumor:*
	  − Eosinophilic granuloma
	• *Traumatic:*
	  − Fracture with callus formation
	  − Radionecrosis
	• *Infectious:*
	  − Pyogenic
	  − Tubercular
	  − Actinomycosis/fungal

Sclerotic Lesions

- *Generalized osteosclerosis:*
  - Fluorosis
  - Osteopetrosis
  - Mastocytosis
- *Focal lesions:*
  - Osteoblastic metastases
  - Healed lesions (fracture, infections, infarct, tumor lesions)
  - Enostosis
  - Lymphoma
  - Fibrous dysplasia
  - Paget's disease.

Lesions Involving Multiple Ribs

- Metastases
- Multiple myeloma
- Lymphoma or leukemia
- Angiosarcoma
- Fibrous dysplasia
- Paget's disease
- Eosinophilic granuloma
- Osteomyelitis
- Fractures
- Brown tumors.

SKULL AND JAW LESIONS

Sclerotic Lesions of the Skull Vault (Table 10)

TABLE 10: Common causes of sclerotic lesions of the skull vault.

Focal	Diffuse
Benign tumors:	*Malignant lesions:*
• Osteoma	• Osteoblastic metastasis
• Osteochondroma	• Myelofibrosis
Malignant tumors:	*Congenital:*
• Osteosarcoma	• Osteopetrosis
• Metastases	• Pyknodysostosis
• Chronic osteomyelitis	• Engelmann-Camurati disease
• Ischemic necrosis	(progressive diaphyseal
• Radiation osteonecrosis	• dysplasia)
• Fibrosis dysplasia	• Osteopathia strata
• Neurofibromatosis	• Melorheostosis
• Paget's disease	• Van Buchem disease (generalized
• Mastocytosis	cortical hyperostosis)
• Tuberous sclerosis	*Metabolic:*
• Hyperostosis frontalis interna	• Hyperphosphatasia
	• Hypervitaminosis-D
• Hyperostosis interna generalisata	• Idiopathic hypercalcemia
	• Hypoparathyroidism

Contd...

Contd...

Focal	Diffuse
• Cephalohematoma • Subdural hematoma • Meningioma • Hemangioma • Calcified sebaceous cyst	• Pseudohypoparathyroidism • Hyperparathyroidism • Healing rickets • Renal osteodystrophy *Miscellaneous:* • Acromegaly • Fibrous dysplasia • Paget's disease • Hemolytic anemia (thalassemia, sickle cell anemia) • Iron deficiency anemia • Cyanotic congenital heart disease • Fluorosis

Hyperdense Skull Base (Table 11)

TABLE 11: Common causes of hyperdense lesions of skull base.

Focal	Diffuse
• Fibrous dysplasia (Figs. 25A and B) • Meningioma • Sclerotic metastasis • Sclerosis of mastoid in chronic mastoiditis	• Paget's disease • Fibrous dysplasia

Lytic Lesion in the Vault of the Skull (Table 12)

- *Meningocele or meningoencephalocele*: Round midline defect with slightly sclerotic margins involving both inner and outer tables and common in frontal and occipital bone.
- *Epidermoid cyst*: Solitary lytic expansile lesion up to 5 cm with sclerotic margins.
- *Dermoid*: Small radiolucent defect without sclerotic margins usually occurring in midline.
- *Arachnoid cyst*: Smooth defect with thin sclerotic rim.

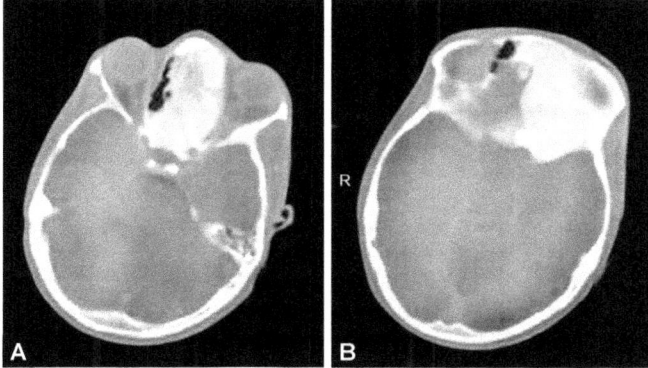

Figs. 25A and B: Axial CT images showing fibrous dysplasia involving the bones of the anterior cranial fossa.

TABLE 12: Common causes of lytic lesions in the vault of the skull.

Tumors		Infection	Miscellaneous
Benign	*Malignant*		

• Meningocele/ meningoencephalocele
• Epidermoid
• Dermoid
• Histiocytosis
• Hemangioma
• Bone tumors
	• Metastases (Figs. 26A and B)
	• Lymphoma
	• Leukemia
	• Multiple myeloma
		• Acute osteomyelitis
		• Tuberculosis
		• Syphilis
		• Fungal infections
			• *Normal variants:*
			  – Pacchonian granulations
			  – Vascular markings
			  – Parietal foramina
			  – Lacunar skull
			• Fibrosis dysplasia
			• Paget's disease
			• Neurofibromatosis
			• Sarcoidosis
			• Burr holes, craniotomies
			• Leptomeningeal cyst
			• Fibrosing osteitis
			• Radiation osteonecrosis
			• Brown tumors of hyperparathyroidism

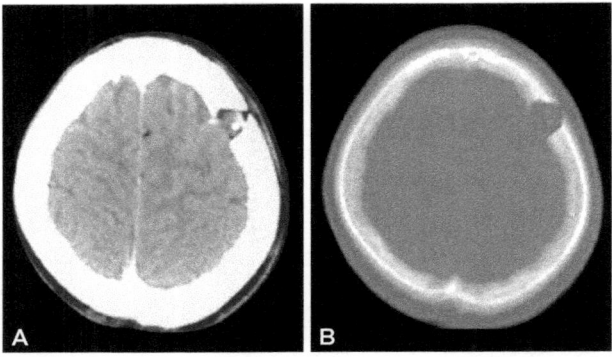

Figs. 26A and B: Axial CT images showing osteolytic metastasis in the left parietal bone.

Lytic Lesions Involving Base of Skull

- Neurofibromatosis
- Acoustic neuroma
- Cholesteatoma
- Glomus tumor
- Chordoma
- Meningioma and glioma
- Carcinoma of nasopharynx, paranasal sinuses (PNS) and mastoid
- Primary or metastatic bone tumor
- Surgical defect
- Histiocytosis
- Aneurysm of internal carotid artery
- Carotid cavernous fistula.

Button Sequestrum

- Eosinophilic granuloma
- Epidermoid cyst
- Tuberculosis
- Radiation necrosis
- Bone grafts undergoing ischemic necrosis
- Syphilis
- Burr holes
- Metastasis (especially breast carcinoma).

Destructive Lesions Affecting the Petrous Pyramid, Middle Ear, and Antrum (Table 13)

TABLE 13: Common causes of destructive lesions affecting the petrous pyramid and middle ear, antrum, and mastoids.

Petrous pyramid	Middle ear, antrum and mastoids

• Neoplasm:
  – Acoustic neuroma
  – Meningioma
  – Glioma
  – Neuroma of the trigeminal and facial nerve
  – Chordoma
  – Glomus jugulare tumor
  – Epidermoid
  – Carcinoma of the nasopharynx
  – Parotid tumor
• Petrositis
• Aneurysm (intrapetrous carotid artery)
• Histiocytosis-X
	• Cholesteatoma
	• Neoplasm
	• Carcinoma
	• Sarcoma
	• Glomus tumor
	• Abscess
	• Granuloma
	• Surgical defect
	• Histiocytosis-X

Lesions of the Orbit (Table 14)

TABLE 14: Common causes of lytic and sclerotic lesions of orbit.

Lytic lesions	Sclerotic lesions

• Neoplasms:
  – Dermoid and epidermoid
  – Lacrimal gland tumors
  – Hemangiomas
  – Retinoblastoma
  – Melanoma
  – Carcinoma—nasopharynx, and paranasal sinuses
  – Optic glioma
  – Meningioma
	• Meningioma en plaque
	• Chronic sinusitis (frontal and sphenoid)
	• Fibrous dysplasia
	• Paget's disease
	• Osteoporosis
	• Histiocytosis-X
	• Craniometaphyseal dysplasia

Contd...

Contd...

Lytic lesions	Sclerotic lesions

- Orbital pseudotumor
- Rare lesions—metastasis, lymphomas, multiple myeloma and primary bone and soft tissue tumor
- Complicated sinusitis with osteomyelitis
- Mucocele
- Histiocytosis-X

Lytic Lesions in the Jaw (Table 15)

TABLE 15: Common causes of lytic lesions of jaw.

Odontogenic lesions	Nonodontogenic lesions
Postinflammatory: • Periodontal abscess • Periapical abscess • Periapical granuloma (Fig. 27) • Periodontal cyst—dental, radicular or apical cyst *Developmental lesions:* • Dentigerous cyst (follicular cyst) • Odontogenic keratocyst (primordial cyst)	*Development lesion:* • Fissural cyst *Infective:* • Osteomyelitis • Actinomycosis *Tumor and tumor-like lesions:* • Simple bone cyst • Aneurysmal bone cyst • Brown tumor • Osteoclastoma • Ameloblastoma (adamantinoma) • Multiple myeloma • Osteosarcoma • Ewing's sarcoma • Burkitt's lymphoma • Metastasis *Miscellaneous:* • Hyperparathyroidism • Fibrous dysplasia • Radionecrosis • Cherubism (hereditary fibrous dysplasia of the jaw) • Histiocytosis-X • Paget's disease • Stafne mandibular defect

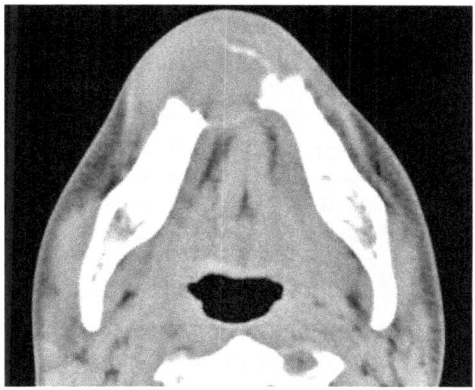

Fig. 27: Transaxial CT image shows giant periapical granuloma of mandible.

Sclerotic Lesions of the Jaw

- *Generalized:*
  - Paget's disease
  - Fibrous dysplasia
- *Focal:*
  - Hypercementosis
  - Osteoma
  - Cementoma
  - Postinflammatory sclerosing osteitis
  - Benign osteosclerosis
  - Odontome
  - Localized fibrous dysplasia
  - Pindborg tumor—calcifying epithelial odontogenic tumor.

Salient Features of the Jaw Lesions

Periodontal Abscess

It is characterized by a lytic lesion in the periodontal region with blurring and loss on lamina dura.

Periapical Abscess

It is seen as a radiolucent defect at the tooth apex with loss of lamina dura and adjacent osteomyelitis.

Periapical Granuloma

It is seen as an ill-defined, lucent lesion at the tooth apex with thin sclerotic rim contiguous with intact lamina dura.

Periodontal Cyst: Dental, Radicular or Apical Cyst

- It is characterized by a well-defined, lytic lesion at the apex of the diseased tooth with thin sclerotic rim contiguous with normal lamina dura.
- It is a final sequelae of periapical abscess and granuloma.

Dentigerous Cyst (Follicular Cyst)

- It is seen as a well-defined, unilocular, cystic lesion related to the crown of an unerupted tooth.
- Most common site is the permanent mandibular third molar and maxillary canine.
- It is seen primarily in adolescents and young adults.
- Multiple dentigerous cysts are associated with Gorlin syndrome.

Primordial Cyst

- It is seen as a large, well-defined, unilocular, cystic lesion unrelated to caries or unerupted tooth.
- It is usually seen in relation to the posterior dentition of the mandible.
- Commonly seen in young males but may occur at all ages.

Fissural/Developmental Cyst

These appear as cystic lesions occurring at the sites of fusion of the embryonic processes and therefore can be located in the medial mandibular, medial maxillary, nasopalatine (behind the central incisors in the maxilla) and globulomaxillary (inverted pear-shaped between upper lateral incisor and canine) region.

Ameloblastoma of the Jaw

- It is seen as a multilocular, expansile, lytic lesion with cortical thinning and erosion resulting in *soap bubble appearance*.
- There is characteristic extension of the tumor to the alveolar margin with destruction of the tooth and their supporting bones presenting a *floating tooth appearance*.
- Most common site is the molar region of the mandible.
- The usual age of presentation is middle age.

Burkitt's Lymphoma

- It is characterized by an ill-defined, large lytic lesion usually involving the mandible with destruction of the lamina dura and supporting bone of the teeth resulting in floating tooth appearance.
- New bone formation gives rise to the *spiculated sunray appearance*.
- Secondary spread of the tumor may occur in the adjacent bones of the face and orbit producing gross deformities of the face.
- It is particularly seen in the equatorial Africa as a childhood tumor although no geographical region is exempted.

Hyperparathyroidism

- It is characterized by loss of the lamina dura of the teeth with osteopenia in the jaw.
- *Floating tooth appearance* may be seen in the advanced cases.
- Brown tumors may also be seen.

Radionecrosis

- It is seen as an osteopenic area in the initial stages followed by a mixed pattern of osteosclerosis and lysis.

- Pathological fracture, bone resorption, and sequestrum may be seen.
- Periosteal new bone formation is unusual.
- The appearance may be complicated by superadded infection.

Stafne's Mandibular Defect/Salivary Inclusion Defect

It is seen as a well-defined, lytic area usually at the angle of the mandible and may show communication with the adjacent salivary gland on CT sialography.

Hypercementosis

It is seen as a homogeneously, hyperdense, enlarged tooth with preserved lamina dura and adjacent bones.

Cementoma

- It is seen as hyperdense areas with coarse trabeculations at the apices of the undiseased tooth, especially in the mandible.
- However, it may appear as lytic defect with punctate, irregular calcification related to the apex of the tooth in the early stages due to the presence of the fibrous tissue.

Postinflammatory Sclerosing Osteitis

- It is characterized by hyperdensity in the apical and intradental region in patients with chronic gingival and dental sepsis.
- Associated features include dental caries and apical bone resorption.

Benign Osteosclerosis

- It is seen as a focal area of osteosclerosis adjacent to the roots of the teeth, sometimes with a spiky configuration.
- It forms secondary to dental surgery, extraction or a bridge.

Odontome

- It is a hamartomatous lesion of the tooth with all the dental elements.
- The radiological appearance depends upon the type of odontome.

Complex variety is seen predominantly in females as a lobulated radiodensity with surrounding radiolucent zone, usually in the molar region in the secondary dentition.

Compound variety is seen as an aggregate of multiple, small denticles with a marginal zone of lucency and are commonly seen in the canine region and may prevent the normal dental eruption.

BONY SPINAL LESIONS

Expansile Lesions of the Vertebra (Table 16)

TABLE 16: Common causes of expansile lesions of vertebra.

Benign	Malignant
- Osteochondroma - Osteoblastoma - Giant cell tumor - Osteoid osteoma - Aneurysmal bone cyst - Hemangioma - Hydatid cyst - Paget's disease	- Metastases - Multiple myeloma - Plasmacytoma - Chordoma - Angiosarcoma - Osteosarcoma - Chondrosarcoma - Lymphoma/leukemia

Lesions Involving Multiple Vertebrae (Table 17)

TABLE 17: Common causes of lesions involving multiple vertebrae

Contiguous	Noncontiguous
- Pott's disease - Pyogenic discitis - Osteochondroma - Chordoma - Aneurysmal bone cyst - Multiple myeloma - Hydatid disease	- Metastases - Multiple myeloma - Plasmacytoma - Lymphoma - Hemangioma - Paget's disease - Eosinophilic granuloma - Angiosarcoma - Pott's disease

Differential Involvement of the Part of Vertebra (Table 18)

TABLE 18: Common causes of lesions involving body and posterior elements of vertebrae.

Body	Posterior elements
• Giant cell tumor • Hemangioma • Hydatid • Chordoma • Paget's disease • Eosinophilic granuloma • Multiple myeloma • Plasmacytoma • Angiosarcoma • Fibrous dysplasia	• Osteochondroma • Osteoblastoma • Osteoid osteoma • Aneurysmal bone cyst • Metastases

Differential Diagnosis of Selected Craniovertebral Anomalies

Anomalies of the Occipital Bone

- *Occipital condylar hypoplasia:* The odontoid seldom extends into the foramen magnum.
- *Occipital vertebra:* Seen in various forms:
    - Tertiary condyle
    - Paracondylar and epitransversary process
    - Posterior (Kimmerle's anomaly) or lateral ponticles.

Anomalies of the Atlas and the Axis

- *Atlantooccipital fusion (atlas assimilation):* It may occur with varying degrees of fusion between the occipital condyles and the body and lateral masses of the atlas.
- *Anomalies of the arch of Atlas:* Dorsal arch may be totally absent or may have variable defects or clefts most commonly in the dorsal midline referred to as the *anterior* or *posterior rachischisis*.

- *Atlantoaxial fusion malsegmentation:* The lateral masses of the atlas and the body of the axis fuse to form a complex that has a butterfly shape in multiplanar images of the region.
- *Odontoid bone (hypoplastic dens):* The dens of the axis is hypoplastic and is seen as a small bony protuberance at the site of the normal dens. The posterior arch of the axis is often absent and the atlas is usually subluxated anteriorly.

Atlantoaxial Subluxation

Atlantodental space, i.e. the space between the posterior cortex of the anterior arch of the atlas and the anterior cortex of the dens >3 mm in adults and 5 mm in children.
- Ankylosing and psoriatic spondylitis
- Congenital craniovertebral junction anomaly
- Down syndrome
- Morquio syndrome
- Pseudogout
- Retropharyngeal abscess
- Rheumatoid arthritis
- Trauma.

Discal Calcification

- Acromegaly
- Ankylosing spondylitis (AS)
- Degenerative disk disease
- Hemochromatosis
- Hyperparathyroidism
- Idiopathic
- Ochronosis
- Poliomyelitis
- Pseudogout
- Transient calcification
- Spinal ankylosis for any reason [congenital, diffuse idiopathic skeletal hyperostosis (DISH), surgical].

Enlarged Intervertebral Foramina

- Congenital absence of pedicle
- Lateral meningocele
- Neurofibroma and neuroma
- *Rare tumors*: Chordoma, dermoid, lipoma, lymphoma, meningioma, and neurofibroma
- Vertebral artery aneurysm.

Vertebral Pedicle Erosion or Destruction

- Metastasis
- Benign bone tumor (aneurysmal bone cyst, giant cell tumor, and hemangiopericytoma)
- Congenital absence
- Eosinophilic granuloma
- Granulomatous disease
- Intraspinal disease
- Multiple myeloma
- Syringomyelia.

Solitary Dense Pedicle

- Osteoblastic metastasis
- Osteoid osteoma
- Osteoblastoma
- Secondary to spondylosis
- Secondary to congenitally absence or hypoplastic posterior arch elements.

Pott's Disease (Figs. 28 to 30)

It can be divided into four categories depending upon the initial site of infection:

1. *Paradiskal* is the most common type and is characterized by osteolytic destruction of the vertebral endplates of two adjacent vertebrae with early destruction of the intervening disk.

2. *Central* is characterized by osteolytic lesion in the central part of the vertebral body resulting in early collapse.
3. *Anterior subperiosteal* is characterized by tuberculous process starting and spreading under the anterior longitudinal ligament with destruction of the anterior part of the body of multiple, contiguous vertebra.
4. *Appendicular or neural arch* is characterized by destruction of the pedicles or laminae (rare type).

Features common to all the above types include:
- Irregular osteolysis with minimal sclerosis and periostitis
- Large pre- and paravertebral soft tissue abscess and granulation with calcification
- Extension of the pathologic process may be seen extending into the spinal canal
- Extension of the abscess may be seen into the adjacent psoas muscle and posterior abdominal wall
- Resultant spinal deformity is marked.

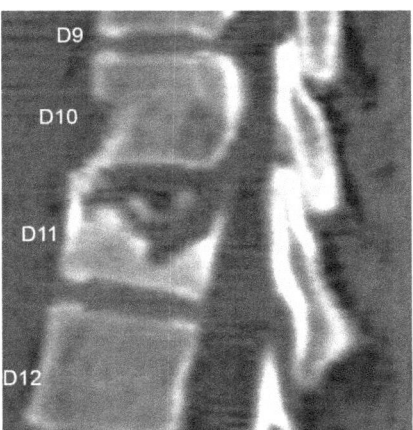

Fig. 28: Sagittal CT image showing central and prevertebral type of Pott's spine.

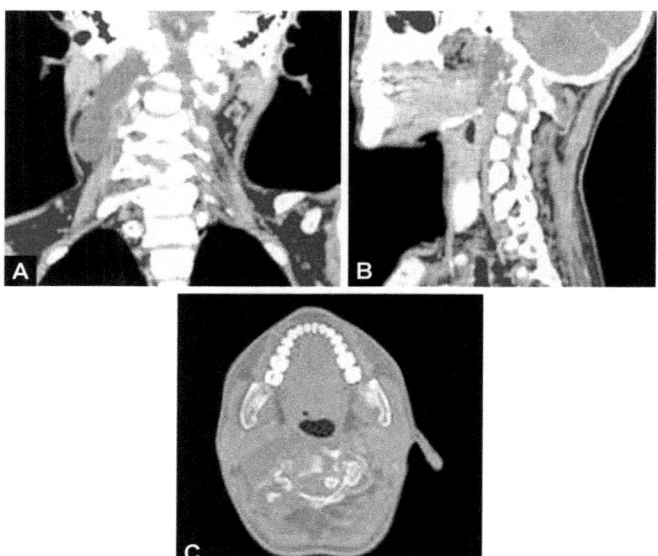

Figs. 29A to C: Coronal, sagittal and axial CT images showing Pott's spine presenting with a neck abscess.

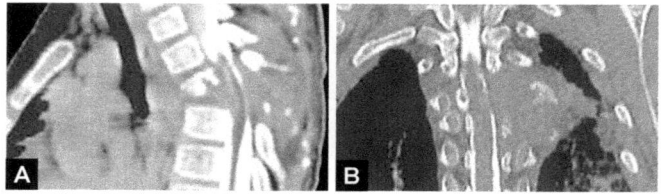

Figs. 30A and B: Pott's spine with epidural abscess and thecal sac compression.

Pyogenic Spondylitis

- It is characterized by osteolysis of the vertebral endplates with destruction of the adjacent disk in the late stages; posterior elements are usually spared.

- Marked reactive sclerosis and osteophyte formation is characteristic of pyogenic process.
- Pre- and paravertebral soft tissue abscess is usual, but calcification and size is much less as compared to the tuberculous spondylitis.

ARTHRITIS

The role of CT imaging is:
- To diagnose
- To evaluate the activity of the disease
- To monitor the effect of therapy.

Computed tomography provides greater details than conventional radiographs, especially in the central skeleton, but is equally useful at the peripheral joints. With good multiplanar reconstruction images and multislice spiral CT (MSCT), it can provide greater overview of the joint diseases in all the three dimensions.

The basic parameters that are of significance in interpreting the images in arthritis are as follows:
- Patterns of osteopenia
- Joint effusion and joint space narrowing
- Erosions, cysts, geodes, and bone resorption
- Changes in the ossification centers and small bones
- Periosteal new bone formation
- Malalignment, subluxation, dislocation
- Disorganization
- Ankylosis
- Soft tissue swelling, atrophy, and calcification
- *In the spine features are noted in the:*
  - Vertebral body
  - Intervertebral disks
  - Apophyseal joints
  - Atlantoaxial joint
  - Paravertebral region.

Osteopenia

- It is associated with several arthritides as inflammatory arthritis (periarticular osteopenia), neuropathic arthropathy, and dialysis arthritis. Subchondral osteoporosis occurs in rapidly developing processes such as septic arthritis.
- In chronic arthritis, osteoporosis proceeds to uniform bone atrophy with a thin, sharp cortex.
- Arthritides like gout, psoriatic arthritis, Reiter's arthritis, and pigmented villonodular synovitis are characterized by lack of osteoporosis.

Joint Effusion (Fig. 31)

- It occurs in early synovial disease and can be detected on CT by its fluid or hemorrhagic attenuation with displacement of the fat planes.
- There may be edema in the adjacent musculature.
- As the amount of fluid increases, joint space widening occurs and in extreme cases particularly in the hip and shoulder in children, dislocation may follow.
- Effusions at the proximal interphalangeal (PIP) and metacarpophalangeal (MCP) joints are typical of RA of the hands.

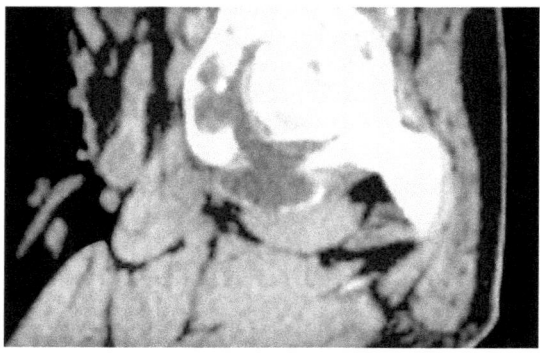

Fig. 31: Oblique coronal CT image showing arthritis with joint effusion.

Joint Space Narrowing

- It is caused by cartilage atrophy or destruction. Cartilage atrophy may also result from disuse.
- Rheumatoid arthritis typically results in uniform joint space narrowing, whereas OA shows narrowing, that is most marked in the weight-bearing areas, which is the medial compartment in the knee joint and superiorly in the hip. All the three compartments are uniformly narrowed in the RA.
- Arthritis in the Paget's disease also shows uniform joint space narrowing.

Erosions, Cysts, Geodes, and Bone Resorption

- These characterize some arthritides, whereas some are typically nonerosive.
- The absence of erosions in the hands is typical of Jaccoud's arthritis, Reiter's syndrome, and systemic lupus erythematosus (SLE).
- Rheumatoid erosions tend to be fuzzily marginated without a sclerotic margin. Erosions are initially located at the bare areas. There may be compression erosions resulting in *ball-in-socket* configuration. Erosions may occur at the tendinous insertions.
- In infectious arthritis, erosions occur in contact areas.
- Later in the chronic disease, the subchondral bone is eroded and destroyed.
- Sarcoidosis can also result in bony erosions in the vicinity of the joint. The margins are poorly-defined and there is an increased trabecular pattern of the bone.
- Hemophilia in the knee is characterized by large erosion in the intercondylar notch of the femur, as well as along the articular surface, owing to hemorrhage.
- Gouty erosions tend to have a well-defined sclerotic margin with a characteristic overhanging edge.
- They can be expansile. The first metatarsophalangeal (MTP) joint is a typical location.
- Erosions in OA also have well-defined margins.

- Synovial fluid is forced through a defect in the articular cartilage to form a cyst, which though may enlarge rarely result in expansion of the cortex. Large cysts are known as *geodes*.
- Osteoarthritis in the hands shows central erosions in the distal interphalangeal (DIP) joints.
- Fungal infections also cause erosions in joints without any other obvious changes.
- Irregularities of the articular surface can also be caused by osteochondritis dissecans.
- Pigmented villonodular synovitis results in well-marginated erosions on both sides of the joint with preservation of joint cartilage and bone density.
- *Resorption of bone* is seen in various conditions, especially in collagen diseases. It is a characteristic of the neuropathic arthropathy. Resorption of part or entire humeral head may occur.
- Tapering of one side of joint is seen in the hands and feet, along with exaggerated concavity of the opposite side, giving *pencil-in-cup* appearance. Resorption and dislocation at multiple joints of the hand cause shortening and deformity of the fingers, resulting in the *main-en-lorgnette* or *opera glass* hand of end-stage RA.
- Resorption of the distal end of the clavicle may occur following trauma or in hyperparathyroidism and RA. Terminal phalangeal tuft resorption occurs in several conditions including scleroderma and hyperparathyroidism.

Changes in the Ossification Center and the Small Bones

- Such changes are seen in juvenile rheumatoid arthritis (JRA), juvenile articular infections, and hemophilia with changes in the time of appearance and fusion of the epiphyseal ossification centers.
- A characteristic appearance includes enlargement, irregularity of contour, squaring, osteoporosis, and coarsening of the trabecular pattern of the epiphysis. In addition, alteration in the length of the extremity may occur.

Musculoskeletal System

- Hemophilia also shows squaring of the inferior margin of the patella.
- Bony proliferation of the epiphyseal ossification centers is seen in dysplasia epiphysealis hemimelica, or Trevor's disease.
- Avascular necrosis of the epiphyses may begin as a subchondral radiolucent fracture line. It then proceeds to sclerosis and deformity. Later collapse and cyst formation may occur. Legg-Perthes disease is a specific type of AVN that occurs in childhood. AVN of the small bones occurs frequently, and various eponyms have been used. For example, Koehler's disease is AVN of the navicular bone.

Subchondral Sclerosis and Osteophytes

- Subchondral sclerosis is characteristic of OA (Figs. 32 and 33).
- Rheumatoid arthritis in the weight-bearing areas develops secondary OA with subchondral sclerosis after cartilage destruction.
- Reactive osteitis of the sesamoid bone may be a cause of pain.
- Sclerosis around a joint may also be seen in melorheostosis.

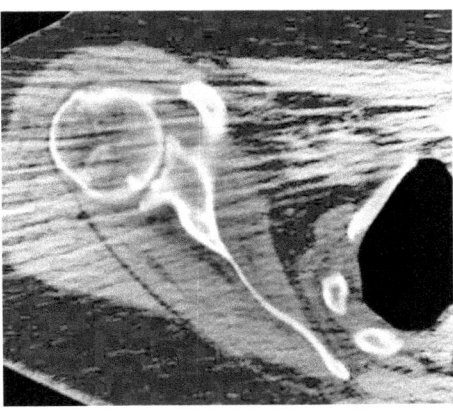

Fig. 32: Transaxial CT image shows osteoarthritis at shoulder joint.

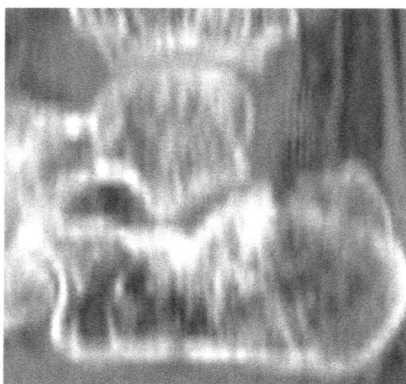

Fig. 33: Sagittal multiplanar reconstruction CT image shows subchondral sclerosis in a case of subtalar osteoarthritis.

- Osteophytes at joint margins are a characteristic feature of OA. They extend horizontally from the articular margins. The cortex of the osteophyte is continuous with that of the adjacent bone. The interior of the spur consists of trabeculae and fatty marrow, often covered with cartilage or periosteum.
- Hook-like osteophytes are characteristic of hemochromatosis and calcium pyrophosphate dehydrate (CPPD).

Periosteal New Bone Formation

- It may be seen in the reactive inflammatory arthritides and is rare in adult-onset RA but in JRA it is typical.
- Reiter's syndrome also characteristically exhibits thick, fluffy periosteal new bone.
- Septic arthritis and osteomyelitis also exhibit periosteal reaction.
- Ankylosing spondylitis may be associated with irregular new bone formation at entheses.
- Fluffy periosteal new bone formation at the base of the distal phalanx of the great toe can be seen in Reiter's syndrome and psoriatic arthritis.

Musculoskeletal System

- Periosteal reaction is a characteristic feature of pulmonary hypertrophic osteoarthropathy.
- Various tumors in the vicinity of the joints are also associated with periosteal new bone formation like osteoid osteoma.

Malalignment, Subluxation, and Dislocation

- *Malalignment* may be seen as deviation, flexion or hyperextension.
- Ulnar deviation of the fingers at the MCP joints is typically seen in RA, SLE, and Jaccoud's arthritis. In RA, ulnar deviation is irreversible and is associated with erosions. In the last two conditions, the reverse is true.
- Deformities of flexion and hyperextension include the *Boutonnière* (flexion at the PIP and hyperextension at the DIP joint) and *swan-neck* deformity (hyperextension at PIP and flexion at the DIP joint). The former is seen in RA, SLE and Jaccoud's arthritis. Interference with the growth plate from injury or a disease process results in deformities.
- *Subluxation and dislocation* result from progression of malalignment, from large effusions, pyogenic arthritis or erosions and destruction of the bone ends. Large effusions of the shoulder or hip in infants result in dislocations.
- Carpal malpositions occur in RA and JRA.
- Elevation of the humeral head owing to the erosion of the rotator cuff tendon occurs in RA.
- Displacement can also occur at the epiphyseal cartilage plate, as in slipped capital femoral epiphysis.

Disorganization

- Disorganization of a large joint is typically seen in neurotrophic arthropathy.
- Fragmentation of bone, dislocation, and soft tissue debris occur. The fragments may later fuse into a bony mass.
- *Arthritis mutilans* refers to destructive end-stage arthritis of the hands and feet. It may result from RA, JRA, psoriatic arthritis, leprosy, and diabetes mellitus (DM).

Ankylosis

- Interphalangeal bony ankylosis is more common in JRA and in psoriatic arthritis.
- Carpal and tarsal fusion can be seen in adult and JRA.
- Ankylosis of the hip and knee is most commonly seen in JRA.
- In the sacroiliac (SI) joints, the inflammatory arthritides can ankylose the synovial-lined lower two-thirds; whereas in DISH, ligamentous ossification can fuse the upper third.

Distribution and Sequence of Changes

- In the hands, the DIP joints are often initially involved in primary OA and psoriatic arthritis.
- The PIP joints are typically involved with RA.
- Calcium pyrophosphate dehydrate (CPPD) has a tendency to involve the radiocarpal compartment of the wrist, whereas gout tends to involve the carpometatarsal joints of the foot.
- Primary OA often involves the first carpometacarpal joint.
- Bilateral symmetrical involvement is characteristic of RA, whereas gout is sporadically distributed.
- Bilateral symmetrical involvement of the SI joints is typical of AS.
- Demonstration of early erosions is an indication to change therapy.
- The evolution of changes is important, e.g. in pyogenic arthritis with rapid progress, destruction precedes osteoporosis; whereas in tuberculous arthritis, the reverse is true.

Soft Tissue Swelling, Atrophy, and Calcification

- Soft tissue debris is characteristic of a neuropathic joint.
- Clubbing of the terminal phalanges is seen in hypertrophic osteoarthropathy, acromegaly, and hyperparathyroidism.
- Soft tissue swelling representing tophi is seen in gout.
- Soft tissue nodules may be seen in RA, amyloidosis, thyroid acropachy, and xanthoma.

Musculoskeletal System

- Diffuse swelling of the entire digit (*sausage digit*) can be seen in psoriatic and infectious arthritis as well as in macrodactyly.
- Diffuse soft tissue enlargement of the entire limb may be seen in plexiform neurofibromatosis.
- Soft tissue prominence with calcification may be seen in vascular malformations and hemangiomas.
- Rheumatoid arthritis has a typical early distribution of soft tissue swelling about the ulnar styloid process and the PIP joints, and later at the MCP joints. Soft tissue mass in the popliteal fossa may represent Baker's cyst, tumors, and aneurysms of the popliteal artery.
- *Soft tissue atrophy* is seen at the terminal phalanges in scleroderma. Atrophy of the thenar and hypothenar muscles, giving a concave rather than convex hypothenar border is seen in SLE.
- *Soft tissue calcification* may be metabolic calcifications, calcinosis (subcutaneous calcification) or dystrophic calcification.
- Metabolic calcifications are seen in chronic renal failure (CRF), hypo- and hyperparathyroidism. Calcinosis is seen in scleroderma and CREST syndrome. Dystrophic calcification is seen in gouty and tumoral calcinosis.
- Hydroxyapatite deposition disease (HADD) is a cause of calcific tendonitis, bursitis, and periarticular calcification.
- Vascular calcification occurs most frequently in atherosclerosis, DM, and renal osteodystrophy.
- Hyaline articular cartilage and meniscal calcification are characteristics of chondrocalcinosis (CPPD).
- Synovial osteochondromatosis is a condition of intra-articular calcific bodies resulting from synovial chondrometaplasia.

SPINE

The vertebral *marginal changes* can characterize several processes.
- CT shows osteophytes as linear osseous structures adjacent to the vertebral body. Posterior osteophytes may encroach on the intervertebral foramina, and may cause radiculopathy. They may even encroach on the spinal canal. Some osteophytes are

1 mm, removed from the actual vertebral corner and are termed as *traction spurs* and indicate segmental instability.
- *Thin marginal* syndesmophytes are calcification of the outer fibers of the annulus fibrosus and the inner fibers of the longitudinal ligament. They are characteristics of AS and reactive spondylitis. They can be seen on CT as a thin line adjacent to the vertebral body.
- *Thick nonmarginal* syndesmophytes are seen in psoriatic arthritis and Reiter's syndrome. They extend from the midvertebral bodies.
- Diffuse idiopathic skeletal hyperostosis has a characteristic appearance of ossification of the anterior longitudinal ligament with a thin radiolucent line of separation from the vertebral body margin. Rarely, the posterior longitudinal ligament may also calcify.

Changes in the shape and density of the vertebral bodies occur in various conditions:
- In late AS, squaring of all the vertebra and syndesmophytes formation produces a *bamboo-spine*.
- Biconcavity of the vertebral bodies is seen in sickle cell disease and homocystinuria.
- Collapse of vertebral bodies can occur from osteoporosis and tumor metastases. Wedge-like collapse can be caused by trauma and metastases. Wafer-like collapse can be caused by metastases or eosinophilic granuloma.
- *Osteopenia* can be seen in metabolic bone disease, along with flattening of the vertebral bodies. Focal endplate depressions are seen due to Schmorl's nodes.
- *Osteosclerosis* can occur in various forms as: *rugger jersey* spine of renal osteodystrophy, the *picture frame* appearance of Paget's disease and *bone-in-bone* appearance of osteopetrosis tarda. Diffuse sclerosis is seen in osteoblastic metastases, Hodgkin's disease, and third-stage Paget's disease.

The *intervertebral disk* may show loss of height, contain gas or calcification. Localized narrowing at one or more spaces

may be caused by herniation of the nucleosus pulposus, disk degeneration, infection, congenital anomaly or atrophy accompanying fusion of the segmental apophyseal joints.
- Chronic discitis and tuberculosis also result in reactive sclerosis. Generalized disk space narrowing with associated disk calcification is suggestive of ochronosis.
- Localized calcification of a disk may be idiopathic, post-traumatic or infectious.
- The presence of air in the disk *vacuum phenomenon* is a sign of disk degeneration.
- The *apophyseal joints* of the spine may show narrowing and erosions in RA and AS, which progress to fusion. AS involves the lower spine, whereas RA predilects the cervical spine. Apophyseal joint fusion is accompanied by atrophy of the corresponding intervertebral disk. Osteoarthritis of the facet joints cause spur formation and hypertrophy which can encroach the intervertebral foramina and lateral recesses.
- The *atlantoaxial articulation* is a critical area because of the subluxation occurring in several conditions. The most common cause is RA and is also commonly seen in Down syndrome. In RA and JRA, erosions, destruction, and fractures of the odontoid process may occur, as well as a large mass of pannus may form that encroaches the neural canal.
- The *paravertebral area* can be involved by thick syndesmophytes in psoriatic arthritis and Reiter's syndrome. A soft tissue mass can occur in association with various diseases including inflammatory and extramedullary hematopoiesis.
- A calcified paravertebral mass is typical of the tuberculous spondylitis or Pott's disease.

Differential Diagnosis of Intra-articular Loose Bodies

- Osteochondritis dissecans
- Synovial osteochondromatosis

- Trauma
- Septic or tubercular arthritis (sequestrum)
- Degenerative joint disease
- Pseudogout (CPPD arthropathy)
- Neurotrophic arthropathy (hypertrophic form)
- Degenerative disease with detached spur
- Avulsion fracture
- Intra-articular tumoral calcification (chondroma, sarcoma).

Differentiating Features of Pyogenic and Tubercular Arthritis (Table 19)

TABLE 19: Characteristic features of pyogenic and tubercular arthritis.

Features	Pyogenic	Tubercular
Joint effusion	Larger and more common	Smaller
Marginal sclerosis of erosions	Present	Usually absentt
Periostitis	Present	Usually absent
Sequestrum	Present	Usually absent
Ankylosis	Bony	Fibrous
Bone deformity	Uncommon	Common (hypertrophied condyles, mortar, and pestle appearance)

SOFT TISSUE LESIONS

Soft Tissue Calcification (Table 20)

- *Calcification (structure-less density):*
  - Metastasis
  - Calcinosis
  - Dystrophic
- *Ossification (organized with trabeculae and cortex):*
  - Myositis ossification
  - Tumoral ossification

TABLE 20: Common causes of soft tissue lesions.

Soft tissue	Fatty	With calcific density
• Edema (Figs. 34A and B) • Hematoma • Abscess/nodular fasciitis (Fig. 35) • Infestations (cysticerci) • Capillary hemangioma • Arteriovenous malformation • Hemangiopericytoma • Angiosarcoma • Desmoid/fibromatosis • Lymph nodes • Fibrosarcoma • Fibrohistiocytoma (Fig. 36) • Neural tumors (Fig. 37) • Leiomyoma/rhabdomyoma • Leiomyosarcoma/rhabdomyosarcoma	• Lipoma (Figs. 38 and 39) • Liposarcoma • Sebaceous cysts • Dermoid (Fig. 40) • Epidermoid	• Healed lesions (hematoma, abscess, cysticerci) • Cavernous hemangioma • Calcifying aponeurotic fibroma • Myositis ossificans • Lymph nodes • Tumoral calcinosis • Extraosseous bone forming tumors (osteosarcoma, Ewing's sarcoma) • Metastases

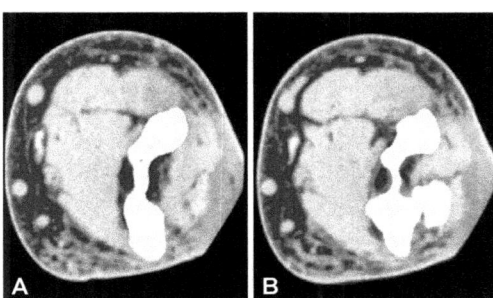

Figs. 34A and B: Axial CT images showing edema in the subcutaneous fat.

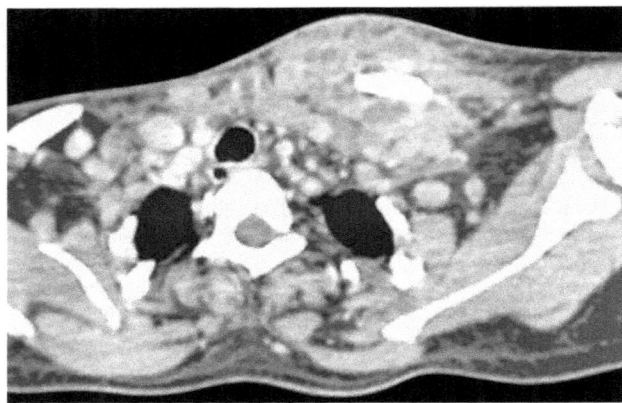

Fig. 35: Axial CT image showing soft tissue abscess to the left of midline.

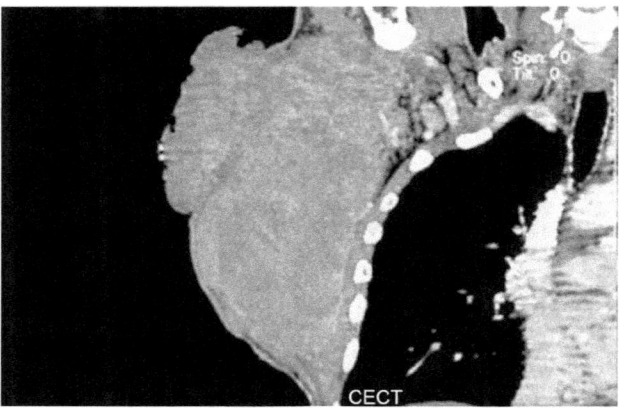

Fig. 36: Coronal CT image showing a large soft tissue sarcoma along the upper part of thoracic wall on the right side.

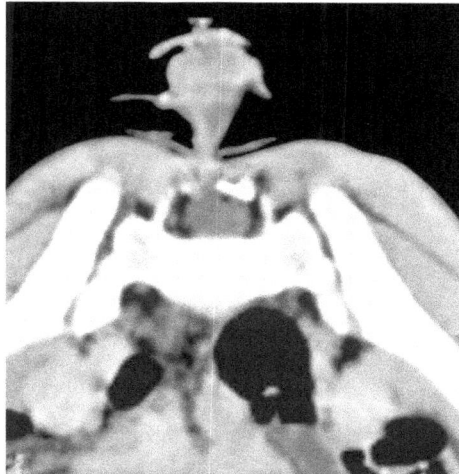

Fig. 37: Axial CT image in prone position showing soft tissue mass in the midline associated with spina bifida in the sacral region.

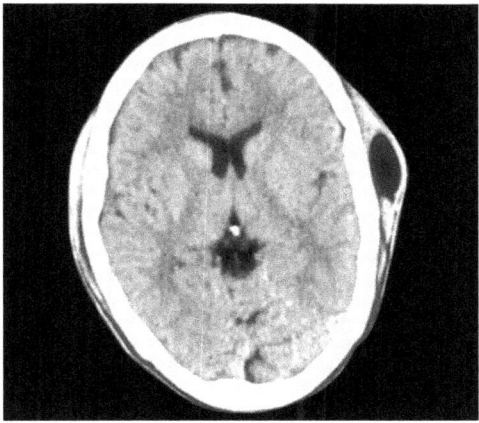

Fig. 38: Axial CT image showing lipoma of scalp in the left frontoparietal region.

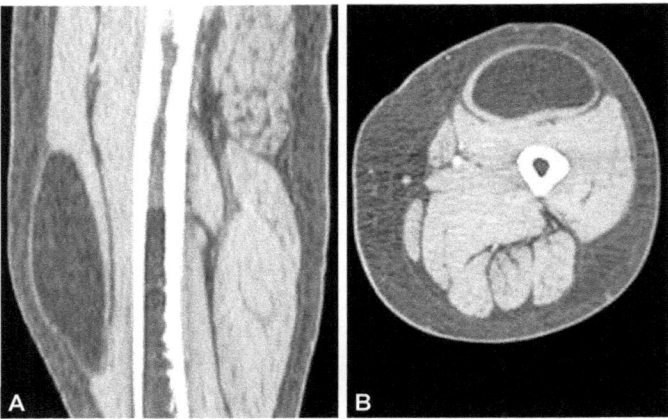

Figs. 39A and B: Sagittal and axial CT images showing intramuscular lipoma of the thigh.

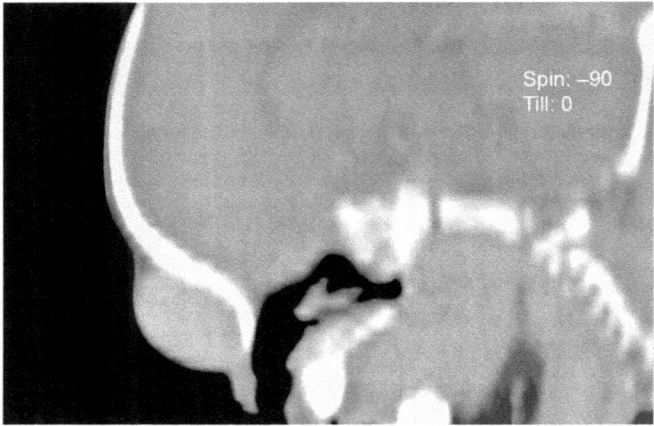

Fig. 40: Sagittal CT image showing a nasal dermoid.

Differential Diagnosis of Bony and Soft Tissue Lesions (Table 21)

TABLE 21: CT differential diagnosis of bony and soft tissue lesions.

Diseases	CT findings	Other findings
Fracture	<ul><li>*Direct signs:* Visualization of fracture</li><li>Accompanying hematoma</li><li>*Indirect signs:* Air-fluid levels</li><li>Subcutaneous emphysema of orbit and face</li><li>Pneumocephalus</li><li>Herniating polypoidal soft tissue mass/fat on the roof of maxillay sinus in blowout fracture</li></ul>	<ul><li>History of trauma</li><li>Postoperative changes may present with bony defect/soft tissue changes</li><li>*Complication:* Cerebrospinal fluid (CSF) leak</li></ul>
Hemorrhage	Diffuse/polypoid mucosal thickening with air-fluid level	History of bleeding disorders, anticoagulation and barotrauma
Sinusitis	<ul><li>*Acute:* Mucosal thickening, air-fluid level</li><li>*Chronic:* Persistent mucosal thickening with inflammatory polyps, partial/complete opacification of sinuses, reactive sclerosis of sinus wall, secondary osteomyelitis with focal thickening and destructive changes in wall</li></ul>	<ul><li>Most common cause of sinus opacification</li><li>Commonly viral infection with superadded bacterial infection Allergic sinusitis associated with bilateral symmetrical mucosal thickening and sinonasal polyps</li></ul>

Contd...

Contd...

Diseases	CT findings	Other findings
Fungal sinusitis	Nodular mucosal thickening affecting multiple sinuses, hyperdense secretions and calcification	• *Common organisms:* Mucor and *Aspergillus* • Primarily diabetic and immunocompromised • Similar presentation with other granulomatous infections and inflammation
Inflammatory polyps	Up to 1 cm in diameter and blends with adjacent mucosal thickening	Most common complication of chronic sinusitis. In children associated with cystic fibrosis and Kartagener's syndrome
Retention cyst	Spherical/dome-shaped low density smooth-walled mass. Maxillary sinus most commonly affected	Caused by inflammatory obstruction of seromucinous gland
Mucocele	• Nonenhancing low-density expansile mass with bony erosion and sclerosis • Most commonly in frontal sinus • Extension into orbit, sphenoid sinus and skull base	Caused by inflammatory obstruction of ostium of sinuses (rarely post-traumatic/neoplastic). Pyoceles are infected mucoceles
Antrochoanal polyp	Mucous mass (10–20 HU) originating in maxillary sinus extending through enlarged and eroded ostium into ipsilateral nasal cavity and through choana into nasopharynx	Focal, reactive mucosal process of maxillary sinus usually without signs of chronic/allergic sinusitis

Contd...

Contd...

Diseases	CT findings	Other findings
Papillomas	Multiple areas of nodular mucosal thickening in sinuses or nose	These are benign epithelial growths which may be polypoidal or papillomatous
Squamous cell carcinoma	Poorly marginated soft tissue mass with extensive destruction of adjacent bone. Regional lymph nodes (retropharyngeal, submandibular and jugular) are involved in 15% cases at time of diagnosis. Invasion of pterygopalatine fossa, orbit, maxillary alveolar ridge, hard palate, buccal space, middle cranial fossa and/or nose occurs frequently. Majority of lesions arise from maxillary sinus; 15% from ethmoid sinus and rarely from sphenoid and frontal sinus	Most common tumor of sinuses and nose (80–90%) cannot be differentiated from adenocarcinoma (in wood workers and cabinet makers), adenoid cystic carcinoma and mucoepidermoid carcinoma on CT. Presents with signs and symptoms of obstructive sinusitis. *Staging*: • *T1:* Tumor limited to antral mucosa • *T2:* Bony destruction limited to hard palate/lateral wall of nose • *T3:* Tumor invades posterior antral wall, orbital wall, anterior ethmoid sinus or skin • *T4:* Tumor invades orbital contents, cribiform plate, posterior ethmoid, sphenoid sinus, nasopharynx, masticator space, or skull base
Lymphoma	Often bilateral soft tissue mass associated with bone destruction	Rare. Usually non-Hodgkin's lymphoma. Concurrent generalized lymphoma is uncommon

Contd...

Contd...

Diseases	CT findings	Other findings
Metastases	Solitary/multiple osteolytic/osteoblastic lesions. May be associated with soft-tissue component	*Common primary sites*: Kidney, lung, breast/prostate
Wegener's granulomatosis	<ul><li>Usually bilateral mucosal thickening and soft tissue nodules with predilection for maxillary sinus and nose</li><li>Extensive bony destruction can occur without soft tissue masses</li></ul>	Necrotizing vasculitis involving upper and lower respiratory tracts and kidneys. *Midline granuloma*: Ulcerating granulomatous masses with bony destruction indistinguishable from Wegener's granulomatosis but limited to nose, hard and soft palate and adjacent sinuses
Bone lesions	<ul><li>*Fibrous dysplasia*: Expansile predominantly sclerotic bone lesion encroaching on sinuses</li><li>*Neurofibromatosis*: Enlarged facial bones with soft tissue masses (neurofibromas) which may erode the adjacent bones</li><li>*Paget's disease*: Obliteration of sinuses with thickened and sclerotic bone</li><li>*Osteoma*: Polypoid bony mass protruding into frontal/ethmoid sinuses which is partially (cancellous)/completely (compact) ossified</li></ul>	<ul><li>*Eosinophilic granuloma*: Lytic lesion sometimes with tooth floating in space</li><li>Giant cell tumor, giant cell granuloma, aneurysmal bone cyst and Brown tumor of hyperparathyroidism: locally destructive, often expansile lytic bone lesions</li></ul>

Contd...

Contd...

Diseases	CT findings	Other findings
	- *Ossifying fibroma*: Lobulated expansile lesion in maxilla with central calcification (localized form of fibrous dysplasia) - *Odontoma:* Well-circumscribed lesion containing undifferentiated dental tissues evident as radiopaque material - *Dentigerous cyst*: Bone cyst containing the crown of an unerupted tooth - *Keratocyst*: Bone cyst without tooth material *Radicular cyst*: Around the root of a devitalized or carious tooth - *Residual cyst:* Sequelae of extracted tooth - *Fissural cyst:* Expansile cyst located in midline or between the lateral incisor and the canine tooth. Arise from the epithelial remnant of an existing fissure or suture	*Ameloblastoma*: Unilocular or more commonly multilocular lytic lesion, often with coarse trabecular structure. - Large tumors cause cortical expansion or breakthrough and may be associated with large soft tissue masses - *Plasmacytoma*: Must be considered in differential diagnosis of an expansile, lytic and destructive lesion - *Osteosarcomas*: Arise often from alveolar ridge and present with bone destruction, new bone formation and large soft tissue mass - *Chondrosarcomas*: Often present as multilobulated, sharply demarcated lytic lesion with characteristic chondroid matrix calcification - *Ewing's sarcoma*: Permeative bone destruction, periosteal reaction and large soft tissue component

Differential Diagnosis of Joint Diseases (Table 22)

Diagnosis of articular disease primarily made on conventional radiography. CT useful to assess the extent of both bone and soft tissue involvement.

TABLE 22: CT differential diagnosis of joint diseases.

Joint involved	CT features	Comments
Sacroiliac joint	• Widening of SI joints commonly found in traumatic diastasis and primary and secondary hyperparathyroidism • Unilateral widening of SI joint associated with erosions, destruction, and sclerosis suggests infection. • Widening of SI joint also in early erosive stage of ankylosing spondylitis, enteropathic spondyloarthropathy, Reiter's syndrome, bilateral symmetrical involvement of psoriasis, and rheumatoid arthritis. These conditions progress to joint space loss and fusion • Unilateral involvement suggests pyogenic/degenerative joint disease. • *Pyogenic sacroiliitis*: Usually in intravenous (IV) drug abusers. CT demonstrates associated	• *Normal joint space*: 2–4 mm; ligamentous portion more variable and wider. • SI joint difficult to evaluate on plain radiographs alone. • Sacroiliitis can be differentiated on basis of both distribution and morphology of articular changes. • *Ankylosing spondylitis and enteropathic spondyloarthropathy*: SI joints with poorly defined erosions, adjacent sclerosis, joint space narrowing and intra-articular osseous and ligamentous ossification • *Psoriasis and Reiter's syndrome*: Bilateral, asymmetric SI joint involvement with extensive sclerosis particularly on ilium side and occasional fusion

Contd...

Musculoskeletal System

Contd...

Joint involved	CT features	Comments
	• Soft tissue abscess and associated erosive and sclerotic joint changes • *Degenerative joint disease*—Above 40 years. Narrowing of joint space, sclerosis, smooth subchondral margins and anterior osteophytes progressing to complete bridging anterior of SI joint. Rarely small subchondral cysts simulating erosions • *Gout and pseudogout*: rarely involves joint space	• *Rheumatoid arthritis*: Late SI joint involvement with superficial sclerosis and minimal sclerosis. Joint ankylosis does not occur. • In primary and secondary hyperparathyroidism: Subchondral bone resorption with symmetric widening of SI joint and adjacent sclerosis
Osteitis condensans ilii	Symmetric triangular sclerosis of inferior aspect of ilium not associated with any SI joint involvement	*Differential diagnosis:* Sacroiliitis of psoriasis and Reiter's syndrome
Pelvic trauma	• Unilateral SI joint dislocation associated with fracture of ipsilateral superior and inferior pubic rami—malgaigne type fracture • SI joint dissociation with fracture of contralateral pubic rami—bucket handle type fracture	All conditions with at least two complete disruption of pelvic ring require open/closed stabilization to prevent pelvic collapse

Contd...

Contd...

Joint involved	CT features	Comments
Hip trauma	CT helps in accurate depiction of fracture-dislocation—size of intra-articular fragments, fracture fragment displacement, and congruity between femoral head and acetabulum	Osteochondral fractures of femoral head frequently associated with hip dislocation. These avulsion fractures are difficult to differentiate from AVN on conventional radiography
Avascular necrosis	CT less sensitive than nuclear magnetic resonance (NMR) or MRI. In normal hip, asterisk-like condensation of bone noted in femoral head due to crossing of tensile and compressive trabeculae. This is smudged in AVN by focal sclerosis and bone resorption. This reaches articular surface in late stages	*Common causes*: Fracture, steroid therapy, sickle cell disease, collagen vascular diseases. *Five stages*: 1. Minimal focal sclerosis and osteopenia 2. Distinct sclerosis and focal lucency/cyst formation 3. Subchondral lucency (crescent sign) without collapse of femoral head 4. Subchondral fracture/flattening of femoral head 5. Marked collapse of femoral head with secondary arthritic changes
Knee	CT useful in detection of intra-articular loose bodies in osteochondritis dissecans, osteochondromatosis, and arthritic disorders. It also helps in defining the degree of cortical depression and fracture fragment	Magnetic resonance imaging superior for ligamentous, cartilage, and meniscal pathology. Spontaneous osteonecrosis of knee involves weight bearing surface of medial femoral

Contd...

Musculoskeletal System

Contd...

Joint involved	CT features	Comments
	displacement which help in selection of treatment modality in trauma cases	condyle and osteochondritis dissecans involves nonweight bearing portion of this condyle in intercondylar notch area
Ankle and foot	CT helps in assessing the fragment displacement and joint involvement and to identify the number and position of loose fragments. It may depict subtle fractures and subluxations. Accompanying soft tissue injuries like trapped soft tissue structures and lacerated ligaments and tendons	
Tarsal coalition	• CT can diagnose tarsal coalition that may be complete/incomplete and osseous/cartilaginous/fibrous • Most common between calcaneus and navicular, then talus and calcaneus, least often between calcaneus and cuboid. • Fusion between talus and calcaneus most commonly occurs at sustentaculum tali. Reformatted coronal images are most useful to demonstrate this coalition	Secondary degenerative changes like close apposition of involved joints, sclerosis of articular margins, and cortical irregularities. Hypoplasia of talar head/talar beak arising characteristically at talonavicular joint. This talar beak has to be differentiated from more common common talonavicular joint capsule talar spur that originates at the more and hence is not directly contiguous with the distal articular surface of talus

Contd...

Contd...

Joint involved	CT features	Comments
Shoulder	CT can demonstrate Hill-Sachs compression fracture and Bankart lesion in recurrent anterior dislocation. CT arthrography may demonstrate pathologies of glenoid labrum	
Elbow and wrist	CT identifies subtle fractures and subluxation not recognized by conventional methods. Fracture complications like nonunion and AVN can also be seen	
Temporomandibular (TM) joint	TM joint is divided by a disc which can be anteriorly dislocated. This can be seen on CT due to high CT density of 60 HU	However, MRI is investigation of choice as it depicts other joint pathologies as well.

Differential Diagnosis of Soft Tissue Lesions (Table 23)

TABLE 23: CT differential diagnosis of soft tissue lesions.

Diseases	CT findings	Remarks
Cyst	Well-marginated homogeneous mass of water density. High density if here is hemorrhage or infection. No contrast enhancement	Cystic lesions can be synovial cyst, distended bursa or ganglion

Contd...

Contd...

Diseases	CT findings	Remarks
Lipoma	Well-defined homogeneous mass of fat density (–50 to –100 HU) without contrast enhancement. Thin septations, vessels or calcifications or ossifications can be found. Lipomas located close to bone may incite a localized hyperostosis. Invasion into surrounding tissue or areas of soft tissue in the lesion may suggest possibility of liposarcoma	Most common benign soft tissue tumor. More common in females between 3rd and 5th decade. Variants of fatty tumors include symmetric lipomatosis hibernoma and lipoblastoma, lipoma arborescans, and macrodystrophica lipomatosa
Hemangioma	Inhomogeneous, usually well-defined mass that may contain phleboliths. They have a density of 30–40 HU and markedly enhance following intravenous contrast administration. Occasionally metaplastic ossifications are found within the lesion. When adjacent to bone erosions and solid periosteal reactions are occasionally observed	Most common vascular tumor with predilection for the skin. Deep soft tissue hemangiomas are usually asymptomatic until early adulthood, when other conditions such as consumption coagulopathy, cardiac decompensation, and massive osteolysis of Gorham or Maffucci syndrome can be associated
Lymphangioma	Similar to hemangioma but without phleboliths and less contrast enhancement	Rare

Contd...

Contd...

Diseases	CT findings	Remarks
Neurofibroma and neurolemoma	Well-defined, homogeneous lesions that increase in attenuation after contrast administration	Solitary neurofibromas are most common between 3rd and 5th decade. No difference between benign and malignant lesions on imaging
Other benign soft tissue masses	Well-defined homogenous soft tissue masses with usually moderate, uniform enhancement	Fibromas, giant cell tumor of tendon sheath, rhabdomyomas, and myxoma are common tumors
Fibromatosis	Variety of benign fibrous proliferation presenting as poorly-defined homogeneous soft tissue lesion. May mimic a malignant lesion because of infiltration in surrounding tissue. Recurrences are frequent	Desmoid—arising in abdominal and extra-abdominal musculature. Recurring digital fibromas in the finger and toes of infants. Palmar and plantar fibromatosis involving respective fascia
Liposarcoma	Well- or poorly-defined heterogeneous mass with a variable amount of fatty tissue. Because of their fibrous, myxomatous, and vascular elements they have a higher attenuation than lipomas and enhance with intravenous contrast	Common soft tissue malignancy of idle age and elderly frequent involvement of lower extremity

Contd...

Contd...

Diseases	CT findings	Remarks
Malignant fibrous histiocytoma	Well- or poorly-defined in homogeneous soft tissue mass with necrotic areas and considerable contrast enhancement. Erosion/destruction of adjacent bone can be seen. Intratumoral calcification can be seen	Most common primary malignant soft-tissue tumor. Occurs at all ages, most common around 50 years. Slight male predominance. Lower extremity is the most common location
Rhabdomyosarcoma	Fairly well- to poorly-defined soft-tissue mass. Erosion or invasion of the adjacent bone common. Necrosis, hemorrhage, and cystic degeneration can lead to inhomogeneous appearance	Occurs usually under the age of 50 years in adults tumor is usually located in deeper tissues of the extremities and torso. In children tumor predominates in the head, neck, and urogenital tract
Synovial sarcoma	Relatively poorly-defined, usually inhomogeneous mass with calcifications in 30% and erosion/destruction of adjacent bone without reactive sclerosis in 25 of cases	Most frequently seen in thigh and lower extremity, male predominance. Calcified metastases are not uncommon, especially in the lung
Other malignant soft tissue sarcomas	Well- or poorly-defined mass lesions that may erode or invade the adjacent bone	Metastasis, melanomas, lymphomas, extraosseous plasmacytoma, angiosarcoma, clear cell sarcoma are common ones

Contd...

Contd...

Diseases	CT findings	Remarks
Abscess	Poorly-defined, isodense or slightly hypodense mass or more commonly, well-defined cystic lesion with a relative thick wall and occasionally septations. The attenuation value of the liquefied content usually exceeds 25 HU. Enhancement of nonliquefied components after contrast administration. Presence of soft tissue gas in the absence of surgical or percutaneous interventions is rare but virtually diagnostic	Common causes of soft-tissue abscesses include trauma, iatrogenic interventions, intravenous drug abuse, spread from a contiguous infection, and septic embolism
Hematoma	Homogeneous enlargement of the involved muscle, which might be hyperdense in the acute stage. In the subacute stage, the hematoma might be poorly-defined and is either isodense or slightly hypodense. When completely liquefied the hematoma has a homogeneous density that is lower than muscle and may be surrounded by a pseudocapsule which enhances after contrast administration	Soft-tissue hemorrhage occurs spontaneously following trauma or surgery, with a variety of bleeding disorders, and during anticoagulation therapy. Bleeding into tumor or abscess is quite common also

Contd...

Contd...

Diseases	CT findings	Remarks
Aneurysm/ pseudoaneurysm	Round soft tissue density with occasionally curvilinear calcification in the vicinity of major artery. Inhomogeneous appearance when partially thrombosed. Intravenous contrast administration is diagnostic	Popliteal artery aneurysm is the most common aneurysm found in the extremities and presents as a pulsatile mass

Differential Diagnosis of Spinal Fractures (Table 24)

TABLE 24: CT differential diagnosis of spinal fractures.

Diseases	CT findings	Remarks
Impacted compression fracture	Double rim along the anterior upper and lower edges of the vertebral body is characteristic. Endplate may appear irregular or abnormally dense, the spinal canal and the roots of the arch are intact	Characteristically a hyperflexion fracture involving the anterior column of thoracolumbar region. The middle and posterior columns remain intact. Seen on plain films as a wedge-shaped deformity
Incomplete burst fracture	Both anterior and posterior portions of the endplate are fractured. Widened of the anteroposterior diameter of the vertebral body. Posterior fragments protrude toward the spinal canal but the roots of the arch remain intact	Axial compression fracture involving both anterior and middle columns. The posterior osteoligamentous column remains intact but the spinal canal is narrowed. Exclusion of complete burst fracture is usually possible only by means of CT

Contd...

Contd...

Diseases	CT findings	Remarks
Complete burst fracture	Fracture of the vertebral arch and dislocation and/or subluxation of the facet joints. Bone fragments in the vicinity of the vertebral body and the arch. Spinal canal is often constricted by bone fragments or traumatic disk herniations	Axial compression fracture with additional shearing and flexion forces involving all three columns. Increased interpedicular distance may be seen already on plain film
Chance fracture	Thin slices demonstrate fracture within the vertebral body and bilateral lack of contact between facet articulations	Rare fracture of all three columns due to hyperflexion with a pivotal point in front of the spinal column. Usually best seen on lateral plain films
Flexion distraction	Fragmentation of the injured vertebral bodies, dislocation of facet joints, and fractured in the spinous processes and arches	Hyperflexion injury with compression of anterior column and distraction of the two other columns. Lateral plain films show a wedge-shaped vertebral body, kyphosis and distraction of the spinous process. CT is used to define the anterior edge of vertebral bodies and to detect intracanalicular bone fragments

Contd...

Musculoskeletal System

Contd...

Diseases	CT findings	Remarks
Translation injury	Subluxation is demonstrated as a slight ventral elevation at a level of the inter-vertebral space associated with lack of contact between intervertebral facets. Fracture dislocation of facet joints is common. A stratified fracture through the vertebral body may not be visible without sagittal reconstruction	Laterally inflicted trauma that subluxes or dislocates all three columns and usually causes immediate paraplegia
Atlanto-odontoid subluxation	The dens is centrally located relative to arch of the atlas	Forcible hyperflexion can rupture the transverse ligament. Lateral plain film shows an atlantoaxial joint space more than 3 mm wide. This can be due to nontraumatic causes like rheumatoid arthritis
Rotatory atlantoaxial dislocation	Rotational malposition of dens relative to arch of the atlas. May be associated with avulsion fracture of the dens and dislocation of one or both atlantoaxial articulations	Rupture of the capsule of anterior atlantoaxial joint, caused by forcible rotation of the head
Fracture of the atlas	Jefferson fractures involve both anterior and posterior arches of atlas. Compression hyperextension fractures involve the posterior arch of the atlas. Fracture	Incomplete ossification of the ring of the atlas is common and should not be diagnosed as fractures. Horizontal fractures may not be seen on CT

Contd...

Contd...

Diseases	CT findings	Remarks
	through the lateral mass is due to lateral flexion and compression	
Fracture of dens	Transverse nondislocated fractures are only detected with thin sections. Dislocated transverse fractures and diagonal fractures are easily seen on CT	Dens is involved in 10% of all cervical spine fractures. Therefore the occipitocervical junction should be examined in connection with any CT examination of cranial injuries
Fracture of arch of axis	These fractures run perpendicular to the CT scanning plane and are readily demonstrable. *Type 1*—hairline fracture through the arch only. *Type 2*—fracture associated with ventral dislocation of the body of the axis. *Type 3*—same as type 2 with additional dislocation of the intervertebral joints	Hyperextension injury commonly seen in the traffic accidents victims. Often associated with other injuries of the occipitocervical junction. Type 1 fractures are stable, whereas type 2 and type 3 are unstable

Index

Page numbers followed by *f* refer to figure and *t* refer to table.

A

Abdomen 327
Abdominal lesions, common causes of 327*t*
Abdominal wall 331
    anterior 332*f*
    lesions 327, 328*t*
    metastases 327*f*
Abscess 47, 205*f*, 215, 225, 228, 300, 352, 370, 534
    amebic 340
        hepatic 352*f*
    cerebellar 140*f*
    chronic 204
    epidural 504*f*
    formation 188*f*
    large retroperitoneal 403*f*
    loculated 224*f*
    mediastinal 304
    neck 504*f*
    pancreatic 375
    pelvic 436
    periapical 496
    periodontal 495
    perirenal 426*f*
    prostatic 438
    psoas 404*f*
    pyogenic 340
        brain 93
    renal 426, 426*f*
    retropharyngeal 228*f*
    soft tissue 518*f*
    spinal
        cord 111
        epidural 123
Acavernous angioma 48*f*
Achalasia 294
Achondroplasia 127
Acoustic canal
    internal 150*t*
    stenosis, bilateral external 134*f*
Acoustic schwannoma 15*f*, 81, 150
Acquired cystic disease 420
Acquired immunodeficiency syndrome 27, 40, 102
Acquired toxoplasmosis 100
Actinomycosis 456
Adenocarcinoma 136, 262
Adenoid 206
    cystic carcinoma 253
Adenoma 144, 263, 338
    proximal tubular 422
Adenomatous hyperplasia 240, 247
Adenomatous polyp 379
Adhesive otitis media, chronic 140
Adnexa 442, 446
Adnexal lesions, common causes of 446*t*
Adnexal torsion 449
Adrenal adenoma 412, 412*f*
Adrenal carcinoma 412
Adrenal enlargement, causes of 411
Adrenal hyperplasia 413
Adrenal lesions 410
Adrenal paraganglioma 414
Adrenoleukodystrophy 22, 64, 98
Aeroceles 49
    multiple 20*f*
Agger nasi cell 210, 213*f*

Air
 bronchogram, differential
  diagnosis of 283
 cells, opacification of 138
Alagille syndrome 155
Alexander's disease 21, 22, 25, 64, 96
Alexander's dysplasia 153
Allergic alveolitis, extrinsic 275
Allergic bronchopulmonary
  aspergillosis 280*f*
Allergic sinusitis 185
Altered globe size 163
Alveolar cell carcinoma 263, 284
Alzheimer's disease 77, 98, 104
Ameloblastoma 198, 457*f*
Aminoaciduria 21, 65
Amyloid angiopathy 74
Amyloidosis 237, 308, 358, 361
Anaplastic carcinoma 248
Anaplastic ependymoma 96
Aneurysm 17, 70, 71*f*, 82
 malformation 3
Aneurysmal bone cyst 129, 199,
  458, 458*f*
Angioblastoma 456
Angiofibroma 216
 juvenile 206
Angioimmunoblastic
  lymphadenopathy 311
Angioma 7
Angiomyolipoma 422, 422*f*
Angiosarcoma 371
Ankle
 and foot 529
 joint effusion 483*f*
Ankylosis 512
Anomalies, duplication 430
Antral polyp, benign 192*f*
Antrochoanal polyp 189, 522
Antronasal fungal polyposis 200*f*

Aorta
 aneurysm of 296
  ascending 292
 atherosclerosis of 409
Aortic aneurysm 301, 409
Aortic arch aneurysm 297*f*
Aortic dissection 409
Apical meningocele 152, 159
Aplasia 156
Apophyseal joints 515
Appendix, mucocele of 393, 394*f*
Arachnoiditis 121
Arch of atlas, anomalies of 500
Arch of axis, fracture of 538
Arnold-Chiari malformation 30, 36
Arterial infarct 37
 right cerebral acute 38*f*
Arteriosclerosis 67
Arteriovenous malformation 27, 82,
  87, 168, 258, 260, 427
Arthritis 505, 506*f*
 mutilans 511
Articular disease, diagnosis of 526
Asbestosis 276, 319
Astrocytic hamartoma 164, 181
Astrocytoma 12, 54, 88, 96, 111
Ataxia-telangiectasia syndrome
  77, 80
Atheroma 7
Atlantoaxial articulation 515
Atlantoaxial fusion malsegmentation
  501
Atlantoaxial subluxation 501
Atlanto-occipital fusion 500
Atlanto-odontoid subluxation 537
Atlas assimilation 500
Atlas fracture 537
Atrophic fatty pancreas 374*f*
Atrophy 35
Auditory canal, internal 83
Autoimmune labyrinthitis 146
Axonal injury, diffuse 76, 78

Index

B

Baker's cyst 513
Bamboo spine 514
Bartholin's cyst 441, 443
Basal cell carcinoma 136
Basal cisterns, effaced 78
Basal ganglia 8*f*, 51*f*
    diffuse hypodensities 23
Basilar artery 56*f*
Bifid facial nerve 156
Bile pseudocyst 340
Biliary cystadenoma 339, 347
Biliary lesions 362, 364
    common causes of 362*t*
Biliary pseudocyst 353
Biliary tract lesions 362
Biloma 340, 353
Bing-Siebenmann dysplasia 153
Binswanger's encephalopathy 104
Bladder 430
    calculi 431
    carcinoma 433, 433*f*
    endometriosis 431
    fungal ball in 432
    intraluminal pseudomasses of 434
Blood dyscrasias 75
Bochdalek's hernia 298
Bone 454, 454*t*
    adamantinoma of long 456
    angiosarcoma of 459
    avascular necrosis of 459
    cyst, simple 487, 487*f*
    destruction 184*t*, 199*t*
    island 460
    lesions, primary 194*t*
    neoplasm
        benign 453
        malignant 453
    resorption of 507, 508
    sclerosis with periosteal reaction 455
    small 508
    temporal 132, 148*t*
    tumors 456
        salient features of 456
Bone-in-bone appearance 514
Bony labyrinthine anomalies 154*t*
Bony lesion 132, 132*t*, 452, 453, 524
    spinal 499
Bony lytic metastases 63*f*
Bony texture, abnormal 195*f*
Bony type disease 133
Borrelia burgdorferi 103
Borreliosis 103
Bowel lesions, small 382, 383
Bowel loops, floating 402*f*
Bracket calcification 4*f*
Brain 1, 13*t*, 26, 69
    abscess 101
    causes of 18*t*
    lesions 12, 37, 37*t*, 69
        nontumoral 20
    nodules, innumerable small enhancing 26
    normal aging 104
    occipital horns 35
    parenchyma, parasagittal 25
    pseudomasses of 18, 18*t*
    tumors 74
        causes of 17*t*
Brainstem
    glioma of 55, 56*f*, 82, 84
    hypodensity 23
    lesions 76
Branchial cleft cyst
    first 231, 251
    second 218, 224, 228
Breast carcinoma 474*f*
Brodie abscess 455, 460
Bronchial atresia 313

Bronchiectasis 315
Bronchiolitis
   acute 317
   constrictive 316
   obliterans 316
      organizing pneumonia 318
   obliterative 316
Bronchogenic carcinoma 264, 410*f*
Bronchus, carcinoma of 295
Buccal space 225
Budd-Chiari syndrome 342
Buphthalmos 175
Burkitt's lymphoma 497
Burst fracture
   complete 536
   incomplete 535
Buschke-Löwenstein tumor 395
Butterfly glioma 26
Button sequestrum 470, 492

C

Caffey's disease 455
Calcific pancreatitis, chronic 373*f*
Canavan disease 21, 22, 25, 64
Canavan-van Bogaert disease 97
Candida 249
Capillary angioma 47
Capillary hemangioma 169
Capsuloma 425
Carcinoma 365, 385
   bronchus 296*f*
   cecum 390*f*
Caroli disease 340, 351, 364
Carotid artery 217, 224
Carotid sheath mass 220*f*
Carotid space 219
Cartilage tumors 454
Castleman's disease 310, 406
Catscratch fever 249
Cavernous angioma 47, 70, 72

Cavernous hemangioma 168, 371
Cavitary prostatitis 437
Cavitating lesion 255
   causes of 265*t*
Cavum septum pellucidum 17
Cavum velum interpositum 17
Cavum vergae 17
Cell carcinoma
   large 262
   small 262
   transitional 424, 424*f*
Cellulitis 173
Cementoma 498
Central dot sign 351
Central nervous system 27
   tumors 96*f*
Central pontine myelinolysis 105
Centrilobular emphysema 282
Cerebellar atrophy 77
Cerebellar hemisphere 43*f*, 77
Cerebellar vermis 77
Cerebellopontine
   angle 83
      masses, differential
           diagnosis of 81, 81*t*
   left 15*f*
Cerebellum 82
   astrocytoma of 84
Cerebral atrophy 77
Cerebral edema 78
   diffuse 25
Cerebral hemisphere, left 70*f*
Cerebral infarction 92
Cerebral lesions, deep 76
Cerebral neuroblastoma, primary 90
Cerebritis 94
Cerebrospinal fluid 44*f*, 83, 182
Ceruminoma 136
Cervical
   carcinoma 445
   fascia 225
      deep 229

Index

space, posterior 228, 229t
thymic cyst 238
Cervix 441
Chance fracture 536
CHARGE syndrome 155
Chest 255
Chloroma 120
Cholangiocarcinoma 365
Cholangitis 364
Cholecystitis 365
    acute 367f
Choledochal cyst 340, 364
    large 365f
Choledocholithiasis 363f
Cholelithiasis 367
Cholesteatoma 134, 141, 141f
    acquired 141
    congenital 81, 142
    primary 152
Cholesterol granuloma 17, 143, 151
Chondroblastoma 148, 152, 458, 461
Chondroma 198, 237
Chondromesenchymal hamartoma 203, 204f
Chondromyxoid fibroma 461
Chondrosarcoma 152, 199, 258, 461
Chordoma 7, 209, 464
Choriocarcinoma 292, 446
Choroid plexus
    carcinoma 54, 85
    papilloma 12, 53, 85, 96
Choroidal detachment 164, 178
Choroidal hemangioma 165, 180
Choroidal melanoma 165
Choroidal nevus 181
Choroidal osteoma 164, 181
Chronic injury 113
Cirrhosis 359
Cluster sign 353
Coal miner's pneumoconiosis 308
Coal workers' pneumoconiosis 278, 321

Coalescent mastoiditis 141
Coats' disease 164, 176
Cocaine 75
Coccidioidomycosis 270
Cochlea 146t
Cochlear aplasia 155
Cochlear hypoplasia 155
Cockayne syndrome 25
Codman's triangle 484
Codman's tumor 461
Cold abscess, calcified 484f
Colitis cystica profunda 390
Collagen diseases 508
Collagen vascular disease 279
Collapse
    wafer-like 514
    wedge-like 514
Coloboma 177
Colon mass, ascending 332f
Colonic lesions 389, 435
    common causes of 389t
Colonic tuberculosis 399f
Colonic wall thickening, lesions with 389
Compression fracture 535
Concha bullosa 210, 211f
Congenital disorders 25
Constrictor muscles 215
Contour abnormalities 361
Cord contusion 113
Corduroy appearance 469
Corpus callosal agenesis 30
Corpus callosum 26
    absence of 36f
    agenesis 35
    dysgenesis 30, 36
Cortical contusions 76, 77f
Cortical dermoid 464
Cranial fossa
    bones of anterior 491f
    lesions, middle 15

Craniopharyngioma 6, 12, 61, 62f, 92
Craniovertebral anomalies,
  differential diagnosis of 500
CREST syndrome 513
Crohn's colitis 392
Crohn's disease 383, 387, 387f
Cryptococcosis 42
Cumbo sign 260
Cyst 339, 507, 530
  adrenal 411
  apical 496
  arachnoid 17, 45, 46f, 83, 120, 490
  bony 225
  bronchogenic 259, 264, 293, 296, 303f
  choroid 181
    fissure 45
    plexus 45
  colloid 49, 238, 239, 247
  congenital 234, 235, 369
  corpus luteal 447
  dental 225, 496
  dentigerous 496, 525
  dermoid 171, 224, 490
  developmental 496
  duplication 383
  ejaculatory duct 438
  enteric 398
  enterogenous 49
  ependymal 45
  epidermoid 120, 151, 152, 224, 465, 490
  esophageal duplication 293
  fissural 496, 525
  follicular 447, 496
  gastric duplication 377
  hepatic 339, 349, 350f
  leptomeningeal 17
  lymphoepithelial 231
  maxillary dentigerous 189
  mediastinal 302
  mesenteric 398, 398f
  mesothelial 398
  omental 398
  pancreatic 374
  parapelvic 418
  parathyroid 242
  pelvicalyceal 417
  periodontal 496
  peripelvic 418
  pineal 17, 91
  pleuropericardial 292
  porencephalic 43, 44f
  post-traumatic 271
  primordial 496
  prostatic 437
  pyelogenic 417
  radicular 496
  residual 525
  retention 222, 437, 522
  sebaceous 17, 329
  simple 417
  springwater 292
  subchondral 467
  supratentorial
    midline 17
    paramidline 17
  theca lutein 447
  thymic 302
  thyroglossal 224
    duct 245
  trichilemmal 17
  unicameral 487
  urachal 329
  utricular 438
Cystadenocarcinoma 347, 450
Cystic bronchiectasis 282, 282f
Cystic glioma 55f
Cystic hygroma 223, 286, 293
Cystic lesions 184
  multiple 449

Cystic lymphangioma, large 226f
Cystic pulmonary diseases 281, 281t
Cystic schwannoma 304
Cystic tumors 303
Cysticercosis 103
Cystitis
    cystica 432
    emphysematosa 432
Cytomegalovirus 2, 3, 9, 249
    congenital 10f

D

Dacryoadenocystitis 175
Dandy-Walker
    syndrome 30, 31f
De Quervain's thyroiditis 246
Degenerative disease 104, 124
Dehiscent jugular bulb 158
Dementia, subcortical 77
Demyelinating disease 20, 22, 22t, 29
Demyelinating disorders, congenital 96
Demyelinating lesion, causes of 21t
Dens fracture 538
Dermal sinus, dorsal 114
Desmoplastic fibroma 464
Desquamative interstitial pneumonia 278
Destructive lesions 493
Diaphragmatic hernia 302, 267f
Diaphyseal achalasia 477
    progressive 149
Diastematomyelia 109, 110f
Diastrophic dysplasia 126, 127
Diffuse hepatic lesions, differential diagnosis of 359, 359t
Diffuse liver diseases, common causes of 355t
Discal calcification 501

Discal disease 122
Disk herniation, postoperative 126
Double-target sign 353
Down syndrome 25, 501, 515
Dromedary hump 421
Drug abuse 75
Duodenal diverticulum 384f
Duodenum 382f
    adenocarcinoma of 385f
Dwarf cochlea 156
Dyke-Davidoff-Masson syndrome 77, 79
Dysplasia
    epiphysealis hemimelica 509
    multiple 154f

E

Ear 132
    lesions, differential diagnosis of 132
Echinococcal cyst 339, 370
Eclampsia 75
Ectatic carotid artery 220
Ectopic pancreas 380
Edema, nonenhancing 38f
Effusion 151
Eggshell calcification 307
Elbow
    and wrist 530
    tubercular osteomyelitis of 483f
Emboli 270
Embryonal cell carcinoma 292
Embryonal rhabdomyosarcoma 144
Emphysema 315
Emphysematous cholecystitis 365
Empyema 49
Encephalitis, acute disseminated 68, 105
Encephalocele 208
Encephalomalacia 43

Encephalomeningocele 204
Enchondroma 464
Endocrine neoplasia, multiple 248
Endodermal sinus tumor 292
Endolymphatic sac
　lesions 146
　tumors 146
Endometrioma 448
Endometriosis 328
Endophthalmitis 165, 177
Endosteal hyperostosis 148
Engelmann-Camurati disease 489
Eosinophilic gastritis 380
Eosinophilic granuloma 144, 146, 197, 470
Ependymal enhancement, causes of 27*t*
Ependymoma 57, 84, 89, 96, 111, 119
Epidural lesions 16
Epidural lipomatosis 120
Epiphrenic esophageal diverticulum 295
Esophageal masses 296
Esophagus, distal carcinoma of 297*f*
Esthesioneuroblastoma 187*f*, 202
Etate crible 22
Ethmoid bulla 210, 212*f*
Ethmoid infundibulum 212*f*
Ethmoid mucocele 190*f*
Ethmoid sinus, left 190*f*
Ethmoid sinusitis 188*f*
Ewing's sarcoma 199, 465, 466*f*, 474
Exostoses 137
Expansile bony lesions, common causes of 453*t*
External ear 132*t*, 154*f*
　lesions 132*t*
Extramedullary hematopoiesis 299
Extraparotid lesion 231
Extrapyramidal disorders 77
Eye, thickened coats of 165*t*

F

Facial nerve
　anomalies 156*t*
　anterior migration of 157
　duplication of 156
　hypoplasia, congenital 156
　neuroma of 144
　schwannoma 150
Fahr's disease 3*f*, 25, 80
Fahr's syndrome 2
Falcine lesions 16
Fallen fragment sign 487
Fatty infiltration, diffuse 356, 357*f*
Feeding vessel sign 258
Femur, distal 472
Fetal lobulations 421
Fibrin balls 323
Fibrinoid leukodystrophy 96
Fibroid 445*f*
Fibrolamellar hepatocellular carcinoma 337, 344, 345*f*
Fibrolipomatosis 416
Fibromatosis 532
Fibrosarcoma 466
Fibrosing alveolitis 274
Fibrosing mediastinitis 314*f*
Fibrosing mesenteritis, chronic 399
Fibrosis, retroperitoneal 408
Fibrous cortical defect 466
Fibrous dysplasia 137, 148, 194, 195*f*, 458, 467, 491*f*
Fibrous histiocytoma, malignant 473, 533
Fibrous tissue tumors 454
Fibrous tumor, malignant 325
Fibrous type disease 133
Filum terminale 116
Fistula 436
Flexion distraction 536
Fluid lesions 184

Focal bacterial nephritis, acute 426
Focal basal ganglia, bilateral 23
Focal caliectasis 417
Focal fatty infiltration 341, 355
Focal hepatic lesions 335
    common causes of 335t
Focal hepatic metastasis 346f
Focal interhemispheric blood 71
Focal lesions 488
Focal nodular hyperplasia 338, 349
Foley's bulb 434
Follicular carcinoma 248
Foramen magnum 15
Foreign body 164, 318
Fracture 521
Frontal horns, abnormal 30
Frontal sinus 185f
    extension 210
    mucocele of 190f
Frontoethmoidal encephalocele 209f
Fucosidosis 65
Fungal infection 192f, 310
Fungal sinusitis 199, 200f, 522
Fungiform papilloma 191

G

Gallbladder 362
    carcinoma 365
    fundus of 366f
Gangliocytoma 89
Ganglioglioma 58, 89
Ganglioneuroma 89
Gardner's syndrome 479
Garre's osteomyelitis 455, 467
Gartner's duct cyst 441, 442
Gastric adenocarcinoma 379f
Gastric bezoar 382
Gastric carcinoma 378
Gastric diverticulum 378
Gastric lesions 377, 377t
Gastric varices 377, 381
Gastroesophageal junction mass 378f
Gastrointestinal lesions 377
Gastrointestinal tumors 473
Genioglossus muscle 221
Geniohyoid muscle 221
Genitourinary lesions 414
Germ cell tumor 59, 258, 287, 292
Germinoma 12, 59, 91, 447f
Gerota's fascia 426
Giant apical air cell 159
Giant cell
    astrocytoma, subependymal 55, 56f
    tumor 137, 198, 458, 468
Giant hypertrophic gastritis 381
Giant osteoid osteoma 475
Giant periapical granuloma 495f
Glioblastoma multiforme 26, 88
Glioma 6, 96
Gliomatosis cerebri 55
Gliosis 87
Glomus jugulare tumor 82, 145, 145f, 493
Glomus tumor 220, 469
Glomus tympanicum 144
Glycogen storage disease 21, 65, 355
Gorlin syndrome 496
Gorlin-Goltz syndrome 52
Granulocytic sarcoma 120
Granuloma, infectious 255
Granulomatous disease 307
Granulomatous masses 186f
Granulomatous sialadenitis 249
Granulomatous thyroiditis, subacute 246
Graves' disease 174, 245
Gray matter lesions 21
Gut wall signature 383
Gyriform enhancement 26

H

Haller cell 210, 213*f*
Hallervorden-Spatz disease 25, 100
Hamartoma 263
Hand-Schüller-Christian disease 470, 471
Hashimoto's thyroiditis 245
Hearing loss, X-linked congenital mixed 156
Hemangioblastoma 39, 85, 90, 112
Hemangioma 83, 135, 135*f*, 226, 231, 237, 251, 338, 347, 469, 531
Hemangiopericytoma 58, 58*f*
Hematoma 42, 71*f*, 204, 206, 263, 328, 534
    epidural 94
    hypertensive acute 70*f*
    intramural 388
        bladder 434
    subcapsular 341, 354
Hemivertebra 126, 128
Hemochromatosis 356, 360
Hemophilic pseudotumor 470
Hemorrhage 69, 74, 75, 87, 164, 521
    acute 69
    adrenal 411
    benign 74
    chronic 69
    idiopathic pulmonary 279
    intracerebral 94
    intraparenchymal 72
    malignant 74
    perinatal 69, 72
    sinus 193
    subacute 69
    subarachnoid 25, 70, 72, 78
    tumoral 70
Hemorrhagic contusion, coincidental small 24*f*
Hemorrhagic cystitis 432
Hemorrhagic infarction 69, 73
Hemorrhagic ovarian mass 450*f*
Hepatic abscess, large 352*f*
Hepatic adenoma 349
Hepatic adenomatosis 338
Hepatic disease, diffuse 356*f*
Hepatic flexure 399*f*
Hepatic hemangioma, typical 348*f*
Hepatic infarct 355
Hepatic laceration, large 354*f*
Hepatic lesions 335
    differential diagnosis of 337
Hepatic lobe herniation, left 267*f*
Hepatic metastases 408*f*
Hepatic parenchyma 353, 356, 358
Hepatic tumors, common causes of 337*t*
Hepatic venous occlusion 342
Hepatobiliary lesions 335
Hepatoblastoma 347, 348*f*
Hepatocellular carcinoma 337, 344
    diffuse 358, 361
Hepatocellular disease 75
Hepatolenticular degeneration 99
Hernia 331
    femoral 333
    obturator 333
    traumatic ventral 332*f*
    types of 331, 331*t*
Herpes encephalitis 100
Heterotopias 36
Hiatus hernia 294, 295, 301
Hiatus semilunaris 212*f*
Hilar lip 421
Hip, tuberculosis of 484*f*
Histiocytosis 281, 470
Hodgkin's disease 303, 325, 514
Holoprosencephaly 30, 33
Homocysteinuria 99
Huntington's disease 25, 79

Index

Hyaloid detachment, posterior 164, 178
Hydatid cyst 45, 93, 260, 260f, 351
    healing 351f
Hydatid disease 264, 471
Hydranencephaly 35
Hydrocephalus 32, 78
Hydrometra 444
Hydromyelia 110
Hydroxyapatite deposition disease 128
Hypercementosis 498
Hyperdense basal ganglia, bilateral 25
Hyperdense bile 362
Hyperdense brain lesions, causes of 24t
Hyperdense cisterns 78
Hyperdense falx 25
Hyperdense renal lesion 415
Hyperdense skull base 490
Hyperdense vitreous, common causes of 164t
Hyperperfusive hepatic abnormalities, common causes of 343t
Hyperplastic gastropathy 381
Hyperplastic polyp 379
Hypertension, portal 362f, 372f
Hypertrophied column of Bertini 421
Hypochondroplasia 127
Hypodense bony lesions, common causes of 453t
Hypodense lesion, causes of 20t, 27t
Hypopharynx 215
Hypophysitis 187f
Hypoplastic dens 501
Hypoplastic left lamina 110f
Hypoproteinemia 383, 388
Hypothalamic glioma 12

Hypoxic ischemic encephalopathy 67
Hyrtl's fissure 159

I

Idiopathic pulmonary fibrosis 274, 281
Idiopathic skeletal hyperostosis, diffuse 501
Ilium, osteomyelitis of 481f
Ill-defined lytic lesions 453
    common causes of 453t
Infarct, chronic 42
Infection 100
    disseminated 26
    orbital 173
    suppurative 146
Infectious lesions 74
Inflammations 100
Inflammatory disease 74, 431
Inflammatory lesions 83
Inflammatory lymph nodes 290
Inflammatory polyp 379, 522
Infraorbital nerve and canal 211
Infratentorial lesions, differential diagnosis of 84, 84t
Inguinal hernia 334
Inherited disorders 25
Inner ear 148t, 150t, 154f
    cavity of 155
    dysplasia, congenital malformations of 153t
Interclinoid ligaments 5
Internal ear lesions 146
Interstitial disease 272f
Interstitial lung disease 272, 272f
    common causes of 273t
Interstitial pneumonia, nonspecific 278

Intervertebral foramina, enlarged 502
Intra-articular loose bodies, differential diagnosis of 515
Intracerebral hemorrhage, hypertensive 70
Intraconal lesions 165*t*
Intracranial calcification 1, 4*f*, 5*t*, 12*f*
   causes of 1*t*, 3*f*
Intracranial lipoma 4*f*
Intracranial masses 19, 19*t*
Intracranial pressure, elevated 167
Intradural lipoma 117
Intrahepatic hematoma 341, 353*f*, 354, 354*f*
Intraosseous ganglion 471
Intraparenchymal hemorrhagic lesions 69
Intraparotid lesion 229
Ischemia 388
Ischemic encephalopathy 25
Ivory vertebra 486

J

Jaccoud's arthritis 507
Jaw 494
   ameloblastoma of 497
   lesion 489
      salient features of 495
      sclerotic lesions of 495
Joint
   diseases, differential diagnosis of 526, 526*t*
   effusion 506, 506*f*
   space narrowing 507
Jugular diverticulum 158
Jugular foramen agenesis 158
Jugular vein 217
   internal 224
Juxtacortical chondroma 486

K

Kartagener's syndrome 522
Keratocyst 525
Keratosis obturans disease 133
Key-hole appearance 30
Kidney, right 419*f*
Klippel-Feil syndrome 126, 127
Knee 528
   right 460*f*
Koehler's disease 509
Krabbe's disease 21, 22, 63, 97

L

Labyrinthine aplasia, complete 155
Laceration 341
Lacrimal gland
   lesions, malignant 164
   tumor 173
Lamellar concha 210, 211*f*
Lamina papyracea 212*f*
Langerhans cell histiocytosis 91, 276
Laryngeal space, causes of 234*t*
Laryngocele 236
Left orbit, coronal anatomy of 161*f*
Leigh disease 25, 66, 99
Leiomyoma 296, 379, 384
Leiomyosarcoma 296, 380, 384
Leptomeningeal carcinomatosis 113
Lesion 238, 264
   benign 255, 256*t*
   causes of enhancing 27*t*
   congenital 312
   developmental 255
   dural 16
   enhancing 24
   malignant 255, 256*t*
   miscellaneous 138
   nonenhancing 24

of spleen, common causes of 368*t*
of vertebra, causes of expansile 499*t*
orbital 161, 164
peripheral 263
  cavitating 268*f*
retroperitoneal 403
tumor-like 29, 456
vascular 17, 255
ventricular 29
Letterer-Siwe disease 470, 471
Leucinosis 99
Leukemia 51, 286, 372, 425, 471
  acute 472
  chronic 472
Leukodystrophy disease 22*t*
Leukoencephalopathy 12*f*
Ligament 129
Ligamentum flavum
  hypertrophy 124, 130*f*
  ossification of 129
Lingual thyroid 233
Lipoblastoma 302
Lipoma 7, 12, 38, 86, 92, 218, 219*f*, 301, 329, 339, 380, 387, 392, 397, 472, 531
  chordoma 83
Lipomatosis 301
Lipomyelomeningocele 116
Liposarcoma 397, 532
Lissencephaly 9
Liver 351*f*, 357*f*, 358*f*
  causes of 361*t*
  cirrhosis of 344*f*
  disease, diffuse 355
  fatty 360
  infarction 342
  infiltrating mass in 357*f*
Lobar nephronia 426

Lobe
  right 352*f*
    frontal 72*f*
    temporal 51*f*
Local pleural masses 321
Lowe's syndrome 163
Lucent bone lesions 454, 454*t*
Ludwig's angina 222
Lumbar hernia 331
Lung
  adenocarcinoma of 263*f*
  right 261*f*
  tissue, normal 255
  zones in 259*t*
Lyme disease 101, 103
Lymph nodes 215, 242
  calcified 307
  enhancing 310
  hypodense 308
Lymphadenopathy 243
Lymphangiectasia 429
Lymphangioma 168, 215, 225, 231, 251, 286, 371, 398, 531
Lymphangiomatosis 429
Lymphangitis carcinomatosa 274
Lymphectasia, retroperitoneal 404*f*
Lymphocele 429
Lymphocytic interstitial pneumonitis 281
Lymphocytic thyroiditis, chronic 245
Lymphoma 50, 86, 90, 146, 171, 202, 207, 217, 254, 269, 284, 285*f*, 286, 309, 372, 376, 380, 386, 425, 523
  diffuse 359, 361
  of bone, primary 487
Lymphomatous adenopathy 405*f*
Lymphosarcoma 284
Lytic lesion 453, 456, 488, 490, 492-494

common causes of 452t, 456t, 491t
of jaw, common causes of 494t
of orbit, common causes of 493t
of rib, common causes of 488t
well-defined 452

M

Macrocystic tumor 376
Macrophthalmia 164, 175
Macular degeneration 165, 181
Madelung's deformity 477
Madura foot 472
Maduramycosis 472
Maffucci syndrome 465
Malakoplakia 432
Maple syrup urine disease 99
Marchiafava-Bignami disease 105
Massive fibrosis, progressive 259, 283
Masticator space 225
 causes of 225t
Mastoid lesions, causes of 138t
Maxilla
 carcinoma of 203f
 osteomyelitis of 480f
Maxillary dentoalveolus 211
Maxillary ostium 212, 212f
Meatus, middle 211
Mediastinal lymphadenopathy 307, 307t
Mediastinal masses 285, 301
 anterior 286, 286t, 290t
 middle 293
 posterior 298
Medullary carcinoma 248
Medullary cystic disease 420
Medulloblastoma 52, 84, 96
Medulloepithelioma 181

Melanocarcinoma 74
Melanoma, malignant 136
MELAS/MERRF syndrome 66
Ménétrier's disease 377, 381
Meningioma 6, 12, 52, 81, 85, 89, 96, 117, 150, 164
Meningitis 101, 159t
Meningocele 204, 208, 304, 490
 dorsal 114
Meningoencephalocele 490
Mesenchymal bladder tumors 432
Mesenchymal hamartoma 339, 349
Mesenchymal tumors, retroperitoneal 406
Mesenteric fat stranding 400f
Mesenteric lesion 396, 396t
Mesenteric mass, large 396f
Mesenteric panniculitis 399
Mesoblastic nephroma 425
Mesothelioma 324, 401
Metabolic disorders, congenital 99
Metachromatic leukodystrophy 22, 25, 63, 98
Metastases 62, 83, 86, 91, 104, 124, 129, 137, 146, 167, 203, 241, 248, 254, 265, 307, 337, 345, 473, 524
 types of 346t
Metastatic disease 358f
 diffuse 358, 361
Metastatic lesions 474
Metastatic lymphadenopathy, bilateral 244f
Metastatic tumor 451
Methyl alcohol 25
Methylmalonic aciduria 25, 98
Michel deformity 155
Michel dysplasia 153
Microcystic tumor 376
Microphthalmia 163, 175
Midbrain 34

Index

Middle ear 138, 154*f*, 493
  causes of 138*t*
  lesion of 138
Mitochondrial encephalopathy 25
Mondini's dysplasia 153, 155
Morgagni hernia 286, 292
Morquio syndrome 501
Moth-eaten lesions 454, 454*t*
Mucinous 450
  adenocarcinoma 258
Mucocele 189, 522
  carotid artery aneurysm 152
Mucoepidermoid carcinoma 253
Mucolipidosis 65
Mucopolysaccharidoses 65
Mucosal disease 392
Mucus retention cyst 189, 204
Müllerian duct cyst 438
Multicentric central nervous system lesion 29
Multicystic dysplastic kidney 419
Multifocal brain tumors 29
Multifocal infarction, subacute 26
Multifocal leukoencephalopathy, progressive 3
Multifocal white matter lesions 22
Multilocular cystic nephroma 416, 419
Multilocular nephroma 419*f*
Multilocular thymic cysts 303
Multinodular goiter 291*f*
Multiple vertebra, causes of 499*t*
Mumps 249
Mural hematoma 383
Musculoskeletal system 452
Myelinating lesion, causes of 21*t*
Myeloblastic leukemia, acute 51
Myeloblastoma 120
Myelocele 109
Myelocystocele 109
Myelolipoma 413

Myeloma, multiple 474
Myelomeningocele 109
Myelopathy, acute transverse 110

N

Nabothian cyst 444
Nasal cavity
  left 186*f*
  right 187*f*
Nasal septum, destruction of 186*f*
Nasal sinus lesions 183, 183*t*
Nasopharyngeal angiofibroma 207*f*
Nasopharyngeal carcinoma 205
Nasopharyngeal lesions
  causes of 204*t*
  common 205*t*
Nasopharyngeal mass 216*f*
Nasopharynx 215
Neck 215, 242
  space lesions 220
Neoplasm 107
  benign 255
Neoplastic disease 104, 271
Nephroblastoma 425
Nephroblastomatosis 421
Nephronophthisis 420
Nerve sheath tumors 163, 219
Neural tumors 60
Neuroblastoma 413, 474
Neurocutaneous syndrome 22
Neurocysticercus 40
Neurofibroma 118, 218, 532
  dumbbell-shaped 119*f*
Neurofibromatosis 9, 22, 164, 165*f*
Neurogenic masses 298
Neurogenic tumor 193, 299, 387, 407
Neurolemoma 532
Nodes, calcification in 245
Nodular compensatory hypertrophy 421

Nodular pleura 326f
Nodular regenerative hyperplasia 339
Nonacoustic schwannoma 82
Nonenhancing lesion, causes of 20t
Nonhemorrhagic contusion 21f, 37
Non-Hodgkin's disease 325
Noniatrogenic coagulopathy, causes of 75
Noninfectious disorders 280
Noninfectious granuloma 255
Nonodontogenic lesions 494
Nonossifying fibroma 475
Nonsteroidal anti-inflammatory drugs 478
Norrie's disease 163, 164, 176
Nose 204f

O

Obstructive pulmonary disease, chronic 318
Occipital bone, anomalies of 500
Occipital condylar hypoplasia 500
Occipital lobes 34
Occipital vertebra 500
Occult intrasacral meningocele 114
Ocular metastasis 165, 179
Odontogenic lesions 494
Odontoid bone 501
Odontoma 197, 525
Olfactory fossa depth 210
Oligodendroglioma 26, 56, 89
Olivopontocerebellar atrophy 80
Olivopontocerebellar degeneration 77
Omental lesion 396
    common causes of 396t
Oncocytoma 422
Onion peel sign 260
Onodi cell 210
    right sided 214f

Opacification, common causes of 184t
Ophthalmic vein thrombosis, superior 175
Optic disc
    drusen 182f
    ocular hemorrhage of 182
Optic glioma 12
Optic nerve
    glioma 165, 166f
    left 166f
    meningioma 166f
    right 214f
    tumor 164
    variations 210
Optic neuritis 167
Optic perineuritis 167
Oral cavity 215
    causes of 232t
    lesions of 232, 232t
Oral mucosa 221
Orbital lesions 493
    causes of 161, 162t
Ormond's disease 408
Ornithine transcarbamylase deficiency 98
Oropharynx 215
Os odontoideum 126, 128
Osseous destruction 132
Osseous involvement 132
Ossification center, changes in 508
Ossifying fibroma 148, 194, 196f, 525
Osteitis condensans ilii 527
Osteitis deformans 130
Osteoarthritis 509f
Osteoblastoma 130, 458, 475
Osteochondroma 130, 131f, 476, 477f
Osteoclastoma 468, 468f
Osteogenesis imperfecta 147

Index

Osteoid
    neoplasms 454
    osteoma 478, 478*f*
Osteolytic metastasis 492*f*
Osteoma 137, 196, 197*f*, 479
    frontal 185*f*
Osteomeatal complex
    frontoethmoid recess 212*f*
Osteomyelitis 479
    actinomycotic 188*f*
    acute 479
    chronic 480, 481*f*
    subacute 480
    tubercular 482, 482*f*
Osteopenia 506, 514
    diffuse 472
Osteophytes 509
Osteosarcoma 199, 258, 458, 484, 485*f*
Osteosclerosis 488, 514
    benign 498
Otitis externa, malignant 135, 136*f*
Otitis media
    chronic 141*f*
        granulomatous 140
        suppurative 139*f*, 140, 140*f*
    with mastoiditis 138
Otosclerosis 146
Otosyphilis 146
Ovarian cyst, simple 447
Ovarian cystadenoma 450
Ovarian dermoid 449, 449*f*
Ovary, hemorrhagic lesions of 447

P

Pacchionian bodies 5
Paget's disease 130, 147, 149, 196, 458, 466, 468, 486, 488, 514
Pancreas
    atrophic 373
    fatty 373

Pancreatic adenocarcinoma 375
Pancreatic atrophy, mild 373*f*
Pancreatic islet cell tumor 376
Pancreatic lesion 368, 372, 372*t*
    hypervascular 373
Pancreatic pseudocyst 370, 374
Pancreatitis, acute 375*f*, 397*f*
Panencephalitis, subacute
    sclerosing 68, 105
Papillary carcinoma 247
Papillary cystadenoma
    lymphomatosum 232
Papilloma 237, 523
    inverted 186*f*, 201
Papillomatosis 237
Paradoxical middle turbinate 210
Paraganglioma 82, 119, 220
Paragonimiasis 270
Paralaryngeal space, right 236*f*
Paranasal sinus
    anatomical variants of 210, 210*t*
    carcinoma 202
    development of 209, 209*t*
    lesions 183
Paraovarian cysts, congenital 447
Parapelvic lymphangiectasia 418
Parapharyngeal lesion 215, 215*t*
Parapharyngeal space 217
Paraseptal emphysema 282
Parathyroid gland lesions 238, 238*t*
Parathyroid lesion 239*t*, 242
Parathyroid mass 242
Parenchymal cell tumors 59
Parietal bone, right 476*f*
Parietal lobe, right 24*f*
Parkinson disease 25
Parosteal osteosarcoma 485
Parotid gland 230*f*
    accessory 226
    right 232*f*

Parotid lesions 229
  differential diagnosis of 249, 249t
  space 229
Parotid space, causes of 230t
Parotitis, acute 249
Pars flaccida 142
Pars tensa 142
Pelizaeus-Merzbacher disease 21, 22, 64, 97
Pelvic
  carcinomatosis 435
  edema 435
  fibrosis 435
  hematoma 436
  lesions 430, 434
  lipomatosis 435
  lymphocele 436
  trauma 527
  urinoma 436
Pencil-in-cup appearance 508
Periapical granuloma 496
Pericardial fat pad 292
Perilesional edema 28f
Perinephric lesions 427
  common causes of 427t
Periosteal new bone formation 510
Periosteal osteosarcoma 485
Periportal edema 354
Perirenal pseudocyst 428
Perisylvian region, right 57f
Peritoneal carcinomatosis 401
Peritoneal dissemination and adenopathy 451f
Peritoneal lesion 396, 396t
Peritoneal metastases 402f
Persistent hyperplastic primary vitreous 176
Persistent stapedial artery 158
Petroclinoid ligaments 5
Petrositis, acute 151

Petrous apex lesion, common lesion of 151t
Petrous apicitis 153
Petrous bone, malformations of 159t
Petrous pyramid 493
Pharyngeal lesion 215
  causes of 215t
Pharyngeal mucosal space 215
Phenylketonuria 65
Pheochromocytoma 414
Phleboliths 237
Phthisis bulbi 163
Pick's disease 77, 79, 98
Pilocytic astrocytoma 96
Pineal cell tumors 59
Pineal gland 5, 59f
Pinealoblastoma 96
Pineoblastoma 12, 59
Pineocytoma 59
Pituitary adenoma 12, 60
Pituitary gland 5
Pituitary macroadenoma 61f
Plasmacytoma 198, 486
Pleomorphic adenoma 252
  malignant 230f
Pleura 325
  mesothelioma of 324f
Pleural calcification 318
  causes of 318t
Pleural effusion, loculated 322f
Pleural lesions 318
Pleural lipoma 323
Pleural lymphoma 325
Pleural thickening 326
Pleuropulmonary blastoma 264
Plexiform neurofibroma 165f
Pneumatosis cystoides coli 391
Pneumocystis carinii
  infection 307
  pneumonia 271, 278
Pneumonia 264
  cryptogenic organizing 317

Pneumonitis, hypersensitivity 275
Polka dot appearance 469
Polycystic kidney disease 418
Polycystic liver disease 350*f*
Polymicrogyria 36
Polyp 208, 237, 385
    regenerative 379
Portal vein thrombosis 359
    acute 357
Postinflammatory sclerosing osteitis 498
Poststyloid compartment 219
    causes of 218*t*
Pott's disease 502, 515
Pott's spine 504*f*
    type of 503*f*
Pouch of Douglas 402*f*
Prestyloid compartment, causes of 217*t*
Propionic acidemia 98
Proptosis, left-sided 190*f*
Prostate
    benign hyperplasia of 439*f*
    carcinoma 439
Prostatic calculi 440
Prostatic hyperplasia, benign 439
Prostatic lesions 437, 437*t*
Protruding jugular bulb 158
Prussak's space 142
Pseudocyst, post-traumatic 369
Pseudomembranous colitis 394
Pseudomyxoma peritonei 395*f*, 399
Pseudotumor 169
Psoriatic arthritis 510
Pulmonary artery
    left 261*f*
    right 296*f*
Pulmonary edema 274
Pulmonary infarction 260
Pulmonary lesions 285*f*
Pulmonary metastases 265*f*
    contralateral 324*f*
    multiple 266*f*
Pulmonary nodular lesion 255
Pulmonary sequestration 259
Pulmonary varix 260
Pulmonary vessels, visualization of 283
Pyogenic arthritis 516, 516*t*
Pyogenic spondylitis 504
Pyometra 444
Pyriform fossa, left 235*f*

R

Rachischisis
    anterior 500
    posterior 500
Racing car sign 35
Radiation injury 342
Radiation myelopathy 110
Radiation necrosis 92
Radiation pneumonitis 283
Ranula 222
Rathke's cleft cyst 17, 49
Rectal duplication 389*f*
Rectal lesion 435
Rectosigmoid carcinoma 391*f*
Regional intrathoracic lymph nodes, classification of 304, 305*t*
Reiter's syndrome 507, 510, 514, 515
Renal cell carcinoma 423, 423*f*
Renal cyst, calcification in 415*f*
Renal hamartoma 422
Renal leiomyoma 425
Renal lesions 414, 416
    bilateral 415
    common causes of 414*t*
Renal lymphangiectasia, bilateral 429*f*
Renal pelvis, right 424*f*

Renal pseudotumor 421
Renal sinus
 cyst 418
 lipomatosis 416
Reproductive system lesions
 female 441
 male 437
Respiratory tract infection, upper 241, 248
Reticulum cell sarcoma 487
Retinal angioma 181
Retinal astrocytoma 164, 181
Retinal detachment 164, 178
Retinal dysplasia 176
Retinal telangiectasia, congenital 176
Retinoblastoma 164, 178, 182
Retractile mesenteritis 399, 400f
Retrobulbar soft tissues 186f
Retrolental fibroplasia 163, 177
Retrolental hyperplasia 164
Retromandibular vein 229
Retroperitoneal fibrosis, malignant 408f
Retroperitoneal liposarcoma, large 407f
Retroperitoneal mass lesion 407f
Retroperitoneal sarcoma, large 406f
Retropharyngeal space 227, 227t
Retrosternal goiter 290
Rhabdomyosarcoma 164, 171, 204, 208, 264, 533
Rheumatoid arthritis 237
Rhinocerebral mucormycosis 208
Rib
 chondrosarcoma of 462f
 lesions 488
 multiple 489
Riedel's thyroiditis 246
Ring enhancing lesions 26
 pneumonic for 26

Rosai-Dorfman disease 16
Rotatory atlantoaxial dislocation 537
Rugger Jersey spine 514
Ruptured aneurysms 70

S

Sacral meningocele, anterior 114
Sacroiliac joint 526
Salivary gland adenoma 218
Salivary inclusion defect 498
Salpingopharyngeus muscle 215
Sarcoidosis 146, 174, 275, 275f, 358, 360, 371
Scalp, lipoma of 519f
Scar, postoperative 125
Scheibe dysplasia 153
Schilder's disease 105
Schistosoma japonicum 360
Schistosomiasis 360
Schizencephaly, bilateral 44f
Schizophrenia 98
Schmorl's nodes 514
Schwannoma 85, 118, 169, 302, 395
 malignant 227
Sciatic hernia 334
Scleritis 165, 177
Sclerosing endophthalmitis 177
Sclerosis, multiple 66, 87, 105
Sclerostenosis 148
Sclerotic bone
 disease 455
 lesions, common causes of 455t
Sclerotic lesions 456, 488, 493
 common 148t
 causes of 456t, 489, 493t
Seminal vesicle
 cyst 440
 lesions 440
 neoplasms 440

Index

Seminoma 292
Seroma 406
Serous 450
Sheath meningioma 166
Shepherd's crook deformity 467
Short pedicles, congenital 126
Shoulder 530
    joint 509*f*
Sialadenitis, chronic recurrent 249
Sialosis 250
Sickle cell disease 480, 514
Sigmoid adenocarcinoma 391*f*
Silicosis 277, 307
Sinonasal cavity
    causes of 199*t*
    lesions of 199*t*
    mass lesions of 184*t*
Sinonasal polyposis 191, 192*f*
Sinus
    ethmoid 209
    frontal 209
    inner table of frontal 185*f*
    maxillary 209, 212
    right frontal 197*f*
    sphenoid 209
    straight 33
Sinusitis 521
    acute 184
    chronic 185
Sjögren syndrome 250
Skull base
    common causes of 490*t*
    hyperdense lesions of 490*t*
Skull lesion 489
Skull vault 489*t*, 490, 491*t*
    sclerotic lesions of 489
Small bowel lesions, common causes of 382*t*
Soap bubble appearance 468, 497
Soft tissue 174*f*
    atrophy 513
    calcification 513, 516
    causes of 132*t*
    density 164
    extension 203*f*
    swelling 512
Soft tissue lesions 132, 138, 205*f*, 228*f*, 257*f*, 521*t*
    common causes of 517*t*
    differential diagnosis of 521, 530, 530*t*
Soft tissue mass 131*f*, 519*f*
    benign 532
    common 150*t*
    extradural 63*f*
    lesion 433*f*
    large 186*f*, 466*f*
Soft tissue sarcoma
    large 518*f*
    malignant 533
Solitary dense pedicle 502
Solitary pulmonary nodule 255, 258, 259, 262
    classification of 259*t*
Solitary sclerotic bone lesion 455
Space occupying lesions, causes of 13*t*
Sphenoid bone 195*f*
    osteomyelitis of 187*f*
Spiculated sunray appearance 497
Spigelian hernia 331
Spina ventosa 483
Spinal accessory 243
Spinal arteriovenous malformation 122
Spinal canal stenosis 130*f*
Spinal cord 106
    lesions 106, 107
        causes of 107*t*
        common 109*t*
Spinal fractures, differential diagnosis of 535, 535*t*

Spinal hematoma 121
Spinal stenosis 126t, 127t
   lesions with 126
Spine 513
Spleen
   abscess in 370f
   diffusely hyperdense 368
   tuberculosis of 369f
Splenic hematoma, large 369f
Splenic infarct 371, 372f
Splenic lesion 368
Splenic pseudocyst 375f
Splenosis 401
Split cord 109
Spondylitis 123
Spondylodiscitis 123
Spondylolisthesis 124
Spongiform leukodystrophy 97
Squamous cell carcinoma 135, 143, 216, 262, 269f, 271, 523
Stafne's mandibular defect 498
Staphylococcus 249
Stein-Leventhal syndrome 448
Stewart's granuloma 201
Stomach, diffuse lymphoma of 381f
Streptococcus 249
Sturge-Weber syndrome 2, 9, 11f
Subchondral sclerosis 509, 510f
Subcutaneous edema 408f
Subcutaneous fat, edema in 517f
Subdural hematoma 7, 32, 72, 95
   acute 24f, 32f
Subdural lesions 16
Subependymoma 57
Subfalcine 30
   herniation 32f
Sublingual gland, mucocele of right 222f
Sublingual space 220
   causes of 221t
Submandibular gland, sialadenitis of 223f
Submandibular space 223
   causes of 223t
Subpleural honeycomb cysts 272f
Subtalar osteoarthritis 510f
Suprasellar cystic mass lesion 62f
Supratentorial mass lesions, differential diagnosis of 88, 88t
Swan-neck deformity 511
Swirl sign 69
Sylvian fissure 33
Synovial sarcoma 258, 533
Systemic lupus erythematosus 273, 507
Systemic sclerosis 279f

T

Tail sign 222
Talus, tubercular osteomyelitis of 483f
Tarsal coalition 529
Tay-Sachs disease 65
Tegmen tympani, dehiscence of 159
Temporal lobe
   left 8f
   right 51f
Temporomandibular joint 530
Tentorial meningioma 53f
Teratocarcinoma 287
Teratoma 12, 59, 91, 290, 380
   benign 287
   malignant 287
Testes 441
   ectopic 441
   undescended 408, 441
Tethered cord 115
Thigh, intramuscular lipoma of 520f
Thoracic meningocele, lateral 300
Thornwaldt's cyst 204, 215, 216
Thymic mass, large 291f

Index

Thymolipoma 302
Thymoma 288, 290, 291f
Thymus, normal 286
Thyroid
    adenoma 240, 247
    carcinoma 240, 258
    diseases, differential diagnosis of 245
    gland lesions 238
        causes of 238t
    goiter 246
    granuloma 239
    large carcinoma of 241f
    lesion 239t
        differential diagnosis of 245t
    lymphoma 241, 248
    ophthalmopathy 174
    stimulating hormone 248
Thyroiditis 239
    acute suppurative 246
Tibia
    metaphysis of right 460f
    upper end of 468f, 485f
Tick borne multisystem disease 103
Tight filum terminale 115
Tissue, granulation 143
Tongue 221f
Tooth appearance, floating 497
Tooth-bearing area 211
Toxic
    causes 25
    demyelination 67
    encephalopathy 25
Toxocariasis 164
Toxoplasmosis 40
    congenital 8f
Tracheal bronchus 313
Tracheal stenosis 312, 314
Tracheobronchial tree, lesions of 312
Tracheoesophageal fistula 313
Tracheomalacia 312
Translabyrinthine fistula 159
Translation injury 537
Transtentorial herniation 30
Trauma 340, 528
Tree-in-bud appearance 280
Trevor's disease 509
Trichobezoar 382f
Tubercular arthritis 516, 516t
Tuberculoma 50, 51f, 259
Tuberculosis 249, 289f, 309, 319f, 383, 388
Tuberculous colitis 394
Tuberous sclerosis 9, 10f, 22, 56f, 281
Tubo-ovarian abscess complex 448
Tumor
    benign 338, 456t
    brown 198, 461
    macrocystic 376
    malignant 337, 456t
    microcystic 376
    mucinous 376
    primary 318, 373
    serous 376
    supratentorial midline 12
Tumoral ossification 329
Typhlitis 393

U

Ulcerative colitis 392
Ulcerative proctitis 393f
Umbilical hernia 332f
Unicystic ameloblastoma 457f
Upper lobe, left 261f
Urachal anomalies 430
Ureter, ectopic 439
Ureterocele 434
Urinary bladder 433f
    lesions 430
Urinoma 428

Uterine cancer 446
Uterine collection 444
Uterine leiomyoma 445
Uterine segment, lower 445*f*
Uterus 441, 443
Uveal melanoma 179, 180*f*

V

Vagina and vulva 441
Vaginal atresia 441, 442
Vaginal carcinoma 441, 443
Vaginal embryonal rhabdomyosarcoma 443
van Buchem disease 489
Varix, orbital 168
Vascular anomalies 157*t*
Vascular dementia 77, 79
Vascular disease 67, 104
Vascular malformation 3, 70
Vascular metastasis 310
Vascular scars 337*t*
Vascular tumors, malignant 164
Vasculitis 67, 74
Vein of Galen 33
Vena cava, inferior 409
Venous infarctions 73
Vertebra
    expansile lesions of 499
    multiple 499
    part of 500
    plana 470
    posterior elements of 477*f*, 500*t*
Vertebral body 475
Vertebral neoplasm, primary 124
Vertebral pedicle erosion 502
Vertebrobasilar dolichoectasia 82

Vesical diverticulum 430
Viking horn sign 35
Villous adenoma 395
Virchow-Robin spaces 22, 42
Visceral disease 100
Vitamin K deficiency 75
von Hippel-Lindau disease 420
Vulvar carcinoma 441, 443

W

Waardenburg syndrome 155
Waldeyer's ring 217
Warburg's disease 164
Warburg's syndrome 176
Warthin's tumor 232, 232*f*, 252
Water lily sign 260
Weber Christian disease 399
Wegener's granulomatosis 164, 169, 186*f*, 201, 269, 524
White matter
    diseases, differential diagnosis of 96, 96*t*
    lesions 21
Wilms' tumor 416, 425
Wilson's disease 25, 80, 99, 360

X

Xanthogranulomatous pyelonephritis 427

Z

Zellweger syndrome 66
Zenker's diverticulum 238
Zygomaticomaxillary suture 211

EU GSPR Authorised Reprsentative
Logos Europe, 9 rue Nicolas Poussin
1700, La Rochelle, France
Phone: +33 (0) 6 67 93 73 78
E-mail: contact@logoseurope.eu

www.ingramcontent.com/pod-product-compliance
Ingram Content Group UK Ltd.
Pitfield, Milton Keynes, MK11 3LW, UK
UKHW021829140426
5217IPUK00021B/1343